BOWEN THEORY'S SECRETS

BOWEN THEORY'S SECRETS

Revealing the Hidden Life of Families

MICHAEL E. KERR

Norton Professional Books

An Imprint of W. W. Norton & Company
Celebrating a Century of Independent Publishing

Copyright © 2019 by Michael E. Kerr

All rights reserved
Printed in the United States of America
First published as a Norton paperback 2022

For information about permission to reproduce selections from this book, write to
Permissions, W. W. Norton & Company, Inc., 500 Fifth Avenue, New York, NY 10110

For information about special discounts for bulk purchases, please contact
W. W. Norton Special Sales at specialsales@wwnorton.com or 800-233-4830

Manufacturing by Sterling Pierce
Production manager: Katelyn MacKenzie

Library of Congress Cataloging-in-Publication Data

Names: Kerr, Michael E., 1940– author.
Title: Bowen theory's secrets : revealing the hidden life of families / Michael E. Kerr.
Description: First Edition. | New York : W.W. Norton & Company, [2019] | "A Norton professional book." | Includes bibliographical references and index.
Identifiers: LCCN 2018028077 | ISBN 9780393708127 (hardcover)
Subjects: LCSH: Bowen, Murray, 1913-1990. | Family psychotherapy—Biography.
Classification: LCC RC488.5 .K47 2019 | DDC 616.89/156—dc23
LC record available at https://lccn.loc.gov/2018028077

ISBN 978-1-324-05264-7 pbk.

W. W. Norton & Company, Inc., 500 Fifth Avenue, New York, N.Y. 10110
www.wwnorton.com

W. W. Norton & Company Ltd., 15 Carlisle Street, London W1D 3BS

2 3 4 5 6 7 8 9 0

*This book is dedicated to those who have taught me much about
differentiation of self:
my mentor, Murray Bowen;
my mother, Mary Margaret Costlow Kerr;
my father, Oscar William Kerr Jr.;
my "schizophrenic" brother, Oscar William Kerr III;
my wife, Kathleen Bower Kerr;
and our three children, Melissa Kerr, Rachel Kerr Schmalhofer,
and Brendan Matthew Kerr.*

Note to Readers: Standards of clinical practice and protocol change over time, and no technique or recommendation is guaranteed to be safe or effective in all circumstances. This volume is intended as a general information resource for professionals practicing in the field of psychotherapy and mental health; it is not a substitute for appropriate training, peer review, and/or clinical supervision. Neither the publisher nor the author can guarantee the complete accuracy, efficacy, or appropriateness of any particular recommendation in every respect.

Contents

Acknowledgments ix
Introduction xiii

Part I: Core Concepts in Bowen Theory
1. Systems Thinking 3
2. Evolution and the Emotional System 7
3. The Molecule of an Emotional System 13
4. Patterns of Emotional Functioning 22
5. Differentiation of Self 46
6. Emotional Regression 65
7. Emotional Regression and the Individuality-Togetherness Balance 79
8. Emotional Objectivity 89
9. Emotional Programming 95
10. Chronic Anxiety 108
11. The Multigenerational Family Organism 119
12. Sibling Position 133
13. Emotional Cutoff 143
14. Societal Emotional Process 149

Part II: The Process of Differentiation
15. Key Ingredients in the Process of Differentiation 165
16. Personal Vignettes of the Process of Differentiation 179
17. Clinical Example of the Process of Differentiation 200
18. The Process of Differentiation: Theory, Method, and Technique 211

Part III: Applying Bowen Theory to Families in the Public Eye

19. The Unabomber and His Family   225
20. Gary Gilmore and His Family   239
21. Adam Lanza and His Family   259
22. John Nash: A Beautiful Mind   272

Part IV: Special Applications

23. Unidisease: A Proposed New Concept in Bowen Theory   297
24. Toward a Systems Concept of Supernatural Phenomena   322

Epilogue: Applying Bowen Theory to My Own Family   331
References   355
Index   361

Acknowledgments

The people that I can be quite specific about I will name individually. The first people I would like to acknowledge are the ones at W. W. Norton. My dealings thirty years ago were primarily with Susan Barrows, who encouraged me to write my first book, *Family Evaluation*, coauthored with Murray Bowen. Deborah Malmud, who provided extremely useful advice on my proposal for this book, and her capable assistants have been my main contacts for this time around. Norton has been a fantastic company to work with. The next group I will mention, all residents of the island of Islesboro, Maine, where I have lived full-time since June 2011, comprises Kathleen Kerr, Priscilla Fort, Charles Dupuy, and Dick De Grasse, each of whom read sections of the manuscript and made extremely useful comments. Finally, I dare not list my Bowen theory colleagues lest I forget someone. There are dozens who have been very important. I would also include many of the people I coached in my clinical practice. Watching them apply these ideas in their lives has been invaluable. Absent being able to communicate my various ideas through the years and listening to their responses, I would have been lost. The Bowen network is a collection of individuals, but it is still a team effort. Representing the ideas in Bowen theory, which still occupy the fringes of public consciousness, can be exciting and frustrating. The whole of the Bowen network is definitely greater than the sum of its parts. One other person I want to acknowledge is Ruth Riley Sagar. She was the highly capable administrative director of the Georgetown Family Center during the entire time I was involved there. I could not have accomplished what I did without her alongside, taking care of business. Murray Bowen used to refer to me as his "right arm." Ruth was my right arm. She often had good ideas about how to improve whatever writing I was doing at the moment. Last but far from least are the many scientists who have interacted with members of the Bowen network for many years. They have kept our group honest, reducing the tendency of any of us to drift into the ozone layer on some of our speculations. As Murray Bowen often said, "If you have questions about theory, go back to the rats. The rats don't lie." I won't try to interpret what Bowen meant by that, but it was relevant to the scientists who collect the facts about the flora and fauna, of which *Homo sapiens* is a card-carrying member.

The examples presented in this volume, although derived from actual cases in my practice, are composites. They nonetheless exemplify approaches and dialogue I have found effective in my practice.

BOWEN THEORY'S SECRETS

Introduction

The title of this book, *Bowen Theory's Secrets: Revealing the Hidden Life of Families*, was strongly influenced by reading *The Hidden Life of Trees* by Peter Wohlleben (2015). Quoting from the book jacket: "Trees are like human families: tree parents live together with their children, communicate with them, support them as they grow, share nutrients with those who are sick or struggling, and even warn each other of impending dangers." Forester Peter Wohlleben describes trees as social beings and the forest as a social network. The life of a tree is intricately connected to the lives of other trees in ways most people are unaware. The successful adaptation of a tree to life's challenges cannot be adequately understood without examining its links to its social network, and the same holds for members of human families. How one family member is adapting to life's challenges cannot be adequately understood separate from that individual's relationships with other family members.

Despite Bowen theory being based on research begun more than seventy years ago, the value of viewing human beings as profoundly emotionally driven creatures and human families functioning as emotional units has yet to significantly penetrate the public consciousness. Nor has the view of the forest as a social network penetrated the public consciousness. Both insights are secret, or at least largely hidden from view. This is obviously not the result of a conspiracy to suppress the information but, in the case of the family as an emotional unit, requires a radical and thus difficult shift in conceptual thinking. Most people acknowledge that the family is critically important to human health and well-being, but few are aware of the emotional forces and patterns of interaction in all families that govern whether the unit functions as a resource or stressor for its members.

I want to forewarn readers that I have packed many complex ideas into this introduction, hoping to alert at the outset those unfamiliar with Bowen theory to the breadth and depth of the ideas. Part I of the book explicates the core ideas in the theory. Part II describes the process of differentiation of self, which is the most important application of Bowen theory. People sometimes think of theories as "ivory tower" productions: interesting but not necessarily practical. Differentiation of self is anything but ivory tower; it has a well-tested real-world application. Part III includes four long case presentations of families in the public eye. They each illustrate how Bowen theory can help explain how families—three of which appear fairly normal and one of which does not—unwittingly produce an offspring that chronically manifests some type of severely aberrant behavior. Part IV proposes a new concept to include in Bowen theory and discusses a concept proposed by Bowen that attracted great interest at the time but never materialized as part of the theory. The epilogue describes the application of Bowen theory to understand my family of origin and develop more ability to function as a differentiated "self" in it. My parents raised four sons, three of whom made reasonable life adjustments. The other son committed suicide when he was thirty-five years old. The study of my family illustrates how stressors related to changes in the family relationship system over time better predict the clinical course of schizophrenia (a diagnosis my brother received) than the conventional view of a pathology-driven process with a natural history.

I begin by emphasizing why I think the theory and its applications are important. During a talk delivered at psychiatric grand rounds at Georgetown University School of Medicine in 1976, professor of psychiatry Henry Lederer stated, "Throughout history, mankind has produced *four hundred original ideas*; Murray Bowen has produced one of them." Lederer was referring to Bowen's origination of family systems theory. Bowen later added his name to the theory to distinguish it from theories being developed by others that were also called family systems theory.

Other scholars, such as Ludwig von Bertalanffy (1951) with general system theory and Norbert Wiener (1948) with cybernetics, attempted to extend their systems theories to human behavior, but Bowen was the first to study the family in a live-in setting *and* describe specific factual details about how families function as systems. General system theory, cybernetics, and Bowen theory have systems thinking in common, but they differ radically in that Bowen theory contains unique components derived from the direct study of families. Bowen's research was the basis for concluding that the human family is a naturally occurring system: the interactions of family members add up to a whole that is greater than the sum of its parts. Families merit study as entities in their own right.

Bowen developed and expanded his theory over more than four decades based on research at the Menninger Clinic (1946–1954), the National Institute of Mental Health (NIMH; 1954–1959), and the Georgetown University Department of Psychiatry (1959–1990). Since Bowen's death in 1990, his close associates and others in many locations have continued developing the theory and its applications.

Bowen recognized the need to apply systems thinking to human behavior during the NIMH Family Study Project. The best books about the details of the Family Study Project are Bowen's book of collected papers (Bowen 1978) and The Origins of Family Psychotherapy: The NIMH Family Study Project (Bowen, 2013). This was a long-term study of families having one young adult member diagnosed with schizophrenia. Bowen and his research staff were able to observe family interactions directly, which meant that their data about family functioning were not limited to listening to what family members said about their interactions.

Other pioneering family researchers at the time recognized the need to look at the family as an entity in its own right, often referring to it as a "family organism," but most of these researchers conceptualized their observations by trying to extend Freudian theory to the family, by borrowing ideas from general systems theory, or by combining some systems ideas with existing individual theory. In contrast, Bowen saw the potential for a completely new theory of human behavior emerging from family research. Many of the other family pioneers were more preoccupied with developing a new therapeutic approach to human problems, namely, family therapy, than with developing a new theory.

Bowen recognized early in his research that family relationship processes could not be adequately conceptualized using the conventional cause-and-effect thinking inherent in theories such as psychoanalytic theory. Applying cause-and-effect thinking to human behavior assumes that the principal cause of a person's aberrant behaviors or symptoms resides within the person of the patient, referring to that cause as individual psychopathology, biological defects in the brain, or a combination of the two. Research by John Bowlby (1950) that eventually contributed to his development of attachment theory was occurring at about the same time as Bowen's work. Bowlby was interested in relationship interactions between mothers and their developing children and used cybernetic thinking to help conceptualize the processes. However, the theory he eventually constructed describes the development of attachment disorders, thus placing the problem within the person of the patient, and invokes maternal deprivation as its prime cause (Bowlby, 1969). In contrast to Bowen's theory, Bowlby's thinking remained in the psychoanalytic realm, never letting go of conventional cause-and-effect or maternal deprivation thinking. Descriptions of the interactions of two people each assessed to have an attachment disorder are best characterized as interlocking psychopathology thinking, not systems thinking. The distinction between the two approaches of Bowen and Bowlby may not be immediately obvious to the reader but should become clearer in Chapter 1 of this book.

In contrast to a pathology-driven model, family research discovered that people's thoughts, feelings, behaviors, and problems could not be adequately explained without taking into account the emotional context in which they lived. Systems thinking is necessary to describe the interactions between family members and the impact of those interactions on the internal psychobiological processes and behaviors of individual members. The individual and the family are a reciprocal interaction process: each affects the other. Furthermore, a two-person relationship cannot be adequately explained without recognizing the impact of others on it and vice versa. People often sense the relationship impact but find it difficult to track what unfolds without the aid of systems thinking. The task of letting go of cause-and-effect thinking is a formidable one. Viewing the problem as "in the other" has long been human beings' default mode.

The eight interlocking concepts that comprise Bowen family systems theory are explicated in this book differently from how they are often described. The most important concept is *differentiation of self*. Bowen borrowed the term *differentiation* from biology, but applying it to human emotional functioning and behavior was new. Cell differentiation and integration are key to the adaptive capacities of complex organisms; the differentiation of human beings is key to the adaptive functioning of complex family units. A balance between differentiation and integration is as crucial to the functioning of human families as it is to the functioning of complex systems throughout the natural world.

Philosophers, theologians, psychologists, psychiatrists, neuroscientists, and others have made useful contributions to conceptualizing the self. However, Bowen theory's concept of "self" differs from all previous efforts. Ideas like sense of self and a person's essential being that distinguishes him or her from others are part of "self" in Bowen theory, but they are not the whole story. Note that in the previous sentence and throughout this book, "self" (in quote marks) refers to differentiation of self to distinguish it from other conceptualizations of the self. Bowen theory, which was first published more than fifty years ago (Bowen, 1966), has broadened the conceptualization of "self" and, by doing so, has led to the development of a radically different therapeutic approach to help people improve their emotional functioning.

The uniqueness of Bowen theory's concept of "self" is that it includes how individuals function in relationship systems, especially their most emotionally significant relationship systems. The ability to maintain "self" is a property of the individual, but its robustness is accurately assessed only in the context of an individual's relationship environment. It can be studied objectively by observing facts about the nature of people's interactions. A continuum of gradations exists between a person's capacity to maintain "self" in relationship systems at one end and a person's vulnerability to lose "self" at the other end. People typically can maintain more of a "self" in some relationship systems than in others, such as work versus family.

This new view of "self" and its associated therapeutic approach were outcomes of the NIMH Family Study Project. This development hinged on discovering that a *family functions as an emotional unit*. The emotional functioning of family members is far more interdependent than had been previously recognized. The core of emotional interdependence is that a change in the emotional functioning of one member is predictably associated with reciprocal changes in the emotional functioning of other members. This is an emotionally driven process, not a rationally driven one. People are expressing and being regulated by emotions that flow through the family system in observable ways. The overly helpful person is reacting emotionally to the more helpless-acting person, and vice versa.

Interdependent functioning is not necessarily a bad thing. If a wife falls and breaks her ankle, her husband modifies his schedule to take over functions that his wife would normally do. When her fracture heals, he stops overfunctioning, and she stops underfunctioning and resumes her old roles. This type of interaction has emotional (sympathetic and caring) and rational (it is the principled thing to do) components.

The pattern of overfunctioning and underfunctioning becomes a problem if chronic anxiety intensifies the emotional reactivity (overly sympathetic, overly caring, overly controlling) and drives the relationship interaction. These sorts of anxiety-driven interactions are based not on the realities of people's capabilities but on anxiety and distorted perceptions. The distorted perceptions include those of self and of others. For example, one person is comfortable feeling in control and caring for a partner this person perceives as weaker; the partner feels more comfortable having the other take disproportionate decision-making responsibility and perceiving the other as the stronger one. The roots of these "postures" are anchored in biology but are also powerfully influenced by developmental experiences. Bowen theory refers to these anxiety-driven interactions as immature, in that people feel incomplete if they are not taking care of someone else or being taken care of by someone else. People who assume responsibility for themselves, do not distance from others if they are distressed, and do not anxiously intrude and try to control others are whole or mature people.

Observing these relationship patterns in families and other relationship systems and how anxiety can transform a cooperative interaction into a problematic one raises a question about the nature of the forces that drive or motivate these interactions. Are these processes culturally driven, psychologically driven, feeling driven, or emotionally driven? Bowen theory's answer is, all of the above. The human *emotional system*, which has been shaped by several billion years of evolution, is where the ancient roots of the fundamental motivating forces originated and exist to this day. The emotional system influences and is influenced by feeling states, psychological states, and culture.

One fundamental characteristic of an emotional system is people pressuring one another to think and act alike, particularly when anxiety escalates in a family and other relationship systems. Thinking and acting alike promote a feeling of connection; thinking and acting differently threatens that connection. A feeling of comfortable connection promotes calmness and a state of well-being. By discerning this pressure for oneness and agreement in the families of the Family Study Project, a pressure that was termed "stuck-togetherness" (later described as the *togetherness force*), it was possible to discern differences among people in their ability to think and act for themselves (maintain "self") in the face of the anxiety-driven togetherness pressure.

Certain communications and behaviors function to define and maintain "self" or distinctness within the group; other communications and behaviors function to maintain oneness with the group. Identifying these two classes of behaviors in relationship systems makes it possible to study objectively the capacity to be a "self." Observing facts about how people function (functional facts) in relationship to one another is the basis of the objectivity. For example, an inflexible person who cannot relinquish the position of being in control and a person who cannot relinquish the helpless position are pressuring each other to function in a certain way, which is a product of the togetherness force. Differentiation of self is a counterforce that motivates people to take more responsibility for themselves and respect emotional boundaries, for example, not intruding on others and taking over their decision making. These are observable differences in behavior.

The counterbalancing force to togetherness is individuality, which is also anchored in the emotional system. An expanded definition of *individuality* is that it is a life growth force toward differentiation of self. This expanded definition is important because it indicates that this life force has components based in the emotional system (subcortical) and components that evolved with the evolution of the cerebral cortex (cortical). The cortical components comprise what Bowen theory defines as the intellectual system, which enables human beings to think, reason, reflect, and use those abilities to exert control over some aspects of emotional system functioning. The recently evolved cortical circuits enable more self-regulation, a key ingredient for maintaining "self," particularly in an anxious social context. A well-thought-out principle and long-term view can guide decision making in preference to acting on the feelings and anxiety of the moment and a short-term view. Feelings are subjectively experienced through cortical activity but reflect activity of the underlying and ancient subcortical circuits of the emotional system. Cortical components of differentiation guide actions; subcortical components motivate actions.

Variation in the development of the intellectual system among individuals is central to explaining variation among human beings in their ability to maintain "self" in relationship systems. How well developed an intellectual system becomes begins with the instinctual roots of individuality/differentiation of self, but the many years of a child's development and interactions with the family and other social environments determine how well the intellectual system and associated ability to maintain "self" develops.

Bowen theory contains specific details about how the variation in "self" among people plays out in relationship systems. In contrast to modern neuroscience, Bowen theory permits study of the "self" by observing how people function in relationships. Neuroscientist Antonio Damasio (2010) explained how self comes to mind through the evolution of consciousness; Bowen theory describes how that evolutionary development manifests in relationships.

An associated innovation during the NIMH Family Study Project was a method of therapy for the family unit. In family therapy sessions during the project, the research observers discovered that motivated family members could learn to apply factual knowledge about predictable relationship processes in their family to improve their ability to maintain "self" in the system. When people see the specific (previously unobserved/hidden) processes of how they lose "self" in a relationship, this provides a blueprint that helps them figure out what they need to do to be more of a "self" in the system. The result is that they can be closely involved with others and not have their most thoughtful and objective assessments of the family situation washed out by the family's anxious interactions.

Psychodynamic psychotherapy is useful for helping people define more clearly what they are feeling and their subjective attitudes but is limited by the subjective view of the "patients" regarding what transpires between them and important others in their life. Having a systems lens to view important relationships and using it in real-world current interactions provide a previously unknown alternative for thinking about one's relationships. For example, instead of viewing someone as critical, one can observe this person as anxiously reacting to real and imagined perceptions of others. A principal limitation of individual psychodynamic therapy is that the therapist is not the real mother or spouse. Theory makes it possible to observe previously hidden specifics of our relationships with others, both in the part we play and in the parts others play. Many examples of this are presented in the chapters that follow.

It may seem counterintuitive, but the ability to be an individual while closely involved with others enhances the stability and adaptive capacities of a relationship system. In contrast, when people lose this ability in a system, such as by trying to please excessively to avoid disharmony or rejection or by being reactively oppositional, the system becomes vulnerable to increased anxiety that undercuts cohesiveness and cooperation. Heightened anxiety and relationship instability can fuel the development of physical, emotional, or social symptoms in a family member.

Being more of a "self" begins with using the lens of systems thinking to observe the basic emotionally driven patterns that exist in family relationship systems and one's part in sustaining those patterns, for example, shifting from the cause-and-effect view, "I am overly helpful to you because you are acting helpless," to a system view, "It's a reciprocal process: the more helpless you act, the more helpful I get, and the more helpful I get, the more helpless you act." Blaming others and blaming oneself are the enemies of gaining a systems perspective. Students of Bowen theory sometimes ponder the question of whether we need to see the patterns to get less reactive and more thoughtful or get less reactive to get more thoughtful and see the patterns. No obvious answer exists for this question, but my opinion is that these two processes are intermixed, with each continuously having an impact on the other.

The next part of the effort is translating this new way of thinking into a new way of being. It requires conviction and courage to move toward a new way of being, such as by behaving less "helpfully" or doing less anxiety-driven overfunctioning. It also takes courage and conviction to take more responsibility for underfunctioning behaviors. Conviction and courage are positive emotional states that emerge from trusting the new systems perspective on the problem. Conviction helps override fears about how others might react to change. It took me ten years of working on resolving key aspects of the relationship with my mother for me to finally recognize my subjective view of her being a fragile person and that this had been the major obstacle to my gaining some resolution of my attachment to her. When I did see that, I realized what the typical next step in our emotional dance would be if I responded to her criticism in my usual conflict-avoidant way.

I recognized bits and pieces of my interaction with my mother fairly early into my learning about Bowen theory. This helped me be less reactive to her when she acted upset, but I still had trouble standing up to her inappropriate attacks on me about certain decisions I was making. I still had to make the link to fearing that she would fall apart (and I would have to pick up the pieces) if I challenged her too much. I came to see her as a worthy opponent in the arena of emotions. I came to recognize that viewing her as fragile was a feeling-driven bias, not a fact. It is not surprising to me that it might take a number of years to unlearn some things that had been repeatedly reinforced as she raised me. I am not suggesting she did that consciously. I got free of blame and self-blame by seeing the reciprocity in our interactions. A hallmark of a successful effort to define "self" is that it does not disrupt a relationship but, rather, solidifies it. The change fosters more mutual respect. When I was finally able to take Mother on and back her off, she responded the next day with, "Finally, you told me what you think." It was so true! Our relationship was vastly improved after that encounter, but it took me ten years to get there. Defining "self" in a family or other relationship system puts the concept of differentiation of self into action.

Variation in basic levels of differentiation occurs naturally in the human species. We have always been social, so it would appear that variation emerged in our earliest ancestors. This variation constitutes a range or continuum of human emotional functioning. The basic level of differentiation of self is associated people's ability to adapt to stressful life circumstances. The less adaptive people are, the more at risk they are for clinical problems of all types and an unproductive life course. Where people fall on this continuum reflects the degree to which they can use their intellectual system to distinguish between feeling and intellectual processes. This possibly unique human capacity enables a choice between whether to act on thinking and a long-term view or to act on feelings to relieve the anxiety of the moment. Acting on a long-term view favors less chronic anxiety and a more consistently directed life course. Being a more differentiated person is not about suppressing feelings but about employing an intellectual process that results in more objectivity about emotions and in less perceived threat. As the result of a more realistic assessment of what is occurring and seeing our own part in the process, as well as others' parts, we gain more emotional neutrality. The essence of that neutrality is less blaming and less of the blame-associated negative emotions such as guilt and anger. Using systems thinking to view relationship systems in a more realistic way provides a greater sense of control over oneself, less perceived threat, and more emotional equanimity.

Research on chimpanzees by Sarah Boysen and colleagues (Boysen, Berntson, Hannan, & Cacioppo, 1996) may offer a parallel to using a theoretical concept to process an emotional reaction, causing that reaction to subside. A chimpanzee was presented with two plates holding tasty food items; one plate had many more treats than the other plate. If the animal pointed to the plate holding more treats, the researcher would immediately give that plate to another chimp in an adjacent cage. The pointing chimp would be given the plate with few treats. After hundreds and hundreds of trials, the pointing chimps never learned not to point to the larger reward, even though it always resulted in the same undesired consequence.

These same chimps had already been taught the symbolic concept of simple numbers. The next step in the research protocol was to place a number on each plate, not the treats themselves. This time the chimps learned rather quickly that, by pointing to the plate with the smaller number, they would be rewarded with the larger plate of treats.

My interpretation of this research is that by making direct eye contact with the actual treats, the chimp could not withhold its impulse to point to the larger number of treats. In contrast, when presented with an affectively neutral symbol, they were able to restrain themselves. Perhaps the neutral symbol allowed the chimps to process information in a more emotionally neutral way. This seems a striking parallel to how using a theoretical construct like relationship reciprocity to process stimuli that evoke negative emotions can extinguish learned emotional programming for a threat reaction. Again, this is not about repressing emotion; rather, it is about decreasing emotional reactivity by information processing, which automatically reduces the perception of threat.

I still faced my mother's verbal and nonverbal cues, but seeing our exchange as transpiring *between* us quickly silenced blaming and self-blaming tendencies. I do not think I could have experienced anything like it in a transference relationship with a psychoanalyst. I simply did not know sufficient detail about this interactive process with Mother until I was able to overcome my observational blindness. I was seeing something that I had lived without seeing. I dwell a bit on this because I am fascinated with the brain's routinely untapped potential for self-regulation once new information about a phenomenon emerges into consciousness. Maybe the next important path for human evolution is tapping that potential, and systems thinking can clearly advance that process. Systems thinking can help our species see the world more as it really is rather than how we feel it and perceive it.

One family member having an improved understanding of how the family system functions and his or her part in the system problem allows for more "self" to emerge and an associated reduction in system anxiety. One person's ability to firmly maintain "self" in an anxious system interrupts the infectious spread of anxiety through the system. If people understand how they are part of a system problem—not its cause—they can be more confident that just managing themselves well in tense times will be sufficient to halt escalating chronic anxiety in the system. It is unnecessary and counterproductive to try to change others. Armed with this newly found confidence, we are less on edge about waiting for the next shoe to drop. Self-help books have long espoused the goal of changing ourselves and not trying to change others, but in the absence of systems theory, there is no guiding framework to convince people that changing themselves does not equate with giving in or giving up on a problem. Nothing is more proactive and constructive than changing ourselves in relationship to important others.

The idea of managing self is very different than trying to act calm and nonreactive. When tension rises in a relationship, often one person tries to act calm, tries not to get drawn into a fight, but this person's seeming lack of response and engagement can send the others into a frenzy. Many marriages polarize around one partner being "rational/even-keeled" and the other being "emotional/volatile." Both spouses are equally emotional in these situations but cope with their emotionality in mirror-opposite ways. The sureness and firmness that come from comprehending both sides of a reciprocal interaction and our own part in it is a vast improvement over trying to act calm and being rigidly rational. The associated emotional neutrality expresses itself in verbal and nonverbal cues that are calming to the other person. As I explained with my mother, I was engaging her more fully, no longer retreating, and she respected it.

Human beings have distinguished between rationality and emotionality for centuries, but Bowen theory emphasizes that what people may consider rational is often under far more influence of emotion than they recognize. Bowen theory is unique by placing the emotional functioning of all human beings on a single continuum. People at one end of the continuum generally can recognize thoughts and viewpoints that are strongly influenced by emotions more than by facts about the reality at hand, and people at the other end of the continuum have great difficulty making this distinction or, even if somewhat aware, still succumb to the emotions. People's ability in this regard varies greatly between these extremes. Jonathan Haidt's book *The Righteous Mind* (2012) beautifully describes the powerful, pervasive, and largely out-of-awareness impact of emotion on thinking. Unlike Bowen theory, Haidt does not conceptualize a continuum in this regard.

People's position on the continuum of emotional functioning is regarded as their *basic level of differentiation*. This basic level corresponds with the ability to define "self" in relationship systems. It is not context dependent. People higher on the continuum have a more *solid self*, and people lower on the continuum have a less solid self. (*Solid self* is explained in more detail in Chapter 5.) The family emotional environment during our developmental years and our position in this environment largely determine our basic level of differentiation. Infants are born with a built-in growth force toward individuality and the differentiation of self, but relationship interactions during the child's development largely determine the degree of development of "self." Siblings typically have different interactions within the family, which results in their developing somewhat different levels of differentiation. Variation in this basic level results from a relationship transmission process, not a genetic one.

The average emotional intensity of interactions between one sibling, the parents, and other family members can be quite different (much stronger or weaker, more or less emotionally intense) than that of the other siblings. The higher the average level of anxiety and immaturity of the interactions between other family members and a developing child, the greater that child's difficulty in learning to discriminate thoughts from feelings. Furthermore, some families are more differentiated and higher functioning than others, related to their multigenerational histories. This constrains the basic level of differentiation that all offspring develop, because the basic levels of the parents establish the emotional climate in the family, which has a significant impact on the development of all the children, albeit on some more than others.

The study of my parents' multigenerational families was extremely helpful in making sense of the family I grew up in. In the several generations preceding my immediate family of origin, I could see that some of the families had more stability and fewer serious problems than my family, and some were less stable. I realized that my family experience was part of a multigenerational emotional tapestry that no one family member had caused. It was a calming perspective to gain.

Over time every multigenerational family produces members who are more differentiated, with highly successful life adjustments, and members who are less differentiated, with poor life adjustments. The poor adjustments can manifest in myriad ways. Examining enough generations reveals that every multigenerational family has members at many gradations between the extremes. Bowen theory describes the emotional forces and relationship patterns that generate this variation in basic levels of "self" over the generations. It is not a chance occurrence; there is an order and predictability to it. Some people consider the multigenerational emotional process idea to be fatalistic. This is ironic, because when people study their own families enough to appreciate the impact of multigenerational processes, it helps them get beyond blaming or idealizing their own parents to see a bigger picture.

Differentiation of self involves thinking for oneself, not taking someone else's word for the accuracy of an idea. People increase their level of understanding based on making more and more observations of how the theoretical concepts play out in real life, particularly in their own lives. They increase their level of conviction about Bowen theory by having the courage to act on a system view of human relationships in personal and professional settings and getting the predicted result (or are able to explain the fairly rare exceptions). It is always easier to blame someone else rather than examine our part objectively. The complexity of the variables involved in a relationship system makes it difficult to apply numbers to measure progress on differentiation at this point, but making factual observations, taking action based on those observations, and getting the predicted outcome are certainly within the realm of scientific investigation.

I have often been amazed by situations when something untoward happened in my personal or professional life, and those events provided enough of a wake-up call to recognize that even though I thought I had been functioning as a fairly mature or "differentiated" person, I had been stuck in an anxious togetherness process. Armed with a theory I trusted in rocky times, family upheavals drove me from my complacency. I could then recognize that I had been distancing from others, overly focusing on trying to change them, or lacking the courage to put myself on the line. Such experiences are typically humbling, particularly when you face up to how your own functioning has unwittingly created significant problems for others. Murray Bowen sometimes commented, "Why is it necessary to fall down a manhole to figure out it's not a good idea?" For most of us, manholes rule!

A note of caution as you embark on reading this book: *Bowen theory can be dangerous to your psychological and emotional equilibrium.* Applying systems thinking to human behavior and anchoring the theory in evolution force serious students of Bowen theory to examine carefully their preexisting assumptions about human nature. Hidden or secret forces and patterns come into view. Making Bowen theory one's own requires shifting completely from individually based, cause-and-effect thinking to systems thinking and shifting from focusing mostly on human uniqueness to understanding human beings in the context of nearly four billion years of evolution. Such challenges generate a mental tension that makes it attractive for students to attempt to fit Bowen theory into their existing mind-set rather than to challenge that mind-set. It is common to distort the theory's concepts in this way, but it dilutes the theory's uniqueness and value. We are all fairly addicted emotionally to the correctness of our own thinking, but it is amazing to realize that it is possible to *decouple emotion from thinking* when we recognize that there is a radically different way to look at something. I hope the reader will experience and enjoy a similar amazement.

I also want to note that there are more than seventy diagrams in this book. I have found both in teaching and clinical practice that symbolizing emotional processes, not just describing them verbally, helps many people grasp the ideas a little faster. One man I saw in my practice, however, watched and listened carefully as I drew some diagrams on my office blackboard. When I finished the diagrams, he said, "Dr. Kerr, put yourself in my position. Think how it might feel to see your life reduced to a series of squares, circles, and arrows on a blackboard." His response notwithstanding, applying systems thinking to human behavior is not easy for anyone. Diagrams can be useful, but for some more than for others. Another man in my practice once said, "Dr. Kerr, when my wife and I get into an argument at home, I am able to think about the square and circle on your blackboard and the jagged line in between, and it helps me take a step back." Ideally, people go to the blackboard and draw their own diagrams. A Bowen-theory-based therapist is not trying to "fix" the patient. By representing systems thinking well, the therapist can help family members educate themselves into defining the life problem in a new way. Failing to define a problem objectively is the principal obstacle to solving it.

Finally, perhaps this could go without saying it, but I want to emphasize that I am writing about a theory that Murray Bowen originated. I have repeatedly read all of Bowen's writings, listened to hundreds and hundreds of talks by him, and had myriad one-on-one conversations with Bowen over the twenty-one years of our close relationship in my effort to understand the theory accurately. I have done over thirty-five thousand hours of therapy with about thirty-five hundred families and conducted a wide range of clinical research projects. I have worked hard and with some success to define more of a "self" in my family of origin and nuclear family. This book is *my version* of Bowen family systems theory. I know Bowen would likely write about some things differently than I do, but as far as I can determine, no substantive differences exist between Bowen's thinking and my own. I like to think that I may have extended the theory some, but time and science will determine that. I approach the writing of this book in the spirit Henry Lederer conveyed: Bowen had an original idea. I will do my absolute best to show that is the case.

PART I

Core Concepts in Bowen Theory

A theory that enables us to do new things constitutes knowledge.
—Y. N. Harari, *Sapiens: A Brief History of Humankind*

Bowen had developed eight interlocking concepts in his theory by the time he published his last comprehensive theory paper (Bowen, 1976). I do not present those eight concepts per se in this section on core concepts. My primary intent is to illustrate how the concepts are interconnected and how other ideas in the theory that are not formal concepts relate to these eight concepts. The essence of all the concepts are covered but are organized differently than Bowen presented them:

- Differentiation of self
- Triangles
- Nuclear family emotional system
- Family projection process
- Emotional cutoff
- Multigenerational transmission process
- Sibling position
- Societal regression

CHAPTER ONE

Systems Thinking

Grasping the core concepts in Bowen family systems theory begins with understanding the distinction between systems thinking and cause-and-effect thinking. Figure 1.1 illustrates cause-and-effect thinking. The diagram implies that event B occurs because an antecedent event A has occurred: A causes B. An example of cause-and-effect thinking in human relationships is a husband asserting to his wife, "I feel depressed because you would rather work in your garden than be with me." This statement implies that her actions cause him to be depressed.

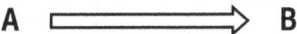

Figure 1.1 Cause-and-effect thinking. *Arrow symbolizes causal connection.*

Figure 1.2 depicts a more complex picture, where A symbolizes the husband and B symbolizes his wife. The process is reciprocal in nature: the wife says it is upsetting for her to be around her husband when he acts depressed and complains about not getting enough attention. She retreats to her garden in response. Systems thinking describes how each spouse changes in response to a process that both unwittingly help create and sustain. They *cocreate* the process.

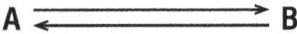

Figure 1.2 Systems thinking. *Arrows symbolize reciprocal interaction.*

Figure 1.3 depicts the shift from cause-and-effect thinking (top) to systems thinking (bottom): the husband's communications, moods, and behaviors trigger a withdrawal response by his wife, and her withdrawal response triggers a depressed mood in her husband. Each contributes equally to an emotional process that alters each other's moods and behaviors. The term *emotional process* refers to the flow of emotions between people. Each person's emotions not only reflect the person's internal states but also change the others' internal states and associated actions. In human beings, the process is primarily mediated by auditory and visual stimuli. The result is that each person changes in relationship to the other people in that relationship.

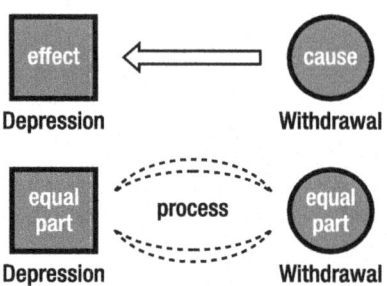

Figure 1.3 *Square symbolizes a male, circle a female. The arrow from the female to the male at the top of the diagram symbolizes that her withdraw causes his depression.* The dashed lines between the male and female in the bottom diagram symbolize a reciprocal emotional process in which neither person causes the other's response.

A key point is that, in the example of the husband and wife, the changes in both partners create and sustain the process—the whole is greater than the sum of its parts. It is nonsense for them to blame each other because they both help create changes in each other, to which they both then react—blaming the other is like reacting to oneself. People see their own behavior in others' reactions. When people comprehend this point, they know that they are best advised to change themselves. A kind of magic in this is that people can work at changing themselves without feeling like they are giving up or giving in. Changing oneself ultimately leads to substantive changes in others as well.

It may seem easy to make this shift in thinking, but it is not. It is difficult for a therapist, and it is difficult for the people a therapist is treating. Both spouses are convinced that the other spouse is causing the problem. It is difficult for many therapists not to feel that one is the perpetrator and the other is the victim. Many people recoil at applying systems thinking to family situations in which physical abuse is occurring. The one being abused is seen as the victim and the abuser is seen as the perpetrator. Viewing the family as a system does not absolve people of responsibility for their actions. Physical abuse is clearly an irresponsible behavior. The anxiety-driven interactions that can culminate in physical abuse are well understood and each member of the system plays a part in the process. Author Marion Collins wrote the following about the physically abusive marriage of suspected murderer Robert Durst: "It started off with verbal abuse, psychological abuse, and emotional abuse and it escalated into physical and economic abuse" (2002, p. 138). His wife Kathy played out the reciprocal opposite side, losing functional differentiation by trying to please, placate, forgive, and eventually distance. Durst's equal lack of "self" manifested in overly controlling possessiveness. It is essential to understand this reciprocal process to address the problem adequately. The ability of someone in the family to make this shift is the primary determinant for the success of the therapy. Invariably, one family member gets it first and changes his or her response, and the others follow. Ideally, the family leader will shift over time among family members.

The husband feels that if his wife were more attentive, he would not feel depressed, which is true; the wife feels if he did not act so depressed, she would not feel overwhelmed and want to distance, which is also true. Both spouses are caught in a process similar to a Chinese finger trap. Each spouse is equally reactive to the other spouse—it takes two to tango. Most people pay lip service to this being is true, but *it is difficult to live it as if it is true*. Importantly, armed with a theoretical framework that describes a reciprocal process and with a persistent effort to apply the idea, most people will eventually see it. Even if just one of the two people sees the "dance," it makes a major difference. The change is both small and profound. The shift from causal thinking to observing emotional process and its impact generates a state of equanimity that produces almost instant changes in an interactive process and its consequent effects on the moods and behaviors of both people.

Cause-and-effect thinking asks, *Why?* Why does the other person treat me this way? Maybe this person has abandonment issues, commitment issues, bonding issues, or anger issues. Cause-and-effect thinking seeks the explanation for another's words and actions within that individual. In contrast, systems thinking does not ask why; it asks *how, what, when, and where*. Such questions enable tracking of the relationship interaction or process and, by doing so, recognizing how each individual's attitudes, thoughts, feelings, and actions are in response to the process. Each individual helps create and maintain the process but does not cause it.

Systems thinking describes *functional facts* about relationship interactions. In the above clinical vignette, it is a functional fact that if the husband says things that blame the wife, she retreats in reaction; it is a functional fact that if she retreats, he makes more blaming comments. Functional facts are easy to observe and document once the observer is thinking systems. Speculations about why the husband makes blaming remarks are subjective and unnecessary. As I discuss in more detail in Chapter 10, the primary social cues that mediate interactions between people are sensitivities to *approval, attention, expectations, and distress.* Such sensitivities are part of all people, but the less "self" people have, the more they are governed by reactions to such real or imagined cues in the relationship system.

The more *undifferentiation,* or lack of differentiation of self, a family system has, the more pronounced the family's continual action-reaction process becomes. It is easier to observe in poorly differentiated families, but it exists to a significant degree in all families. The process may be overt or covert. People who place a premium on getting along can be just as reactive to getting approval as people who argue and yell a lot.

As I describe in Chapter 3, tense two-person systems predictably involve a third person through the process of *triangles* and *interlocking triangles.* The reciprocal interactions described in the above two-person system also occur in all three relationships of a triangle, and each relationship in the triangle affects the other two. If anyone has doubts about the importance of applying systems thinking to human behavior, try to describe triangles without it—it does not work. Freud had the concept of the Oedipus complex, which involved three people—mother, father, and child—but it was an extension of individual, cause-and-effect thinking, not systems thinking. The Oedipus concept does not facilitate tracking an ongoing emotional process and how that process regulates behavior of all three people and the child's development.

One reason it is difficult to apply systems thinking to human behavior is that cause-and-effect thinking is our default mode. It is easier, more automatic, to react to a situation and blame someone for it (or blame oneself, which is an equal problem). If anxiety escalates, it becomes harder to do the type of thinking and reflection necessary to maintain a systems understanding of a situation. Decades of clinical experiences have shown that, with persistence, people can get better at it. It is easier to apply systems thinking to subjects with little or no emotional valance attached: mankind has applied systems thinking with great success in such fields as astronomy, geology, and engineering. But the undertow pulling toward cause-and-effect thinking is magnitudes greater when examining human behavior.

Being able to observe our family as a system is essential for working to increase our level of "self." Being more of a "self" depends on seeing more clearly the ways in which I am not being a "self" and its interplay with others who are having the same problem. Many techniques exist for better managing anxiety, but they do not change our way of thinking—that type of change depends on our ability to make more factual observations of the relationship system.

CHAPTER TWO

Evolution and the Emotional System

Human families, ant colonies, naked mole rat colonies, and the social groups of myriad other species function as naturally occurring systems. Deborah Gordon has written an excellent book about natural systems based on her research on harvester ants. She states, "But nothing ants do makes sense except in the context of the colony" (1999, p. viii). The study of behavior best begins in the context of relationships: discerning how a behavior functions in a relationship system. People often object to being compared to ants or naked mole rats, but this is precisely the message of Bowen theory: human beings have far less autonomy in their emotional functioning than we generally assume. People have more control over automatic reactions to their relationship environments than do ants and naked mole rats—and better differentiated people have more control than do less differentiated people—but, more control notwithstanding, the emotional system is incredibly powerful in human beings.

Living systems are fountains of energy and activity. Bowen theory assumes that the driving forces for this energy and activity reside in the *emotional system*. The emotional systems of *Homo sapiens* and of all other species have been shaped by their long phylogenetic histories. The emotional systems of all the species on the phylogenetic tree are not composed of identical biological systems and mediated by identical communication signals, but there are more common denominators among the seemingly disparate emotional systems of the myriad species on the planet than is generally thought.

Bowen theory uses the term *emotional* more broadly than in common usage. Simple unicellular creatures such as bacteria do not have a brain, but they are capable of *adaptive behavior*—the capacity to change a nonconstructive behavior to a constructive one (Damasio, 2010). Bowen theory considers the intracellular systems that support and motivate adaptive behavior to be part of a bacterial emotional system. It sounds odd to say so, but in Bowen theory emotional *systems* were part of living systems long before what people commonly consider emotions entered the picture.

Interestingly, bacteria are capable of enormously complex social behavior under certain conditions (Shapiro, 1988). Individual bacteria can come together to function like multicellular organisms. When bacteria are in this social mode, study of their relationship systems and mechanisms of communication provides another window on their emotional system functioning. Bowen theory takes this expanded view of emotional systems so as not to foreclose the possibility that, despite the complexity of the human emotional system, it may contain a significant legacy of the more than nearly four billion years of evolution that preceded it.

Human beings are sufficiently steeped in individual, cause-and-effect thinking that it is very difficult to shift to a systems view. It requires letting go of individual thinking. The quote below is from Scott Huler (2004), who describes the long history of the development of the Beaufort wind force scale in the late eighteenth and early nineteenth centuries. The quote captures the change in mind-set that must occur to study the wind, a change strikingly similar to the shift required to see the family as an emotional unit or system.

> There was something about describing the wind that sparked expressive language. . . . And I think the answer is that the wind is invisible. You can't describe it because you can't see it. You can only describe what it does to things that you can see—sails, the sea, trees, roof tiles. To describe clouds, trees, or anything else, you focus in on that specific thing, ignoring everything else. To describe the wind, you do the opposite: you look at everything else. It's mind-expanding. (p. 90)

The flow of emotional forces through a family system is an invisible process, but you infer their presence by their impact on the emotional functioning of family members. Observing the impact of emotional forces, or the "emotional field," on family members is emphatically mind expanding.

An example of an emotional system process inferred from watching its impact on individuals is that of a young adult man who reports that he does not like to visit his parents because they still treat him like a child. "It is like I never left home," he laments. If you ask him, "Do you act like a child?," his response is, "Yes, and that is what I hate most about going home!"

At this point, the man thinks that his parents cause him to act like a child. He is the waving tree that Huler described, but he does not understand the force of the wind that he unwittingly helps create. He has usually not reflected much on his highly sensitized emotional reactions to his parents' facial expressions, tone of voice, and other nonverbal cues. It is not just what they say, although that is in the mix, too. Furthermore, he has not thought much about what his parents react to in his own behavior and demeanor.

Emotions are flowing among the three people in this situation. The threesome creates an emotional field that regulates the emotional functioning of each of them. The process is triggered by the high level of emotional reactivity each person has to the others. All people are reactive to some degree to the various social cues listed earlier in Chapter 1, but the level of reactivity among this threesome is an unresolved legacy from the years of the son growing up in the family. It is a legacy as well of what the parents never resolved with their own parents, but more on that subject in Chapter 11.

A useful perspective for people to develop when are trying to change the type of process described in the above clinical vignette is that *the past does not cause the problem in the present*. The father, mother, and son repeatedly re-create the problem in the present. Correspondingly, changing the process that unfolds in the present is the high road to resolving issues from the past.

This same idea applies to the son's current romantic relationships. People select mates for many reasons, but one of the most important is that they are an emotional fit. The mates then re-create in the present the problems from the past. For example, the son, feeling he did not get adequate acceptance from his parents while growing up, is highly reactive to that issue with his mate. His mate works very hard to make him feel accepted, but the reciprocal interaction of him feeling inadequately accepted and her overdoing efforts to reassure him lead to an unsatisfactory interaction. The problems of the past have been re-created in the present for both partners.

As in the earlier example in Chapter 1 of the depressed husband and his distancing wife, it is impossible to discern when this particular chapter of an old process begins. The son has likely been anxious for weeks anticipating his visit home. The mother has likely been excited about seeing a son she wishes she could see more of. The father may worry about having another visit that does not meet expectations, particularly for his wife. All three people are primed in their emotional reactivity, whether aware of it or not.

The parents meet their son at the airport. When the mother sees her son she greets him warmly and says, "Why don't you have a coat on? You must be cold." The son bristles at this comment. The father stiffens as well but supports his wife, "Yes, your mother is right." The son feels hovered over, not treated as an adult. His demeanor gets subdued, sensitive about his parents thinking he can't make good decisions. His mother says, "Are you sure you feel alright. You don't seem like yourself." His father says, "He'll be fine." His mom retorts, "There you go, minimizing my worries." The son is thinking, "Well, it's only two days here. Then I'll go back home."

Commonly, the mother's worry and hovering are viewed as the problem, by both the son and the father. The father walks on eggshells with the mother, knowing how easily she gets upset about signs she interprets as unhappiness in her kids. He tries to do what it takes to keep her happy. The son is somewhat angry that his father mostly seems to take his mother's side. The son has the same deep desire as his father to please his mother, to keep her happy. It is easier that way. The mother is not to blame. She is one of three equal participants in an automatic emotional system process that is easily activated when the three people are in proximity. Each person has difficulty maintaining "self" in the others' presence.

Gaining an understanding of the emotional system and the eight concepts that currently comprise Bowen theory begins with evolution. The human emotional system is the outcome of an evolutionary process that extends deep into the history of life on Earth. The fundamental forces and patterns that operate in all human families described by the theory are anchored in the emotional system. *The forces and patterns manifest in relationship systems, not just in the internal workings of individuals.* This is a unique aspect of Bowen theory. Neuroscientists study the internal workings of individuals, the interplay among cortical and subcortical processes and larger bodily processes. Neuroscientists are obviously keenly aware that every brain exists in a social context and that the brain is continuously adjusting to environmental inputs.

Only Bowen theorists think that, when they study human relationship systems, they are also studying the emotional system. Relationship systems are extensions of the many emotional systems of individual brains. Bowen theorists study the emotional system as it plays out in human relationship interactions. Neuroscientists know that the skull does not define the boundaries of the human brain and that they need a theory of the social context to fully understand the interplay between the human brain and the social context, and also the interplay of many brains at once. The workings of the brain make more sense when they are understood in the context of the relationship system in which the brain is embedded.

The human emotional system has evolved far more sophistication and complexity than the emotional systems of simple life forms, but the large cerebral cortex and elaborate feeling systems of human beings retain essential connections with parts of the brain that evolved long before the emergence of hominoids, even long before vertebrates. Human beings typically offer psychological and feeling explanations for their behaviors, but those factors do not preclude the behaviors being anchored in the emotional system. For example, how far back in the phylogenetic history of our species must we go to discover the roots of our automatic tendency to distance in face of emotional intensity?

Single-celled organisms could not survive without a distancing mechanism to protect them from adverse stimuli. Such a comparison may seem far-fetched to some, but reflecting on the knowledge of primitive life forms can help us grasp how automatic most of these behaviors are, how little emotional autonomy we really have. People want to believe they exert rational control over their actions, but if that were true, the world would not be in the mess it is in today.

The brain's emotional system or limbic system is subcortical, located under the cerebrum. Figure 2.1 shows four of the several components of this emotional brain: hippocampus, amygdala, hypothalamus, and cingulate cortex. Though not shown in this figure, extensive connections exist between the emotional system and the higher brain, the brain stem, and the body as a whole. The two-way connections extending into the cerebrum make subjectivity part of the emotional system. The extensions into the brain stem make the body as a whole part of the emotional system. Communication pathways have been delineated between the higher brain and every cell in the body, making it plausible that interactions between people can regulate the functioning of each person's genes!

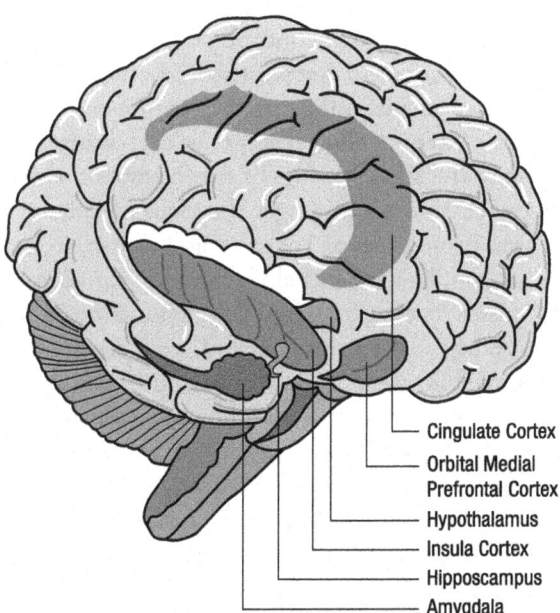

Figure 2.1 *Some components of the human brain emotional system. The front of the brain is on the right. All the labeled components are part of the emotional system except the orbital medial prefrontal cortex. These components occupy parts of the brain that are more ancient evolutionarily than the prefrontal cortex and the rest of the cerebral cortex, long predating the evolution of* Homo sapiens.

Besides studying the many brain systems, neuroscientists also study the body's highly sophisticated regulatory processes that assure the systems work together optimally and adjust to changing circumstances. This research on regulatory processes is important for Bowen theory because the brain's ability to distinguish between feeling and thinking, to be informed by both but able to choose to act on thinking versus feeling, is at the core of theory's concept of differentiation of self.

The oft-uttered phrase, "Can't live with him, can't live without him," targets the powerful impact intimate relationships have on people's health and sense of well-being. Bowen theory conceptualizes the relationship processes that regulate the emotional functioning of individuals, which in turn regulate the internal workings of the brain and the rest of the body. The interactive processes or patterns in relationship systems regulate the emotional reactivity of individuals, and those patterns are also expressions of that emotional reactivity. Just as the cells of the body communicate with one another to preserve bodily homeostasis, people communicate through the five senses to preserve family relationship system homeostasis. Importantly, the metaphor of the wind for an emotional system breaks down in one particular way: the trees, roof tiles, and flag on a flagpole do not generate wind; their movements are strictly reactions to the wind. In contrast, people help to generate an "emotional wind" by their reactions to one another's reactions. Another limitation of the metaphor is that people, unlike smoke coming out of a chimney, have some choice over the extent of their reaction to even a strong anxiety-driven togetherness. Despite the shortcomings of this metaphor, it does capture the mind-expanding process necessary to get the focus off specific individuals in the system who have been diagnosed as causing the problem and onto the system process that all family members help create. You cannot see an emotional system, but you can see its effects on how people function.

What neuroscientists are learning about the emotional system is important for many reasons, but one especially important to Bowen theory is that the scientists are discovering pathways for how the instability in relationship systems translates into emotional reactivity in individuals and associated increases or decreases in functioning. The brain emotional system is significantly regulated by family interactions, and family interactions are significantly regulated by the brain emotional system. The emotional system both as it exists in the brain and as it manifests in a relationship system can be described precisely.

CHAPTER THREE

The Molecule of an Emotional System

A dysfunctional family is any family with more than one person in it.
—Mary Karr, *The Liars' Club*

Triangles are one of the eight concepts in Bowen theory. The triangle conceptualizes a pattern of emotional functioning in relationship systems. As the smallest stable relationship system, triangles are considered to be the molecules or building blocks of an emotional system. If the triangle is the smallest stable system, what is it that makes a two-person system unstable? Observations about the functional facts of triangles were first made at the NIMH. The researchers watched tension grow between family members, and then one member would talk to a member of another family living on the research ward about her angst related to the tense family relationship. This triangled third person would typically respond sympathetically, thus taking a side.

The epigraph above by Mary Karr recognizes the instability of a two-person system. The instability inherent in any intimate relationship is sufficient to render all families, even fairly well-differentiated families, vulnerable to at least some degree of dysfunction at some points in time. When relationships become unstable, some type of dysfunction is usually lurking in the wings.

One explanation for this instability is the consistent clinical observation that human beings have a profound need for emotional closeness but are adverse to too much of it. The phenomenon is a fundamental aspect of human nature and exists in people of all cultures. A threat to closeness triggers feelings of rejection; a threat of too much closeness triggers feelings of being intruded upon, overwhelmed, and out of control. Threats of too much distance and too much closeness activate the stress response. If the threats are prolonged, they generate a chronic stress response that can impair the functioning of any organ and tissue in the body.

While all human beings are vulnerable to experiencing the feelings just described, well-differentiated people manage the closeness-distance dilemma more effectively than do poorly differentiated people. Well-differentiated people are better at rising above the feeling reactions and remaining present and accounted for in a relationship system, even an anxious system; poorly differentiated people are very prone to shut down and distance or to react aggressively.

The formation of a triangle is a "solution" to the instability of a two-person system. *Solution* is in scare quotes because someone pays a price for the triangle—two people gain at the expense of a third. The triangle pattern of emotional process involves two people agreeing that the cause of any tensions between them is not their own immaturities but a third person. In essence, two people align and reject a third. The two people in agreement are the "insiders" in the triangle, and the person blamed for their tensions is the "outsider." The triangle is more stable than a dyad because of the dynamic equilibrium in the triangle. This allows anxiety in the system to shift around through all three relationships and reduces the chances that any one relationship in the triangle will overheat and disrupt.

The triangle can contain more anxiety, but when it is overloaded, one member of the threesome will involve a fourth person, which leads to the formation of *interlocking triangles*. Anxiety can spread infectiously in a group of people through a series of interlocking triangles. This can lead to the formation of strongly biased, polarized subgroups.

An important perspective on this process of subgroup formation is that the beliefs group members hold about themselves and members of the other groups support the polarization but do not cause it. It is an emotional process at its core. It is the coupling of emotion with belief and the compulsion to preserve the alliances within one's own group that make it extremely difficult for either side to grasp the other side's perspective. Any group member who attempts to step outside what can become a highly malignant process is typically labeled as disloyal and often shunned. Triangles and interlocking triangles are the fundamental building blocks or molecules for the formation of we-they groups. Subgroups illustrate how the human need to feel at one with others, a strong affiliation with the group, can trump feelings of empathy for outsiders. The same triangling process that unfolds in family units also unfolds in social units of unrelated people. The less "self" people have, the more dependent they are on affiliation with a group or groups to support their emotional functioning. People with low levels of "self," suffering from depression, with no direction in their lives, may join cult groups and improve their functioning dramatically. Rudyard Kipling's poem "We and They" makes excellent points about the dynamics of subgroup formation and is an enjoyable read (1926).

An important aspect of the dynamic equilibrium of a triangle is that the person in the outside position absorbs the anxiety generated by the triangle. The alliance, togetherness, or fusion of the insiders is comforting to both insiders and calms them. If tensions begin to surface between the insiders, they quickly blame the outsider, such as their child or some other family or group member. The stability of their togetherness depends on being able to externalize their anxieties onto a third person, which manifests in rejection of that person. The rejection can take many forms, such as the insiders overly focusing on what is wrong with the outsider, judging and criticizing that person, whether face to face or behind closed doors. It is easier for people to talk about a third person than to talk personally to each other. Rejection, of course, can also take the form of actively excluding the third person.

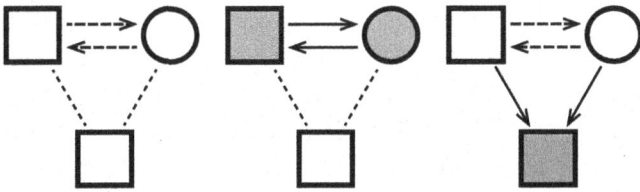

Figure 3.1 *The triangling process.* The black arrows in the diagram on the left symbolize a fairly comfortable human interaction and the dotted lines indicate that there is not an anxious focus on a third person. The jagged line and moderate shading of the people in the middle diagram indicate that both people are more anxious and interacting in an anxious way. The dashed arrows on the diagram on the right symbolize a comfortable human interaction on the surface but with some emotional distance decreasing their anxious focus on each other. The thicker black arrows symbolize an anxious focus on a third person. The heavy shading in the symbol for the person getting the focus indicates high anxiety.

Figure 3.1 illustrates this process. At the left the triangle is dormant: the two people are interacting calmly (symbolized by dashed arrows), which keeps both of them calm. In the center, tense interactions begin to develop between the twosome, and each feels uncomfortable with it (symbolized by thicker dark arrows between them and the shading). At the right, the twosome, now active insiders in the triangle, focus on the third person as the source of their tensions. The third person is in the outside position and carrying the anxiety for the triangle. Bowen theory uses squares to symbolize males and circles for females.

The anxiety generated by the triangle includes the conflicts that could potentially arise between the insiders plus the anxiety the outsider has about being in that position. The most difficult rejection to manage is when a person feels the others prefer each other over him or her, which is what the outside position in a triangle is all about. It can be the basis for jealous, sometimes murderous, rage. Outsiders both generate their own anxiety and absorb anxiety from insiders through their blaming rejection of them.

One strategy outsiders often use to reduce the anxiety they carry for the triangle is to try to change the dynamics of the triangle by maneuvering into a comfortable togetherness with one of the insiders. One way to do this is the outsiders tell an insider a negative story about the other insider. If the negative story is sufficient to persuade the insider to become negative about the other insider, the outsider can often then successfully form an alliance with this insider. That puts the other insider in the outside position, now absorbing the anxiety of the triangle. Predictably, this drives the new outsider to reestablish an inside position, and thus unfolds the dynamic process of a triangle. People can form cooperative alliances based on principles, of course, but that is not a triangle. Triangles represent an anxiety-driven emotional process. Each member of the triangle either automatically seeks relief from anxiety or feels stuck in doing anything about it. A common lament of an acting-out teenager is that his parents are ganging up against him. They are!

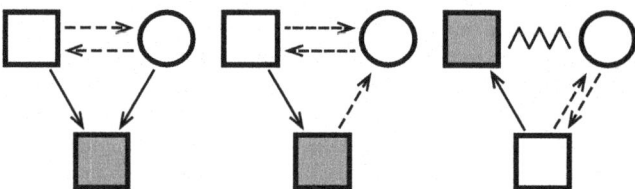

Figure 3.2 *The lines and arrows between people symbolize the same things they did in the previous figure. The arrow from the outsider to one of the insiders in the middle diagram symbolizes his effort to gain an inside position with the insider. In the diagram on the right, the absence of shading in the person previously in the outside position indicates a marked decline in anxiety by gaining an inside position. The shading in the new outsider indicates increased anxiety.*

Figure 3.2 illustrates the success of the outsider forming an alliance with one of the insiders. On the left, the outsider is carrying the anxiety of the triangle. He typically carries it because that position in the triangle is associated with feeling isolated and out of control. In the middle, the outsider persuades one insider to ally with him by telling her a negative story (symbolized by dashed arrow) about the other insider. On the right, the newly persuaded insider becomes negative (jagged line) about the former insider, who now carries the anxiety for the triangle. The arrow between the new insider and the old insider symbolizes new insider's anxiety driven relationship with the previous insider. The interaction between the son and his mother now feels calm and close.

Another example of dynamic equilibrium in triangles is when tensions arise between the two insiders and the most uncomfortable insider initiates closeness with the outsider. The predictable process begins with tension arising between the two insiders. The insiders cope with the rise in tension by using *emotional distance*, another pattern of emotional functioning. Distancing works better for one insider than for the other. One partner experiences the distance as insulation from the other partner's distress. The other partner, who has typically been the one making the most accommodations to preserve relationship harmony, feels blocked from reconnecting with the other partner. She absorbs the anxiety generated by the relationship between the insiders and commonly feels isolated and out of control. The insulating insider is usually blaming the other for the tensions. The other insider is usually feeling inadequate and self-blaming. The uncomfortable insider now initiates closeness with the outsider. The outsider is eager for closeness with one of the insiders and jumps on the opportunity. The previously calmer insider now inherits the anxiety of being in the outside position.

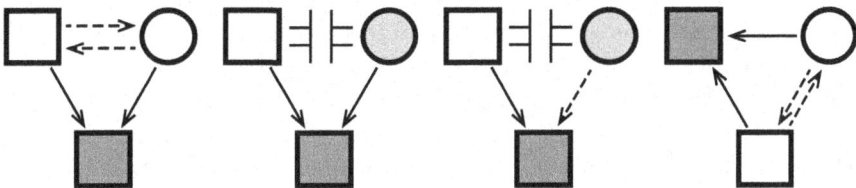

Figure 3.3 The dashed lines between two people and heavy arrows directed by both at the third person on the left diagram symbolize the same things they did in the right diagram of Figure 3.1. Moving from left to right, *the solid lines between two people and empty space indicate increased tension in their interaction and emotional distance.* The absence of shading in the male on the first three diagrams (from left to right) and the light shading on the female in the second and third diagrams indicates she has become an uncomfortable insider having absorbed anxiety for the relationship. On the third diagram from the left, the dashed line from the female to the male indicates her effort to gain an inside position with him. In the diagram to the far right, the former outsider has gained an inside position with the female accompanied by a reduction of anxiety in both of the new insiders. The dark shading in former insider male, indicates anxiety related to the outside position.

Figure 3.3 summarizes this process, which moves from left to right. The first diagram depicts the initial equilibrium. The next diagram depicts emotional distance developing between the insiders in response to tension building up in their interactions. The distance typically works better for one partner (the male in this example) than it does for the other. This motivates the female to initiate closeness with the outsider (third diagram from left). He responds to her overture, and the previously insider male now feels the anxiety of the outside position (diagram on the right).

An interesting variant of the dynamic equilibrium of triangles is two people who can keep their relationship comfortable provided they are not interacting with a third person. This involves each of the insiders putting maximum energy into the other. If a third person enters the scene, say, a friend of the wife, and the wife directs her energy toward the friend, the husband gets upset and criticizes the wife for her inattention to him. (He is usually not that direct.) When the third person departs, the wife invests more energy in her mate again and that calms him. One common strategy for avoiding this situation is for the husband (or whoever is in this position in the triangle) to pressure his wife to cut off contact with her friends. This strategy is an "administrative" solution, not a grown-up solution. In this scenario, each person is having difficulty maintaining "self."

Another facet of the dynamic equilibrium of triangles is illustrated by a common occurrence in my family of origin when I was growing up. (I turn to my family from time to time in the main text of the book to exemplify a theoretical idea. In the epilogue I give a detailed description of my family-of-origin emotional process.) The first step in this process is a state of comfortable closeness between my mother and my schizophrenic brother, with my father in the outside position of the triangle. Then tension develops between Mother and my brother. Mother expresses increasing distress about this, which is a signal that Dad reacts to. He reacts in an attempt to get my brother's behavior to change. Conflict erupts between them. Mother then strategically retreats to the outside position, which has become a more comfortable spot than the inside position. It is a posture of, "Let's you and him fight!" If it begins to border on physical violence between Dad and my brother, Dad involves my oldest brother and establishes another, interlocking triangle (Dad and my two brothers). My oldest brother was never involved in physical conflict with my brother, so his involvement tended to take the pressure off things. This is diagramed in the sequence that follows (Figures 3.4–3.7):

Mother and schizophrenic brother are in the inside positions associated with a low-tension state (Figure 3.4). Dad is in the outside position. He draws comfort from work activities and having a fairly calm spouse, one who is calmed by satisfying her need to be needed.

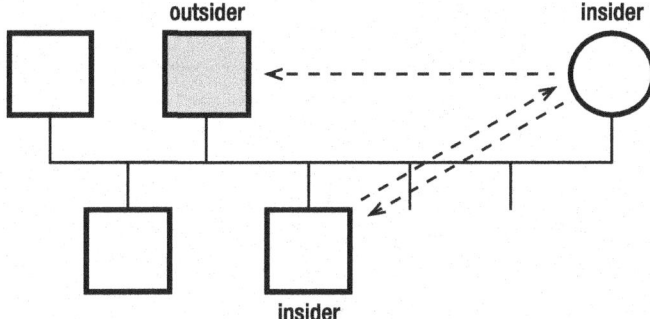

Figure 3.4 *The diagram symbolizes a mother having a son in her first marriage, a firstborn son in her second marriage, and two younger children (identified only by lines, not male or female symbols. The reciprocal dashed arrows between the mother and firstborn son from her second marriage indicates a strong and comfortable emotional attachment. They occupy the insider positions in the parental triangle. The dashed lines leading to the father indicate that he is in the outside position of the triangle. The absence of shading indicates that the triangle is calm and stable at this point in time.*

Tension develops between Mother and my brother (Figure 3.5). Mother sends out distress signals to Dad. He is also highly tuned into her upsets about my brother and anxiously moves in on my brother to get him under control.

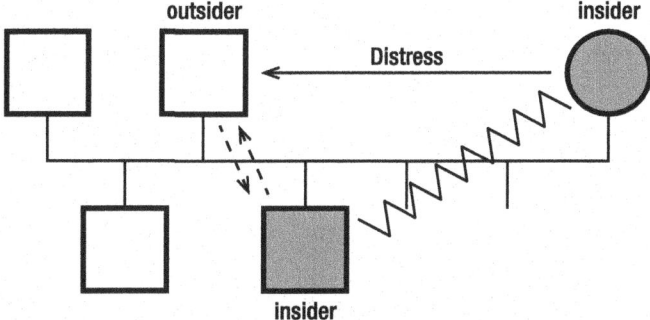

Figure 3.5 *The jagged line between mother and son indicates tension and conflict having erupted in their relationship. The arrow between the mother and father indicates that she is communicating her distress about the relationship with their son to her husband. The arrows between father and son indicate that his wife's distress has triggered his increased focus on the son to get him to change in how he is interacting with his mother.*

Major conflict develops between the two uncomfortable insiders, Dad and my brother (Figure 3.6). Mother is calmed by moving into the now most

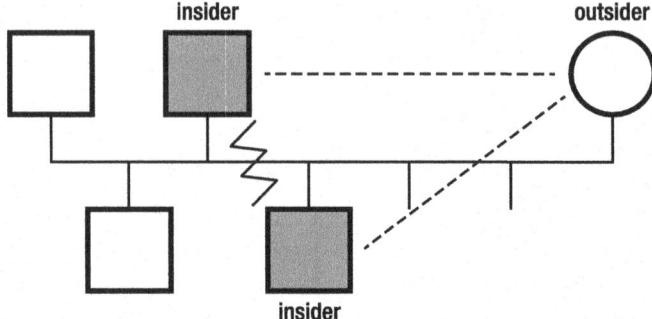

Figure 3.6 *Severe anxiety-driven conflict erupts between father and son (thick jagged line), and mother is calmer. The inside positions in the triangle are now the uncomfortable ones, and outside position the mother has gained is the most comfortable position. The dashed lines indicate mother's distance from husband and son.*

comfortable, outside position. When some degree of physical violence occurs between Dad and my brother, Dad moves to involve my oldest brother, creating an interlocking triangle.

My oldest brother was never involved in physical altercations with my schizophrenic brother, which usually helped family anxiety subside over a day or two (Figure 3.7).

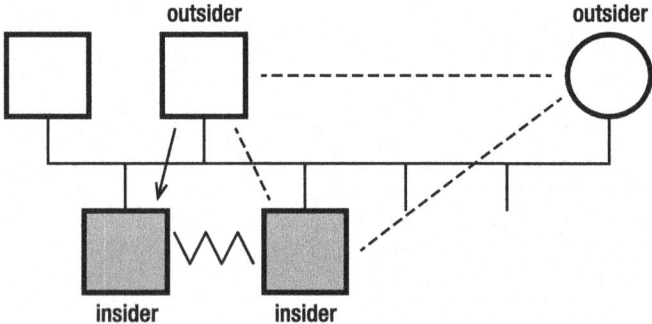

Figure 3.7 *The black arrow between the father and mother's first son indicates the father's anxious effort to involve him in dealing with this son's half-brother. Conflict to a lesser degree shifts to the half-brothers through an interlocking triangle process.*

Learning how to track the paths of triangles rather than getting lost in the content of the moment requires discarding cause-and-effect thinking and employing systems thinking. Figures 3.4–3.7 are intended to aid the reader in thinking about the forces governing human behavior in this very different way. The *why* of each person's behavior does not reside within the confines of each person; each person contributes to and is responding to a larger relationship process.

Triangles are ubiquitous and not pathological. They are ways for a relationship system to compartmentalize anxiety in one part of the system, such that system anxiety impairs the functioning of as few people as possible. However, someone does pay a price for that stability. My schizophrenic brother was not a victim of the triangles but an active participant in them.

One could argue that triangles are rooted in the enormous curiosity we human beings take in one another's lives. A gossip system is a seemingly essential element of all human groups. It can serve a useful purpose. Gossip spreads through triangles. When the emotional valence of the gossip content rises, it becomes more likely to create insiders and outsiders. When two people talk about a third, it is often a subtle line between a constructive process, spreading useful information that enhances the functioning of the group, and a destructive, anxiety-driven process.

CHAPTER FOUR

Patterns of Emotional Functioning

We live our lives in networks of emotional forces that follow triangle patterns.
—Murray Bowen, 1976 interview

This chapter begins with a quote from Murray Bowen that could have also introduced the previous chapter on triangles. It is placed here because it contains the phrase "networks of emotional forces." I emphasize this phrase because, although most people accept that other people's emotional states affect them and that their own emotional states affect others, they think about it in cause-and-effect terms. They worry that they might have caused upset in others or they blame others for causing upset in them. They do not see patterns of interaction in the way described in Chapter 1 on systems thinking. They do not see the flow of emotions back and forth between themselves and others and how that flow regulates each person's emotions and functioning. Cause-and-effect thinking is the principal obstacle to seeing the patterns of emotional functioning that Bowen theory describes.

Triangles are one of four patterns of interaction that Bowen theory describes. All the patterns are anchored in the emotional system. Their activity ranges from almost dormant to extremely active, depending on the level of chronic anxiety in a relationship system. The patterns are key variables for explaining *which* member of a family system develops clinical symptoms. Symptoms can manifest as disorders in the functioning of mind, body, or behavior. The widely accepted medical model views the cause of symptoms as a process residing within the patient. It is easier to think the medical model way because it lets you off the hook in facing up to your own part in the problem. Commitment to this model interferes with people seeing the relationship patterns. It is necessary to let go of individual thinking to shift to relationship thinking. Again, this is not about one person causing a particular symptom in another person; it is about reciprocal relationship interactions and triangles rendering one member of the system more vulnerable to developing some type of symptom. Other factors, such as genes, toxins, and pathogens, have to be at play as well for symptoms to emerge.

If there is obvious turmoil in the family system, people tend to assume that the family turmoil results from distress about the symptomatic person's impaired functioning. This is a half-truth, not the whole story. The role of the relationship system in creating and maintaining the impaired functioning is the other half. A common response to suggesting that the family system has an important role in symptom development is that it is tantamount to blaming the family. People tend to say either that the family has nothing to do with it or that they blame the family for not being loving enough, attentive enough, or involved enough. Systems thinking shows how the family is part of the problem, but interpreting that as blame misses the point.

Murray Bowen liked to say, "The way to prevent schizophrenia is to try to create it." His point was that parents are anxiously trying their best *not* to create it. The anxiety can turn a well-intentioned action into a problem for the child. It is an old adage that it is not what parents say they do that is important; it is what they really do that matters. Anxiety-driven overly zealous efforts to protect children from harm can unintentionally make the children overly dependent on the parents to make decisions for them. Most people know this, but fear trumps wisdom.

Understanding the link between patterns of emotional functioning and clinical symptoms depends on understanding a person's *functioning position* in a family relationship system. The nature of this position in a family system renders the person more or less vulnerable to absorbing system-generated chronic anxiety.

The patterns of emotional functioning are sustained by people's functioning positions in the patterns. Each person's functioning position reflects the nature of the prevailing pattern, and the positions reinforce the prevailing pattern. Examples of functioning positions are the dynamic interplay between inside and outside positions in triangles and the reciprocity between the overfunctioning and underfunctioning positions in a dyadic interaction. The person in the outside position of a triangle absorbs anxiety that the triangle as a whole generates. The absorption of system-generated anxiety results from one member of the system being in a position that generates a greater sense of threat than the positions others occupy. For example, the "outsider" is the member of a triangle most vulnerable to developing clinical symptoms.

Relationship systems, driven by the emotional system, shape the functioning of their members to an extent that people rarely recognize. This process is most extreme in poorly differentiated systems, but it is present to some degree in all families. People often sense the process but struggle to put their finger on it. Theory can help people recognize it. Hypertension is often referred to as the silent killer. Anxiety-driven emotional processes can be silent killers too.

Many people react to Bowen theory by feeling that they are being blamed for the problems of other family members: Do you think I caused my son's schizophrenia, or my husband's heart attack? An important distinction exists between causing something and playing a part in it. Cause-and-effect thinking can foster guilt or denial; systems thinking permits us to be more realistic about our part in an emotional process and others' parts in that process. Seeing a larger picture helps us to address difficult and distressing problems without descending into guilt or denial.

Family process does not cause people to have heart attacks or other problems—many other variables must come into play for these clinical conditions to occur. Systems thinking does not assign cause to any one variable; it is the interaction of all the variables that is important to understand. Bowen theory does assume, however, that the chronic anxiety generated by relationship process disturbances can disturb the balance of relationship processes at many levels, including the family and the body. Ironically, the body's and the family's exaggerated efforts to correct those disturbances can play a critical role in many if not all types of clinical symptoms (I discuss this in more detail in Chapter 23).

Knowledge of the existence of patterns of emotional functioning helps people observe them. However, it takes time for people to convince themselves of the accuracy of the idea and to use that knowledge to rein in the compulsion to assume that a cause for the problem resides within one person. Operationalizing Bowen theory, meaning to live it, depends on being able to see how the processes the theory describes play out in one's own life. Reading about it helps, but it is not enough. The denouement of one's efforts is to use the knowledge gained from new observations to guide changes in one's actions such that they are constructive for self and for others.

Murray Bowen described what he later termed *patterns of emotional functioning* in his first published comprehensive presentation of the theory (Bowen, 1966). He included the patterns in his description of one of the concepts in the theory: relationship system in the nuclear family ego mass. He referred to them in that paper as "three major mechanisms to control the intensity of the ego fusion" (p. 166): (a) marital conflict, (b) dysfunction in one spouse, and (c) transmission of the problem to one or more children. He described a fourth mechanism, emotional distance, as inevitably accompanying each of the other patterns. In Bowen's last comprehensive theory paper, he substituted the phrase "patterns of emotional functioning in a family" for the term *mechanisms* (Bowen, 1976). He labeled the patterns similarly to the first theory paper and described them as operating in nuclear family emotional systems, extended family emotional systems, and social systems. Bowen theory's main point is that marital conflict, dysfunction in one spouse, and transmission of the problem to one or more children are all expressions of the same thing:

undifferentiation and associated chronic anxiety in the nuclear family system. The more it manifests in one area, the less likely it is to manifest in other areas.

Observing what appears to be a finite number of patterns in relationship systems requires viewing group interactions through the lens of systems thinking. This allows the observer to focus on the facts of the *process* playing out between people rather than getting lost in the *content* of that process, for example, staying focused on the fact that people are fighting rather than getting lost in what they are fighting about—issues to fight about come and go; arguing about them is the constant. Another example of seeing process is observing a husband's part in fostering emotional distance in a marriage along with the wife's part in the creating the distance. A next step is to connect the wife's drinking and depression with her isolation and despair in reaction to the intractable distance in the marriage. Watching the relationship interaction and its consequences is process thinking; focusing on drinking and depression as diseases that cause the interaction is content thinking.

Many clinicians think of the process just described as arising from the existence of two problems: the wife's illnesses, and the marital problem. This is multicausal thinking, not systems thinking. Systems thinking sees what is transpiring between people and how the people are functioning emotionally as seamlessly intertwined. The wife's despair and withdrawal play a part in the distance but do not cause it. The distance, which is cocreated, plays a role but does not cause the wife's symptoms. Symptoms affect the relationship, and the relationship affects the symptoms. It is inaccurate to say that either one causes the other, but it is hard to think this way. It gets back to the idea of the whole being greater than the sum of its parts.

These are called *patterns of emotional functioning* because their activity is driven by the emotional system. Bowen's initial reference to the patterns as "mechanisms" is accurate because *mechanism* conveys a different aspect of the patterns. *Mechanism* refers to the function of the patterns. They function to control the intensity of the ego fusion in relationships. It is important to note that Bowen theory no longer uses the term *ego fusion*. It is now termed *emotional fusion*. Psychological processes and feelings contribute to emotional fusion, but fusion is anchored in the emotional system. Intensity describes the degree of chronic anxiety and heightened emotional reactivity that a relationship fusion generates. The patterns function to "bind" the anxiety generated by the fusion.

Figure 4.1 illustrates this idea. The relationship diagram on the left symbolizes the anxiety (shading inside the square and circle) generated in each person consequent to how they are interacting. The diagram on the right symbolizes the people using emotional distance to reduce the anxiety triggered by

Figure 4.1 The shading of each member of the dyad on the left side of the diagram and black arrows between them symbolize anxiety-driven processes in a relationship and anxiety in each person. The diagram on the right symbolizes emotional distance developing between the people, with subsequent reduction of each person's chronic anxiety. The shaded bars between the people symbolize that the anxiety is bound in the emotional distance. The term "bound" conveys that by anxiety expressing itself in the distance maintained by two people, it no longer expresses itself within each individual.

their interactions. Both people experience less internal anxiety in this process, but the anxiety is now evident or bound in distancing behaviors (symbolized by the shaded rectangles in the distance symbol). If people are unable to distance from each other for whatever reason, internalized anxiety reappears.

In a pattern, each person's behavior regulates the other person's behavior in reciprocal fashion. Distancing can occur through physical and emotional means. An example of emotional distancing is people being in physical proximity but avoiding potentially emotionally charged topics. The anxiety is bound in the avoiding of such topics. Another way of describing the binding of anxiety is that the anxiety is integrated into the structure of a relationship.

On many occasions, Murray Bowen stated the following: "If I had to reduce my theory to one basic idea, it would be that it explains how two people can begin their relationship very close, but become increasingly distant over time." One can learn to regain a mature closeness by understanding how each person's immaturity undermined it and then applying that knowledge to change one's part in the process.

In the late 1970s I undertook a detailed study of E. O. Wilson's famous tome *Sociobiology: The New Synthesis* (1975). The studies of the social groups of a wide range of species described in the book reveal the existence of close parallels between the patterns of emotional functioning that Bowen theory describes and the observation of similar patterns in other species. The descriptions support the idea that the patterns described by Bowen theory are a product of evolution and embedded in the emotional system.

In an effort to facilitate a link between evolutionary biologists and Bowen theory's idea of the emotional system, I began in the early 1980s to use terms for the patterns similar to those in Wilson's book and widely used by biologists. The changes I made were the following: referring to marital conflict as *emotional conflict*, dysfunction in one spouse as *dominant-adaptive* (*deferential*) interactions, and transmission to one or more children as *triangles*. I retained the term *emotional distance*. I was not suggesting different patterns, just new terms to describe them. These are summarized in Table 4.1. These modifications do not represent a change in Bowen theory from Bowen's original writings; I offer them as a clarification of the original terminology.

The adaptive or deferential one is the member of the dyad making the most behavioral changes in an attempt to maintain harmony in the relationship. These terms in Bowen theory imply not inferiority in the deferential partner but a functional position that results from a relationship interaction, for example, an emotionally driven process in which one person acts stronger than that person really is and the other acts weaker than that person really is. Such interactions are commonly associated with one partner "overfunctioning" and the other "underfunctioning." The overfunctioner may appear to be the dominant partner, but that is not always the case. The overfunctioner may be adapting disproportionately in the relationship under pressure from the underfunctioner.

TABLE 4.1
Modifications of Bowen's Original Terminology

BOWEN'S 1966 PAPER	MY MODIFICATIONS
Marital conflict	Emotional conflict
Dysfunction in one spouse	Dominant-adaptive (deferential)
Transmission to one or more children	Triangles
Emotional distance	Emotional distance

I chose these new terms for two other reasons as well: (1) to emphasize, for example, that the development of dysfunction in one spouse is the outcome of a sufficiently intense pattern of dominant-adaptive (deferential) interactions in the marriage; and (2) to note that the pattern that can foster dysfunction in a spouse is not confined to the marital relationship but can also operate in other family relationships, such as between a parent and a child.

The triangle is the cornerstone of the four patterns. Triangles are of central importance in Bowen theory because they show how relationships are interlinked. What transpires in a dyadic relationship affects and is affected by what transpires in the other two relationships in the triangle. The marital relationship and the father-child relationship affect and are affected by the mother-child relationship. Figure 4.2 illustrates that any of the three patterns can operate in any of the relationships of a triangle.

If emotional conflict is the dominant pattern between the spouses, marital

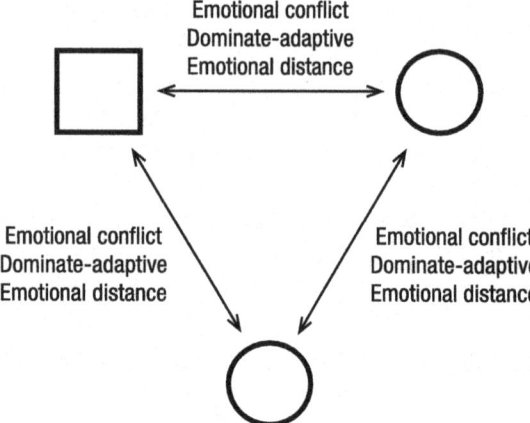

Figure 4.2 *All four patterns of emotional functioning are represented on this diagram.* The bi-directional arrows between people in each of the three relationships indicates three emotionally interconnected relationships functioning in a triangle pattern. The other three patterns can play out in any of the three relationships, such as between father and mother, mother and daughter, and father and daughter.

conflict is the presenting clinical problem. If the dominant-adaptive (deferential) pattern is the principal pattern at work, dysfunction in a spouse will be the presenting problem. Emotional distance consistently operates with both of those patterns. Marital conflict (emotional conflict) and dysfunction in a spouse (dominant-adaptive) are different ways of managing the chronic anxiety generated by the emotional fusion in a marital relationship.

Other factors affect the level of chronic anxiety generated by emotional fusion, such as the number of stressors on the relationship and how isolated the relationship is from other potentially supportive relationships. I now describe the patterns in more detail.

DOMINANT-ADAPTIVE (DEFERENTIAL)

It is important to note that dominant-adaptive (deferential) interactions are very common when the conspecifics of many species are living in proximity. They are the emotional basis of social hierarchies. A stable hierarchy can function to reduce conflict by means of the presence of deferential social behaviors. In human families, the process can be gross or subtle. Dominance hierarchies, some more complex than others, are common in species that routinely live in social groups. Another way to activate dominance hierarchies is to purposely crowd animals that normally live at a distance from one another.

In nature, sometimes conspecifics change from living at a distance from one another to clustering into groups in response to changes in their environment. The change commonly brings out hierarchies. It may be that dominant-adaptive (deferential) interactions are deeply ingrained in many species but are not always expressed.

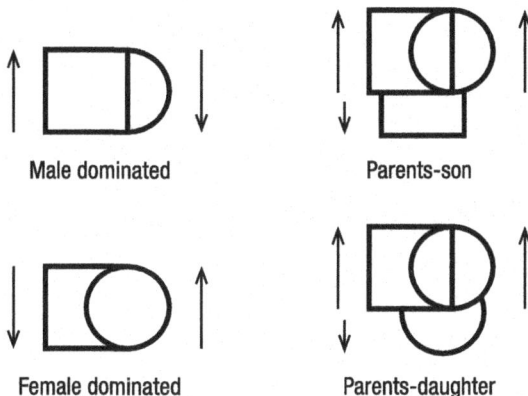

Figure 4.3 *The diagrams on the left side symbolize dominant-adaptive (deferential) patterns in adult-adult relationships. One symbol overlapping another symbol indicates the dominant partner, male dominated at the top and female dominated at the bottom. The arrows pointing up or down on each side of the symbols indicate overfunctioning and underfunctioning in their reciprocal interactions. The diagrams on the right side indicate the pattern playing out between parents and a son at the top and a daughter at the bottom, with overfunctioning and underfunctioning again symbolized by arrows.*

Figure 4.3 shows how Bowen theory symbolizes this type of interaction in human relationships. The left diagrams depict a male-dominated emotional fusion at the top and a female-dominated one at the bottom. Dominant-adaptive (deferential) interactions are usually accompanied by some degree of overfunctioning-underfunctioning reciprocity. In a male-dominated fusion, the male tends to overfunction (symbolized by the arrow next to the male pointing upward), and the female tends to underfunction (symbolized by the arrow next to the female pointing downward). The opposite is the case in female-dominated fusions. The diagram at the top right depicts a parent-dominated fusion with a son, and the one below it, with a daughter. Again, overfunctioning parents and an underfunctioning offspring typically accompany this process.

It is important to note that part of the normal structure of families is that parents are in charge. This involves reality-driven functioning for the child until the child matures sufficiently not to require it. The overfunctioning-underfunctioning reciprocity between the parents and a child, like the case between spouses, is anxiety driven. Parents do more for the child than the child's reality needs require, and the child plays out the opposite of the process.

An overfunctioning-underfunctioning reciprocity does not reflect role differentiation, although it could bear some relationship to it. Role differentiation results from people taking on specialized tasks that render a family or social system more functional and adaptive. It is not anxiety driven but reality driven. In contrast, anxiety drives overfunctioning-underfunctioning reciprocal interactions. The overfunctioner is not necessarily more capable than the underfunctioner. Real differences between people do not account for the functioning positions they occupy. For example, in a male-dominated fusion, the male is calmer when he feels he is in charge. His posture to the other person is emotionally driven, not reality driven. The female may feel calmer at not having to be the primary decision maker. Her posture is also emotionally driven, not reality driven. The potential anxiety of the relationship fusion is bound in the reciprocal interaction. The adaptive (deferential) partner may also go along out of fear of conflict and rejection.

In my early years of learning and applying Bowen theory and watching overfunctioning-underfunctioning reciprocities play out clinically in cases where one spouse had developed psychiatric symptoms, it appeared that it was the underfunctioning spouse who was most vulnerable to symptom development. A cause-and-effect way of thinking about this is that, for example, the person's depression causes the underfunctioning. This triggers the other spouse to take up the slack and overfunction. However, clinical experience indicates that the overfunctioning-underfunctioning reciprocity typically predates the development of symptoms. If the reciprocal interaction becomes sufficiently intense, the underfunctioner begins to report a loss of confidence, indecisiveness, and feeling emotionally isolated. The more people feel this way, which is a consequence of their functioning position in the reciprocity, the closer they move toward clinical depression or some other symptom.

In 1976, I began a study of families in which one member had developed cancer. The research changed my thinking about which member of an overfunctioning-underfunctioning reciprocity is vulnerable to symptom development. In many cancer cases it was the overfunctioning person in the family who developed the cancer. The overfunctioning members would report feelings of being overwhelmed and isolated. They had been working to meet the perceived expectations of others and were driven as well by their expectations of themselves. The families seemed heavily dependent on these people to do what needed to be done to make things better. The overfunctioners were disproportionately carrying family anxiety. The overfunctioners looked dominant, but these were cases of the overfunctioners being pinned down in the one-up position.

More experience with psychiatric problems over time convinced me that it could also be an overfunctioning family member who developed psychiatric and behavioral symptoms. The fact that both overfunctioning and underfunctioning people could develop symptoms of all types led me to the following conclusion: the person most vulnerable to dysfunction in a dominant-adaptive (deferential), overfunctioning-underfunctioning pattern is the one making the most internal adjustments in functioning to preserve harmony. This can happen on either side of the reciprocity. Assessing which spouse is most compromised in functioning by the dominant-adaptive (deferential) relationship process that both spouses create and maintain requires careful examination—appearances can be deceiving. The important point is that an interactive process can result in people getting into positions in a system that eventually impair their functioning.

The most active pattern of emotional functioning in a family can change over time. A dominant-adaptive (deferential) pattern may characterize the early years of a marriage, but this can shift into one of emotional conflict or emotional distance later on. Additionally, more than one pattern can be active in a family at the same time.

EMOTIONAL CONFLICT

Conflict between people is not inherently bad. Legitimate differences between people often merit vigorous exchanges that may help clarify the viewpoints of each person, for both parties. In contrast, emotional conflict implies that the fighting is emotionally driven, not rationally driven. Emotional conflict is anchored in the emotional system. Emotionally driven conflict encompasses biases and feelings as well as emotions.

The following quote by Jonathan Haidt is speculative, but the idea fits with much of human experience: "Reasoning has evolved not to help us find truth, but to help us engage in arguments, persuasion, and manipulation in the context of discussions with others. Confirmation bias is a built-in feature of the argumentative mind" (2012, p. 89). Bowen theory states that when emotions are intensely involved, as they are in the emotional conflict pattern, reason operates in the service of emotion, not in the service of a careful assessment of the facts. As a result, people's alleged attempts to act "reasonable" only fan the flames.

Emotional conflict in a marriage and in a parent-child relationship functions to bind anxiety. Figure 4.4 illustrates this in a marriage. The diagram on

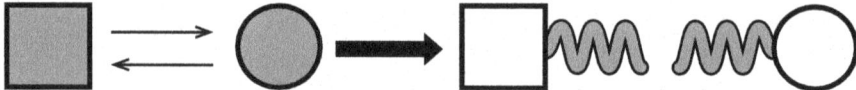

Figure 4.4 *The shading in the male and female symbols on the left (the symbols could be same sex as well) and arrows between them indicate anxious people interacting anxiously.* The absence of shading in the male and female on the right and shading in their conflictual interaction indicates that the anxiety is now externalized into (bound in) relationship conflict and not internalized by either partner.

the left depicts a buildup of chronic anxiety in a relationship that is internalized by both people. The diagram on the right illustrates the externalization of the anxiety into conflict. The empty space between the two conflict symbols represents emotional distance, which is part of the conflict pattern.

People blame each other for the problem, which is calming for both: "I'm not the problem, you are the problem!" But the anxiety is now bound in both people dogmatically adhering to their own viewpoints. The process is fueled, in part, by each spouse's hypersensitivity to being controlled by the other spouse. Each accuses the other of trying to control the relationship. The upside to such a process is that it externalizes the anxiety rather than internalizing it. Consequently, each person becomes less vulnerable to developing mental or physical symptoms related to internalized anxiety. For example, one spouse's depression may improve if the couple starts fighting more. This does not necessarily represent progress because the anxiety and reactivity are the same, just expressed differently. Fighting back can sometimes reflect an incipient effort to carve out a little more "self" in the relationship. As a person gains more objectivity about the relationship process, more "self," this leads to less anxiety and conflict.

Triangles enable two people to bind anxiety through involvement of a third person. This enables them to maintain a more stable closeness. Dominant-adaptive (deferential) interactions bind anxiety by one person absorbing it for the relationship through deferential behaviors. This can maintain a feeling of closeness. It is an alternative to distancing, although some distancing is usually part of the picture, particularly at heightened levels of chronic anxiety. Emotional conflict is a fascinating pattern in that people maintain contact and enforce distance at the same time. Poking at the other gets a reaction and pushes the other away at the same time. Each of the three patterns solves the dilemma posed by the intense need for closeness and equally intense aversion to too much of it. Each pattern solves it in a different way. Up to a point, the patterns stabilize relationships but lead to dysfunction occurring somewhere in the system if sufficiently high levels of chronic anxiety develop.

Conflict arises from neither person having enough "self" not to feel that going along with the other's wants and ideas is "giving in." The mutual defensiveness precludes reasoned compromise and cooperation. Poorly differentiated relationships are vulnerable to the most extreme levels of conflict.

The usual pattern is periods of intense arguing, maybe even fighting physically, followed by periods of distance. People may distance to the point of avoiding all but absolutely essential conversation, and even eye contact for days or weeks. During the distant part of the cycle, people obsessively focus on what is wrong with the other person. The distance may result in both spouses feeling justified to do what they want to do when they want to do it. Then there may be a brief period of making up and closeness. It does not usually take long, however, for even a small issue to disrupt the closeness, and vigorous arguments resume.

Borrowing from evolutionary biology's concept of punctuated equilibrium, I sometimes describe the emotional conflict pattern as "punctuated disequilibrium." *Punctuated* refers to the brief closeness phase. Interestingly, conflictual marriages are often enduring. If one spouse announces he or she wants a divorce, the other spouse is often shocked. "Why in the world would you want a divorce? We've always done it this way!" In other cases, people grow so weary of the fighting that they quit doing it. It is not a solution, however, because emotional distance replaces the more raucous periods.

A common but conspicuously unsuccessful strategy for trying to avoid exhausting arguments is one person trying not to take the bait. This spouse tries hard not to react, no matter how provocative the other's words and actions are. It only makes the one who wants some type of response angrier. The spouse feeling ignored by the seeming lack of response typically escalates attacks on the other spouse until that spouse finally loses it and explodes. Some report more sense of connection when they succeed at provoking the other to explode. "Finally, I know what you feel!"

Myriad issues exist for people to fight about, but, like the other patterns, the content of the issues does not drive the pattern. Emotional reactivity drives the pattern. Feelings of not getting enough attention, of not being adequately affirmed, of expectations unmet, and of being blamed for the other's distress are key elements in triggering the reactivity. The issues that these hypersensitivities inflame commonly center on sex, money, or children. The underlying problem that drives the reactivity is the absence of a sense of comfortable connection, the lack of oneness.

A frequent time for significant emotional conflict in parent-child relationships is during adolescence. A recurrent story is that the mother and son or daughter have had a very close and harmonious relationship during the child's preadolescent years. It is intensely emotionally fused (not well differentiated), but the quality of the relationship has been positive. As the teenager moves into adolescence, however, he or she begins to change, in part, based on biological maturation.

The early adolescent typically wants to be less actively involved with the parents and more focused on peers. The mother most often experiences the change as a threat to the special closeness they have always had. She worries about whether the son or daughter is making good judgments and decisions. The less "self" the adolescent has developed by that point, the more reactive the adolescent is to mother's intrusiveness. Rebellious conflict is a way for the adolescent to distance from the parents.

Adolescent rebellion is reactive distancing, not differentiation. It stems from both parent and adolescent having trouble maintaining "self" in their relationship. It does not indicate that the teenager is developing "self." A vicious action-reaction circle ensues, with the teenager communicating less and less, even lying, to the parents, and the parents being mistrustful and increasingly upset about not knowing what is going on with their child. Paradoxically, even though this process is playing out in an intense emotional fusion between parents and offspring, the teenager often reports not feeling close to the parents. This results not from a lack of parental involvement but from the reactivity that keeps them at a distance. This greatly interferes with parents being a resource for their child. The adolescent will not listen, and the parents cannot stop lecturing, threatening punishments, and the like.

I once treated a family in which all communication with their son was with the father. Mother and son avoided each other as much as possible. The mother said the following about the relationship with the son: "Dr. Kerr, I want you to understand that in my son's preschool years, our relationship was like Velcro. We were like one person. We were so sensitized to each other, however, that our relationship slowly turned from positive to negative."

The father is typically upset with the disharmony between his wife and their teen. He may side with the teenager against the mother, which makes the mother-adolescent conflict worse, or side with his wife, which also makes the conflict worse—the adolescent experiences it as a two against one, which it is. A father's attempts to control the teen's behavior often trigger intense conflict in the parent-child relationship. It can also add to tension and conflict in the marriage if the mother tries to protect the child from what she sees as her husband's harshness. The adolescent exploits the conflict between his parents to get his or her way.

Dominant-adaptive (deferential) and triangle interactions involving parents and offspring are part of the adolescent period as well. Unsure parents alternate between overly controlling behaviors with the teenager and overly permissive ones. One parent may appear to hold the line better than the other, but commonly both parents give in more than they stand firm. None of the three people can maintain "self."

Parents exacerbate each other's unsureness about how to handle the teenager by second-guessing and criticizing each other. The blaming reflects a lack of understanding of the triangle and the part each of the three people play in it. For example, when the father takes sides with the teenager, it is impossible for the mother to take an effective stand with the adolescent. This makes her more anxious and intrusive and the teenager more resistant to cooperating. The father lectures the mother about the need to back off but does not recognize that he is just as much a part of the problem as his wife is. The mother lectures the father about how he should be different as well.

When parent-child relationships have been more mature during the preadolescent years and the teenager has developed more "self" than in the just described examples, little adolescent rebellion unfolds—there is no reason for it. The parents are less threatened by the typical changes in their teen's behavior as teen navigates adolescence, and the teenager also feels confident as well.

However, appearances can be deceiving. Absence of adolescent rebellion does not always indicate that the relationships in the parental triangle are more mature, less fused emotionally. Some adolescents will manage the lack of differentiation from their parents by trying to please, always do the "right thing," and excel in school. These kids commonly view their parents as normal and think that they themselves are the problem if anything goes wrong. They do little if any fighting with their parents but internalize any relationship-generated anxiety. Such kids are often hypersensitive about acceptance in peer relationships as well. The kids have adopted a one-down relationship with their parents, which stems from this type of typically unrecognized dominant-adaptive (deferential) interaction.

Seeing symptoms in an adolescent as relating primarily to the parental triangle distinguishes Bowen-theory-based therapy from conventional therapy. Conventional therapy diagnoses the adolescent and treats the teen with medication and individual therapy. Bowen-theory-based therapy seeks to help the parents understand the workings of the triangle, their parts in it as well as the adolescent's part in it, and tries to help them make changes in themselves. When a family is in anxiety-driven free fall and has drifted off a constructive path, it is unrealistic to expect their dependent adolescent to lead the family out of the morass and back onto a constructive path.

Before leaving this subject it is important to note that factors other than the parental triangle come into play in the functioning of an adolescent, such as peer group influences, but modifying the parental triangle is key to progress. If parents try to control the people their adolescent hangs out with or continually change schools looking for the right fit, they are putting off dealing with the triangle.

TRIANGLE

Bowen modified the phrase *transmission to one or more children* that he used in his first theory paper to *impairment of one or more children* in his second theory paper (Bowen, 1971). In that same paper, he made the *family projection process* a separate concept in the theory because of how important it is in this impairment process. I have included the ideas of impairment of a child and the family projection process under the term *triangle*. As with the new terms I have suggested for the other patterns of emotional functioning, this term is primarily intended as a teaching device, not to replace Bowen's original terms.

The reason for using the term *triangle* to cover impairment of a child and the family projection process is to emphasize that the dyadic interaction between mother and offspring occurs in the context of a triangle. If the dominant-adaptive (deferential) or emotional conflict patterns adequately bind anxiety in the marital relationship, it protects the children to some degree from family anxiety. Clinical observations show that a major chronic dysfunction in one parent or extreme conflict between the parents does not preclude their raising reasonably functional kids. This is not to say that a major dysfunction in a parent has no effect on the kids but that it creates less impairment than child focus does.

The triangle pattern describes how potential anxiety in the marital relationship can shift out of that relationship and into the parents' relationships with the children. Because the mother is usually the primary caretaker for the child, her relationship with the child is usually more emotionally intense than the father's. This makes the mother-child relationship the most direct influence on transmitting the parental undifferentiation to the child. The anxiety flows most through that relationship, but that anxiety is not inherent in the mother. It is a product of the context in which she lives. The relationship with her husband is a critically important part of that context. How he manages himself with the child also has a strong impact on the mother. She is not operating in a vacuum. She is not to blame for child focus. It is not about the mother—it is about the parental triangle and the larger context in which it exists. Make no mistake about it: despite the mother's greater emotional influence on the child, the father participates equally in the parental triangle.

Of course, fathers and mothers influence their children in important other ways besides the emotional process of the parental triangle. The triangle has the most direct effect on the level of emotional maturity the child develops.

Maturity affects how successful kids are at making full use of the skills, interests, and talents that parents, grandparents, and other family members helped stimulate in them. This does not mean that a less well-differentiated person cannot excel in some area.

Figure 3.1 in Chapter 3 illustrates how anxiety shifts out of the marital relationship and into a focus on a child. The child pays a price through the impaired development of "self." It may be a fairly calm and stable triangle for a time—the anxiety is bound in the structure of the relationships—but the child is vulnerable to buildups of anxiety (symbolized by the shading in the child in the right diagram in Figure 3.1) and symptom development at some point. The appearance of significant symptoms shakes the whole triangle.

Another way to talk about the undifferentiation that exists in a marriage is to refer to it as immaturity. Each parent is equally immature. Some characteristics of the immaturity are the following:

1. Feeling-based reactions to a perceived lack of attention and approval from important others trump thoughtful assessments of what is unfolding in the relationship. Automatic feeling reactions lead to short-sighted decisions and actions.
2. Unrealistic expectations of self and others override reason and reflection.
3. Difficulty maintaining appropriate emotional boundaries. For example, if either spouse is distressed, the other takes it personally and either shuts down and distances or gets overly intrusive, often done in the name of "fixing" the problem—it is an emotional reaction designed mostly to relieve the anxiety in the fixer. Feelings, obviously, are not bad, but if they are acted on without thinking, the process sets off an action-reaction process between people and a predictable escalation of chronic anxiety.

If the parents use emotional distance to reduce the tension generated by their immature interactions, a readily available pathway for the tension to take is to infect their interactions with one or more children. The parents' anxious interactions with focused-on kids may range from unsureness and passivity to being overly certain and dogmatic. The child most targeted by this process inherits the parents' immaturities through what Bowen theory terms *emotional programming*. Depending on the intensity of the interactions, one or more children may develop less maturity than the parents through this relationship transmission.

The most focused-on child in a nuclear family is not a scapegoat—that term implies that the child is a victim, but this is an inaccurate characterization. It is important to remember that the child's own immaturity plays a part in sustaining the intensity of the parental triangle. The parents are child focused *and* the child has learned to be parent focused. The emotional programming of the child starts early in life and is continually reinforced until the offspring leaves home. Of course, it may continue into the child's adult life as long as the parents are alive.

As I depict in Figure 9.2, the interactions in one parental triangle in a family may be highly immature and the parental triangle with another child characterized by more mature interactions. In this case, one family triangle is sufficient to manage the family's undifferentiation.

Before going into more detail about child focus in families, here I make a brief excursion into the role of evolution in shaping child focus. It is important to view the processes discussed here from an evolutionary perspective. If people grasp this broader view, they can be more forgiving and tolerant of themselves and others for having limited control over processes that can have adverse impacts on the people they care about the most.

Physician and brain researcher Paul D. MacLean (1990) dates the evolution of the family to when mammals evolved about 200 million years ago. The triad of basic family behaviors he describes comprises (1) nursing in conjunction with maternal care, (2) audiovocal communication for maintaining maternal-offspring contact, and (3) play behavior. The evolution of nursing in conjunction with maternal care made the mother's ongoing relationship with her offspring much more important for the offspring's survival than had generally been the case prior to the emergence of mammals. Mammals (and birds) ratcheted up the degree of interdependency between mother and offspring. Audiovocal communication for mother and offspring to maintain contact is essential to this process. The infant evolved the isolation call, and the mother evolved to be highly responsive to that call. (DePisapia et al. [2013], using functional magnetic resonance imaging technology to assess male and female brain responses to infants' hunger cries, found that women were distracted by the crying far more easily than were men.) Play behavior facilitates offspring interactions in litters and the learning of important social behaviors.

Another important fact is that *Homo sapiens* is among only 6 percent of mammalian species that provide biparental care. This makes a cooperative and enduring relationship between the mother and father important for the care of the young. Human beings have an extremely long developmental period and have a relationship with their parents until each parent dies. In contrast, the predominant social bond in mammalian species as a whole is a mother-offspring relationship that usually terminates at weaning.

The term *symbiotic* is often used to describe the extremely interdependent relationship between a mother and child. Symbiosis is a normal state in the early mother-infant relationship, particularly because human infants are so helpless. The following quote by Diane Ackerman, in a 2012 opinion piece in the *New York Times*, informed by the field of interpersonal neurobiology, poetically describes the mother-infant symbiosis: "Brain scans show synchrony between the brains of mother and child; but what they can't show is the internal bond that belongs to neither alone, a fusion in which the self feels so permeable it doesn't matter whose body is whose."

Observations during the NIMH Family Studies Project (see Bowen, 2013) led Bowen to the conclusion that the relationship between mothers and their young adult schizophrenic offspring indicated that little resolution of the symbiotic attachment had occurred over the many years of the offspring's development. The level of interdependence between mother and dysfunctional adult child Bowen and his research team observed during the project was more extreme than even Bowen had anticipated.

Some might argue that the unresolved attachment between the mother and the adult dysfunctional child is so great because the young adult child is schizophrenic. The mother needs to hover and protect because of the child's limitations. Bowen saw it differently: the unresolved attachment is the substrate on which schizophrenia and other types of major dysfunctions develop.

When a successful emotional separation between mother and a well-differentiated offspring has developed by the time the child leaves home, this renders the young adult largely invulnerable to developing a major clinical symptom during the transition into adult life, and throughout life, for that matter. Emotional separation means much of the fusion or symbiotic interdependence has been resolved between the mother and young adult offspring. Less fusion does not mean lack of closeness; it means that enough maturity exists in both people to permit a stable and open connection throughout life. Considerable variation exists in the human population in the degree of resolution of the original symbiosis with the caretaking figure. This variation is reflected in a continuum of levels of differentiation of self in the populations of all human cultures.

I inserted the discussion about some relevant aspects of the evolution of mammals to highlight that a mother's time and investment in her offspring is deeper than culture. It is wired into her biology and to the biology of her offspring. It is anchored in the emotional system. The evolved importance of the mother-offspring relationship to an infant's survival makes it an easy target for absorbing chronic anxiety from the family system. Furthermore, evolution of a high degree of emotional interdependence between parents to facilitate successful biparental care renders marital relationships vulnerable to generating chronic anxiety. It is not easy to balance autonomy and closeness in a way that works for both people.

Two parents enter into their relationship with equivalent needs for emotional closeness and equivalent aversions to too much of it (I discuss the basis for the equivalence idea in Chapter 5). This makes the relationship vulnerable to emotional distance to reduce the anxiety generated by difficulty striking a balance between these two countervailing vectors of contact and distance. The distance reduces the anxiety of too much closeness, but it also reduces the amount of emotional reinforcement each gains from the marital relationship. The reinforcement is usually at its peak during courtship and the early stages of married life. As responsibilities increase, however, mutual satisfaction can begin to erode. The addition of kids, no matter how much they are wanted, comes with a big load of demands. More mature people can shoulder those demands and maintain decent emotional contact and cooperation in face of those demands; less mature people have a harder time managing.

Chronic anxiety generated in the marital relationship can co-opt a process that nature designed to assure a child's survival. When anxiety generated in the marital relationship cannot be contained there, it can infect the mother's interaction with a child. The basic process is that the mother meets needs for emotional closeness with a child (some details of this were covered earlier in this chapter and will be amplified later in this chapter). The father moves to the outside position in the parental triangle.

The mother's involvement with the child is comforting for her. Commonly, the father supports the mother's overinvolvement with the child, believing she is just being a good mother. The triangle serves the immature needs of the family more than the reality needs of the child (As I described earlier in this chapter, Murray Bowen once said that if there is any bias in his theory, it was to keep the family problem off the back of the child). The focus on the child can be calming to both parents. It is stabilized by the father meeting some of his emotional needs for acceptance and approval through his work and other activities.

The mother's anxious overinvestment in the child can trigger excessive worries in her about the well-being of the child. This is where the family projection process comes in. It starts with the mother's worry about some aspect of the child, such as whether the child is happy. She focuses on the child, looking for and fearing that she will find indications that the child is, in fact, unhappy. If she spots something, or imagines she has, she begins to relate to the child as if he is unhappy. She may talk to her husband about it. He may tell her it is all in her mind but still tends to support her agenda on how to help the child. The child goes along with the mother's projection that he is unhappy because this rewards the child with a calmer mother. The mother is calmer because she sees the anxiety as coming from outside herself: it is the child's behavior that is doing it. Furthermore, the child increasingly looks to the mother to solve any problems that arise, which pressures her to maintain an overfunctioning posture with the child. This type of process interferes with the child's ability to develop "self." The child develops in the context of anxious parents whose interactions with the child are governed by their more immature sides. The child gets enveloped by the emotional intensity and focuses on the parents as much as they focus on the child. This hampers the normal resolution of the original symbiosis and development of "self."

Many family therapists hold the view that, if there is a problem in a child, the parents must have some tensions and conflicts in their relationship. This is true, but it may not always look that way to an observer or seem that way to the parents. The parents may agree that their marriage is just fine. On the surface it is, but it is one side of a triangle. The closeness between the parents in supported by the focus on the child.

A brief clinical vignette can help illuminate some of the points being made about the impairment of one or more children through the triangle:

Two parents were in their early fifties when they sought family therapy after their third daughter and youngest child had a psychotic break during her first year away at college. A family approach had been strongly recommended to the mother as a way of addressing the situation, and she was very receptive to it.

The parents had three daughters, ages twenty-two, twenty, and eighteen. The father was a practicing lawyer, and the mother had developed a successful small business. The mother had occupied an overfunctioning position in the family, and the father was in the reciprocal underfunctioning position. That process was not so extreme that it contributed to any significant symptoms in either parent. The parents thought that their youngest daughter had grown up just fine and were shocked by the psychotic break. With the help of Bowen theory and therapy, the mother gradually assembled a picture of what had contributed to such a serious symptom occurring in their family.

At the time of the youngest daughter's birth, the law firm her husband had helped found was breaking up. He said he was extremely anxious about it for more than a year. The pattern in the marriage had been for the father to vent his anxieties to his wife. She felt a lot of responsibility for helping him manage but also felt overwhelmed and angered by it. The whole process triggered a lot of insecurities in her. The anger related to the wife thinking that her husband should be handling the situation better than he was. She had a way of coming at him that tapped into his deep insecurity. She began to distance from her husband emotionally. He began to drink more.

In retrospect, the wife recognized that taking care of the new baby was incredibly calming for her. It renewed her confidence and sense of competence. The baby, of course, was very dependent on her, but she did not mind it in the way she minded it with her husband. Babies are supposed to be dependent—they cannot help it.

She realized in retrospect that, although the immediate stressor of the husband's professional situation eventually resolved, a powerful overfunctioning-underfunctioning pattern persisted with the youngest daughter. The mother described it as "seamless," meaning that she had no clue about how entrenched the process was.

Interestingly, the daughter explained that she too had no idea what a powerful impact going off to college would have on her. The seamless interaction growing up with her mother hid the fact that she was far more dependent on her to help make decisions than she realized. When she got to college, she felt overwhelmed, isolated, and unable to make even simple decisions. She called home many times before the psychotic symptoms occurred, but the mother realized, again in retrospect, that she and her husband were so anxious when she called that it blocked any useful conversation. The attempts to gain some emotional support from her parents, which she did while also communicating a powerful sense of helplessness, only accentuated her anxiety and sense of isolation. The daughter's helpless signals sent the mother into high gear in an attempt to figure out what she needed to do to fix the problem.

After her hospitalization and emergence from the psychosis, the daughter realized when back living with her parents that she was far more reactive to her mother's approval and her expectations than she had ever realized. It helped her see how much this was true in her other relationships as well.

There were many ups and downs during the course of the family therapy, but the daughter eventually finished college and began teaching. However, she struggled intensely in romantic relationships. Fears of rejection in those relationships triggered a paralyzing level of insecurity in her.

In summary, it is clear in this case how the emotional distance invoked to deal with marital tension rendered the mother vulnerable to getting overly involved with her youngest daughter. The daughter paid a price for it in terms not developing much of a "self." I might add that the mother learned a great deal from applying Bowen theory to understand the family she grew up in. She realized that a triangle involving her own mother and younger sister had powerfully shaped her vulnerabilities to overfunctioning with one of her children. Understanding how patterns of interaction have come down through the generations, seeing how automatic and unseen that they can be, helped her resolve her guilt about the process with the daughter.

EMOTIONAL DISTANCE

Earlier in this chapter I discussed this pattern somewhat, to illustrate the idea of binding anxiety. I also discussed previously how emotional distance could take the form of withdrawing internally or through physical distance. An important distinction is that emotional distance is a reactive process of moving away from someone, as distinguished from a more thoughtful and self-regulated process of pursuing a particular goal. Emotions are also involved in moving toward a goal, but they could be considered positive emotions that are in the service of implementing a thoughtful decision to take certain actions. Decisions are based more on a realistic assessment of a situation and a long-term view.

The pattern of emotional distance is easy to grasp on an intellectual level, but it is very common for a person to be distancing from another person without being aware of it. Alternatively, the person might offer some rationalization for the distance but is underestimating the underlying emotional reactivity involved. The hardest thing to perceive accurately about distancing is its impact on the other person. For example, the other person may have become more irritable or even developed a symptom of some kind in reaction to the distance. The distancing person may justify the distance by blaming it on the other person's irritability, but that reflects losing sight of the reciprocity in the interaction with the other person. Ideally, the person who has been distancing can respond to the other's flare-up of, for example, irritable bowel syndrome by questioning whether emotional distancing from the other had triggered the flare-up.

The example of one person reactively distancing and the other person developing a symptom is one of the most important ideas in Bowen theory: one person's anxiety can express itself in another person's symptoms. The anxiety transfer is not mystical. Distancing gets communicated in subtle and not so subtle ways. Anxiety-driven distancing can manifest, for example, in talking less to a partner, having less eye contact, and being more distracted. A partner can, often unconsciously, respond with an emotional reaction to having less contact that triggers that person's stress response. One woman in my clinical practice was diagnosed with uterine cancer. The shock of the diagnosis forced her to reflect seriously on months of suspicion that her husband was having an affair. And indeed, he was having an affair.

Bowen theory's concept of an "open relationship" is the opposite of emotional distance. An open relationship is discussed at length in one of a series of video interviews I did with Murray Bowen, titled *The Best of Family Therapy*. This videotape, which was made in 1985, is available at www.thebowencenter.org. In an open relationships both parties are able to communicate their innermost thoughts and feelings without fear of hurting the other person. Such a relationship enhances the functioning of both people and is health promoting. In an interview with Bowen, he described four contexts in which an open relationship most often exists: (1) the early mother-infant relationship; (2) courtship; (3) a psychoanalytic relationship; and (4) a fantasied relationship with someone (Bowen & Kerr. 1985).

For reasons I have discussed so far in this book, it is very difficult to maintain an open relationship. An infant grows up. People get married and the realities of life buffet their relationship. It can last with a good psychoanalyst, one who consistently maintains neutrality, as long as people are willing to pay for it. Fantasied relationships seem inevitably to lose their luster over time.

Murray Bowen once said, "There are two ways to deal with anxiety: one is with drugs, the other is with "self;" "self" is better." The interrelationship between "self" and anxiety is detailed in Chapter 7, but this is an important idea here because it is "self" that keeps relationships open and having the anxiety-reducing effects associated with that openness. The less "self" people have, the more emotional distance will come in to play over time.

An attendee at a presentation Bowen was making asked him a question that implied to Bowen that the man thought there was something wrong with emotional distance. Bowen responded by straightening up, holding the microphone close to his mouth, and firmly asking, "Do you think emotional distance is pathological?" Needless to say, the attendee was somewhat taken aback. What I think Bowen was trying to communicate is that to think of reactive distancing as pathological fails to respect the power of the dilemma in all human relationships: the need for closeness coupled with the aversion to too much of it. Both the inability to have a reasonably comfortable emotional connection with another person and the inability to distance emotionally if the relationship becomes overwhelming could impair functioning to the point of symptom development. The most differentiated person on the planet will from time to time emotionally distance to some degree to cope in a relationship system.

To summarize this chapter on the four patterns of emotional functioning, I pose the question, Is it really this simple? This is a serious question. It is unsurprising that many people think that human relationships are so complex that it has to be reductionistic thinking for Bowen theory to place so much emphasis on four patterns of relationship interaction to explain which family member becomes symptomatic.

Besides cause-and-effect thinking, perhaps the biggest obstacle to seeing patterns and their impact is not grasping the evolutionary base of Bowen theory. The rapid evolution of the large cerebral cortex and the emergence of consciousness have made human relationship systems exponentially more complex than the relationship system of any other species. However, that does not mean that fundamental patterns of emotional functioning, ancient automatic processes, have disappeared as a manifestation of the emotional forces that drive human behavior. Nor does it mean that the more recently evolved parts of the brain are not subject to control by more ancient parts. To quote Jonathan Haidt (2012) on this subject:

> Automatic processes run the human mind, just as they have been running animal minds for 500 million years, so they're very good at what they do, like software that has been improved through thousands of product cycles. When human beings evolved the capacity for language and reasoning at some point in the last million years, the brain did not rewire itself to hand over the reins to a new and inexperienced charioteer. (pp. 45–46)

Haidt's point about automatic processes running the human mind does not conflict with the most recently evolved parts of the cerebral cortex, the *intellectual system*, having the capacity in some areas to control automatic processes. This capacity to self-regulate is embodied in the concept of differentiation of self. Differentiation of self is one way to talk about the concept of free will. People's basic level of "self" correlates with their capacity to be present and accounted for in a relationship system and use their fact-based reasoning process to self-regulate behavior sufficiently to not get swept up in the inevitable infectious spread of anxiety through a system. One person with sufficient importance to the system is enough to halt the spread of anxiety. The reduction of anxiety results in less intense activity of the patterns of emotional functioning in a system and, consequently, less chance of the impingement of the functioning of one member of the system to the point of serious symptom development.

CHAPTER FIVE

Differentiation of Self

Bowen theory's concept of differentiation of self is the most misunderstood of the eight concepts in the theory—probably also the most important. Many years ago, a well-known family therapist said, "Poor Murray Bowen, he differentiated from his family; now he has no family!" It was said as sort of a joke, but it betrayed an underlying confusion that most people in the family movement had at that time about differentiation. The difficulty in understanding is also captured in the discussion of the presentation Murray Bowen made about his own family at a national meeting of family therapists in 1967. The presentation described the theory base that guided Bowen and the steps he took in his effort to function as a more differentiated person in his own family of origin. The discussants were baffled by how doing what he described could possibly have a constructive impact for himself or his family.

A big part of the problem in understanding differentiation is that it is necessary to grasp Bowen theory as a whole to do it, particularly the concept of the family as an emotional unit. Confusion about the idea prevails to this day. A few years ago, I received a letter from another well-known pioneer in the family movement asking me to explain what Bowen meant by differentiation of self. The man was a very fine therapist.

One factor that generates bewilderment about differentiation is Freudian theory, which still dominated thinking during the heady early years of the family movement. Many people in recent years have criticized Freudian theory and disavowed it, but many people to this day carry around its basic ideas in their heads, whether aware of it or not. An individual-based model works against understanding differentiation. Freud advocated for the need to express repressed feelings in the therapeutic process. Many people, then and now, perceive differentiation, a key aspect of which is using the higher brain to regulate the emotional brain, as tantamount to the repression of feelings. On the contrary, it is not repression at all.

Another still widely accepted idea that contributes to the confusion is the view that adults suffering from various types of emotional and psychological problems did not get enough love and attention as children. If this were one's model for explaining insecurity, poor self-worth, and the like, differentiation of self in relationship to such a person would seem to be exactly the wrong approach. How can a therapist remaining emotionally separate and objective, as Bowen theory suggests, be useful? Deprived people are supposed to need love, attention, and acceptance to make up for what they feel they never got enough of growing up. It is difficult for people to fathom a cornerstone of differentiation that it can be useful to another person to be both separate from and emotionally connected to that person.

Obviously, love and attention are comforting, and people typically yearn for it, particularly when in distress. There is, however, more to the story of being truly helpful and useful to others. The Sandy Hook shooter Adam Lanza, a very anxious kid and frequently in turmoil, drowned in the flood of love and attention his mother provided. Most people who read the descriptions of the Lanza family relationships recognize the intense involvement between Adam and his mother—it is way too obvious to miss—but many people are puzzled by why it did not seem to help Adam. Given the puzzlement, many people invoke mental illness as the cause of Adam's severe impairment. From a Bowen theory perspective, in contrast, Adam's core problem was that he could not develop any semblance of "self" in the anxious emotional environment of an incredibly overfunctioning mother, a father who blindly supported her efforts, and Adam's own dependence and underfunctioning. The parents thought they were doing everything they could, but the missing ingredient was differentiation of self, in the parents as well as in Adam.

The existence of different levels of differentiation of self among people explains a basis for the easily observed individual variation in emotional functioning that exists in all multigenerational families and in all cultures. The concept describes how well an individual and family system are functioning emotionally. The most important variable that affects a person's level of emotional functioning is the interplay between the intellectual and emotional systems. Except in acute emergency situations, when automatic and immediate emotional reactions can be lifesaving, if emotional reactivity frequently overwhelms reasoned, reflective, and long-term thinking, then emotional functioning regresses. If reason, reflection, and long-term thinking can stem the flood of emotional reactivity when that is important to do, emotional functioning increases.

The capacity to maintain a "self" in relationships is a very powerful anxiety reducer. This effect derives from the interplay between the intellectual system and the emotional/feeling system. (I use both the terms *emotional/feel-*

ing system and *emotional system* because the emotional and feeling system processes are so intertwined. Feelings are a person's subjective experience of the activity of the emotional system.) Reflection and objectivity guide responses versus knee-jerk reactivity and associated feelings states. One family leader's ability to maintain a "self" when the family is dealing with significant stressors can halt the infectious spread of chronic anxiety through the system.

Saying that parts of the more recently evolved cerebral cortex can regulate emotions and associated feeling states generated by more evolutionarily ancient parts of the brain does not mean that cognitive processes and behaviors are ever devoid of emotional influence. It is important to note as well that emotions do not just reside in the brain but interact with the rest of the physiology in the body, including cellular physiology.

Feelings are the conscious awareness or subjective experience of some aspects of emotional system activity. Neuroscience research in recent decades has shown that feelings are enormously important for normal cognitive functioning and that influence often occurs out of awareness (Eagleman, 2015). Based on learning over time what we do and do not value, feelings add value to one choice over another, thus enabling us to make decisions. Feelings enable us to care enough about a certain choice to act on it. Emotion/feeling motivates us to act. Life experience continually updates the brain through the emotional/feeling system as to what we do and do not value. This helps us prioritize information for making a decision, thus increasing the efficiency of the brain. Absent this interaction of newer and older brain systems, it is extremely difficult if not impossible to make decisions based on higher cortical processes alone.

As important as the emotional/feeling system is to enhancing cognitive functioning, neuroscientist Jaak Panksepp (1998) points out that the useful interchange between cognitive and emotional processes is optimally balanced only in nonstressful circumstances. During emotional turmoil, the influence of subcortical circuits on the higher reaches of the brain are stronger than the other way around, making it difficult for the higher parts of the brain to control emotion/feeling-charged impulses. When this occurs, reasoning is co-opted by emotionality. Not only is reasoning impaired, but feelings dictate behavior. This is reflected in the sacrifice of principle and associated actions to relieve the anxiety of the moment. A long-term view of the consequence of one's actions does not surface in consciousness or, if so, is quickly dismissed.

Following on Panksepp's description of how difficult it can be for people to ride herd on the feeling responses, one of the most important core ideas in Bowen theory is that people vary in their ability to distinguish between the feeling process and the intellectual process. The more people can distinguish the functioning of the two systems, the more choice they have about acting on the feeling or the thought when that is important to do. Panksepp states that chimpanzees, human beings, and a few other species have self-awareness, but *Homo sapiens* has *awareness of awareness*. David Eagleman (2015) describes this phenomenon as the brain being able to see itself. This ability seems to have emerged in evolution along with consciousness. In line with Panksepp's and Eagleman's ideas, Damasio (2010) states that human beings can have thinking with emotions, in parallel with emotions, and can even control emotions. People can be conscious of thinking and emotions at the same time. Despite thinking, emotions/feelings are still present. The ideas of these three neuroscientists are consistent with Bowen theory's contention that human beings can distinguish thoughts from feelings and use that capacity to choose between them. Most people can cite examples of their feelings compelling one set of actions and their rational mind suggesting a very different set.

Human beings are capable of reflecting on a belief, value, or attitude and determining whether it is firmly anchored in fact or largely feeling governed. The human brain has the capacity to discern the difference between a thought based more on fact, for example, that human beings are far more alike than different from one another, and a thought based more on feeling, for example, racist thoughts.

Poorly differentiated people are not good at acting based on long-term reward versus automatically opting for instant gratification. Their generally overly reactive feeling system trumps their poorly developed intellectual system. Reasonably well-differentiated people may feel like taking the easy way out, feel like acting to relieve the anxiety of the moment, but can fall back on fact and principle, consider the long-term consequences of a particular action, and stay the course. It is also important to note that it is possible for people to stay on a disciplined course for totally emotional reasons, such as not wanting to risk disapproval. A person's powerful drive for success may be primarily emotionally driven.

Bowen theory uses a number of criteria to assess emotional functioning: the type of work people have done and how well they have performed it; educational achievements or lack thereof in light of opportunities; health history; and assessment of how stable their relationships have been. No one piece of data is sufficient to assess a person's or family's level of emotional functioning. This is because it can be uneven; for example, a person who excels academically and occupationally may have a very difficult time in personal relationships, especially intimate ones. A family's level of emotional functioning is estimated from the assessments of all of its members. The overall family assessment is necessary because the patterns of emotional functioning in a family system can result in one person functioning well at the expense of another person doing poorly, such as experiencing overfunctioning-underfunctioning reciprocity in a marriage or chronically being in the outside position of a triangle.

Summarizing, a well-differentiated person operates with a good balance between intellectual and emotional functioning, with the two as a working team. This will reflect in fewer life problems both personally and in the family. Lower-level emotional functioning or poor differentiation manifests in difficulties in many areas of life. Anxiety-driven emotionality poorly counterbalanced by reason, reflection, and principle is a prescription for a rocky life course. People seem to have known this throughout recorded history, but Bowen figured out how the family a person grows up in unwittingly creates variation in the emotional functioning of the offspring and how multigenerational families create an even wider range of variation in their many descendants. The understanding of how the processes that create variation unfold provides a blueprint for individuals to work on increasing their levels of "self."

Before describing the specifics of how Bowen theory conceptualizes the processes that create individual variation in differentiation of self, an attention-getting quote by whale scientist Roger Payne can add some perspective: "The human brain is the most unsuccessful adaptation ever to appear in the history of life on earth. What we call intelligence may only be a form of vandalism, just mischief on a grand scale" (quoted in Ackerman, 1991, p. 144).

A way to interpret Payne's statement is that the excessive influence of the emotional brain and associated narrow-mindedness, for example, thinking of oneself as the center of the universe, has made human survival on the planet and the survival of a multitude of other species extremely precarious. Human beings seem flawed in their ability to adapt to the realities of their natural environment. We do not do well with excess. Murray Bowen once opined that the big brain of human beings has grown like a weed, like kudzu, and could lead to the extinction of our species (personal communication in 1982).

This vise-like grip that emotions often have on cognitive processes, generating beliefs and biases that have no basis in fact, is included in Bowen theory's concept of *pseudo-self*. In the postgraduate training programs over the years at the Bowen Center for the Study of the Family, trainees have been challenged with the task of identifying their most important beliefs and reflecting on where they came from. The trainees orally present their "belief papers" to the other trainees and the faculty. Bowen originated the idea of this exercise, intended as a stimulus for trainees to sort out the distinction between "solid self" and pseudo-self in themselves and others.

Pseudo-self is made up of principles, beliefs, philosophies, and knowledge that people acquire because the important groups they are part of consider the beliefs and other ideas to be correct. Pressure from a group to incorporate its ideas comes in many forms and with varying degrees of intensity. One powerful reason for people to incorporate and espouse the right thing to believe is to enhance their image and sense of belonging to the group. James Henry and Patricia Stephens (1977) consider anxiety over one's status in a social system—where one fits on the hierarchy—to be as powerful a motivator of human behavior as anxiety triggered by threats to important attachments. A preoccupation with status is in line with the concept of pseudo-self.

Pseudo-self is negotiable in a relationship system, meaning a person will disavow or discard a belief or principle in face of emotional pressure to do so. An example would be a father who loaned one of his cars for an extended period to his adult son. The son did not take very good care of the car, and this did not sit right with the father. The father held a principle that the son had a responsibility to take good care of the car since it belonged to someone else. He discussed this with his wife, but she urged him to try to understand their son better and cut him some slack. In response to his wife's attitude, the father ignored his principle and stopped pressuring the son. He did not follow through on insisting that the son return the car. He explained his change in position as based on fear of his wife's disapproval and his son's possible rejection of him. A belief anchored in solid self does not evaporate in face of emotional pressure such as this. Principles anchored in solid self can change, but based only on intellectual reasoning and careful consideration of other alternatives.

A hallmark of pseudo-self is people pretending to be something they are not. This can involve deceiving others and themselves. People can feel and act stronger or weaker than they really are, feel more or less attractive than they really are, and have inflated or deflated self-worth. A man I once saw in family therapy had hidden his deep financial debt from his wife and professional colleagues and eventually resorted to kiting checks to maintain the cover-up. He explained that his actions were like putting up a mask in front of his face to retain his status with people. It would have been more painful to remove the mask than to continue using it. Yet the scheme eventually collapsed.

Knee-jerk opposition to others' points of view is another manifestation of pseudo-self: having so little solid self that agreeing with or cooperating with another person who has a different viewpoint is untenable—accepting the other's viewpoint equals giving up. Oppositional behavior provides the illusion of an emotional boundary, albeit a reactive one, between self and others. This is typically a key dynamic in intensely conflicted relationships.

If one's status is so important, why is one person in a reciprocal relationship vulnerable to functioning in an inadequate position? People often explain it as the prospect of rejection and conflict being more frightening than deferring to preserve harmony and an associated feeling of connection. Many people are prone to look at an overfunctioning-underfunctioning relationship as one person exerting power over the other person. It is not that simple when examined as a relationship process. The underfunctioning one is freed from the anxiety of responsibility and decision making, and the overfunctioning one is freed from the anxiety of not being in control and in charge. Furthermore, underfunctioners may feel at their core that they are the cause of the problem in the relationship. An overfunctioning person often thinks the underfunctioner is the cause of the problem as well.

Another feature of pseudo-self is holding discrepant beliefs. This occurs because the beliefs are acquired through relationship pressure to adopt them coupled with the person's deep desire for acceptance and connection. They are not acquired through intellectual reasoning and careful consideration of facts that support or refute them.

The holding of discrepant beliefs is similar to doublethink, a term George Orwell introduced in his 1949 book *Nineteen Eighty-Four*. Doublethink is "the capacity to engage in one line of thought in one situation (at home, in another group, in private life) without necessarily sensing any conflict between the two" (McArthur, p.321). One similarity of this quote to pseudo-self is its emphasis on context dependence. The content of pseudo-self plays out in the higher brain, but it is an emotional process at its core. Psychologists describe not sensing any conflict in the lines of thought as a lack of cognitive dissonance. I suggest that the need for attention, acceptance, and meeting perceived expectations is so powerful in human beings that the feeling system bypasses or overwhelms the important process of cognitive dissonance in rational thinking.

Solid self is strongly related to the human intellectual system, which endows us with the capacity to think, reason, and reflect. Bowen theory considers the intellectual system to be that part of human beings that makes us unique in nature. Although strongly related to a well-functioning intellectual system, the capacity for solid self may be rooted in emotions that come into play if an intruder animal steadily encroaches on another animal's territory. At some critical point, the encroached upon animal stands its ground and fights vigorously to preserve its boundaries. This is similar to a person who has been yielding to the anxiety-driven pressure from the family or another relationship system to think, feel, and act in specific ways. Finally, this person states firmly, "I am unwilling to do this any longer." Bowen theory refers to such a stand as an "I-position." Such I-positions are not taken in anger or to oppose the other but reflect a firmness born of conviction.

Solid self reflects a functional intellectual system. It enables a person to withstand pressure from the emotional/feeling system. Solid self is made up of firmly held convictions, principles, and beliefs that are formed slowly during development. The contents of solid self are never changed by coercion or persuasion, such as the case with pseudo-self. They can be changed only from within self. The convictions, principles, and beliefs anchored in solid self can be expanded and added to during adult life, but the basic capacity to be a "self" usually does not change appreciably after a person leaves home.

It is possible to increase solid self some as an independent adult through a structured, theory-guided effort (this process is discussed Chapters 15-18). Unusual life circumstances may also increase solid self, such as seemed to be the case with a man I met after he had been a prisoner of war in Vietnam for over seven years. He coped with that experience by learning as much as he could about the thinking and life experience of every other prisoner. His perspective on the human condition broadened as a result, and this likely contributed to his having a bit more solid self.

The intellectual system is a function of the brain and presumably is composed of a number of brain systems. It may have some overlap with intelligence, but it is not the same thing. After several decades of research, cognitive psychologist Keith Stanovich (2009) helped clarify Bowen theory's distinction between the intellectual system and intelligence. He made two particularly important points that are relevant to Bowen theory: (1) individual differences in the capacity for rational thinking exist in the human population, and (2) these individual differences do not correlate with intelligence. Intelligence tests do not measure a person's capacity for rational thinking, meaning that a person can have a high IQ but be highly prone to less than rational thinking.

Stanovich focused on cognitive processes, not the role of emotion in affecting a person's ability to think, reason, and reflect. He made several interesting points with his cognitive model that parallel Bowen theory: problems in rational thinking arise when (1) cognitive capacity is insufficient to override automatic responses, (2) the necessity to override is not recognized by the person, and (3) the "simulation processes" do not have access to the mindware necessary for the synthesis of a better response than the automatic one. Keith Stanovich coined the term *mindware*, which refers to mental knowledge and procedures used to solve problems and make decisions. In the chimpanzee example described in the introduction, the chimps had learned the mindware of simple numbers to represent phenomena in the real world.

All three of these obstacles to rational thinking are consistent with Bowen theory, but Bowen theory conceptualizes their occurrence differently. In the first case, it is the emotional/feeling system overwhelming an inadequately developed intellectual system that interferes with rational thinking. In the second case, pseudo-self, which at its core is emotionally driven, interferes with the capacity to recognize discrepancies in one's thinking and beliefs and thus lack the motivation to modify those thoughts and beliefs. In the third case, the simulation processes, which mean the ability to consider alternatives consciously, lack the kind of mindware that systems thinking, seeing reciprocity, and seeing triangles provide as an alternative to a cause-and-effect and blaming response. Systems thinking permits seeing the world more closely to the way it really is than cause-and-effect thinking allows.

Before leaving this discussion of Stanovich's research, it is important to clarify that the capacity for rational thinking is an aspect of the ability to function as a "self" but is not the whole story. Quoting Bowen from the epilogue of *Family Evaluation*: "The 'self' is composed of constitutional, physical, physiological, biological, genetic and cellular reactivity factors, as they move in unison with psychological factors" (Kerr & Bowen, 1988, p. 342). Bowen's quote indicates that differentiation of self is conceptualized as much more than a psychological process. However, the most effective way to increase one's capacity to function with more differentiation is a psychological one that depends on rational thinking as applied to factual observations generated by a disciplined effort to apply systems thinking to relationships. Clinical observations support that even a small increase in a person's capacity to function with more "self" in important relationship systems results through top-down pathways, brain to other organs, in changes at a biological level.

The prefrontal cortex seems to be particularly important in the functioning of the intellectual system. The following quote from John Hughlings Jackson, the father of English neurology, is about how self evolves—though based on knowledge of the brain at the time of Queen Victoria, it is consistent with modern neuroscience: "The CNS has a hierarchical organization that reflects evolutionary history. Ascending levels show increasing integration and coordination of sensorimotor representations. The highest-level coordination, which allows the greatest voluntary control, depends on prefrontal activity. Self is the manifestation of this highest level of consciousness" (1932, p. 41). Jackson suggests that the evolutionary development of the prefrontal cortex is necessary for the emergence of self, but this is not to say that self resides in the prefrontal cortex (Meares, 1999). Emotions and other physiological processes are involved in a person's capacity to function as a "self."

As described earlier, a person's level of solid self is best assessed by how that person interacts in emotionally significant relationship systems. Recall the father who loaned his son the car. The vulnerability of his principle was not evident until anxiety built up in the triangle with his wife and son. Had his principle been anchored in solid self, he would have been less fearful of his wife's and son's reactions to his clear statement about what he believed, what he would do, and what he would not do. I-positions can have a long-term calming effect on a system because they halt the infectious spread of anxiety through a relationship system. Less differentiated people are vulnerable to taking reactive I-positions, which typically polarize the system and intensify anxiety. The position comes across as dogmatic rather than principled. I-positions rooted in solid self may spark disagreement, but that is different than emotionally governed polarization.

Solid self is not a structure in the brain—it is a function of the brain (and associated bodily systems). It resists relationship pressure for two reasons: (1) its contents have been carefully thought out, thus trusted sufficiently to become convictions; and (2) the type of family emotional climate that permits the development of a well-functioning intellectual system does not program intense emotional reactivity into the person. For example, people with good levels of solid self are not immune to disapproval, but they are not so reactive to it that it floods their intellectual system and dictates their behavior.

Before discussing the interplay of solid self and pseudo-self, another term to define is *no-self*: a person who is unable to differentiate between the feeling and intellectual systems. This does not result from a structural defect in the brain but is a functional dysfunction. The intellectual system is dysfunctional because it developed little during the person's development. Again, this is not about intelligence, as very smart people can be poorly differentiated. Ted Kaczynski, the "Unabomber," is a perfect example of a person with a very high IQ who was poorly differentiated. People are born with the potential to develop solid self, but development of "self" depends largely on the character of family relationships during the years a child is maturing. The emotional climate of the family in relationship to that particular offspring may not be conducive to developing a reasonably well-functioning intellectual system. Another example of a no-self was a young schizophrenic woman who could describe the chain reaction flow of emotional reactivity in her family but so deeply blamed herself for it happening that her feeling system totally interfered with her having any objectivity about it and reflecting on it usefully.

People with no-self have little if any resistance to the anxiety in the relationship systems that surround them. Their own anxiety contributes as well to the anxiety in the system. They commonly withdraw in some fashion to protect themselves when system anxiety is high, such as into psychosis, or externalize the anxiety into the environment, such as with sociopathic behaviors. Bowen theory can help people see underneath clinical dysfunctions, such as psychosis or antisocial acts, and discern that a person's real vulnerability is based on the absence of solid self.

The levels of no-self, pseudo-self, and solid self in a person's makeup govern the degree of *emotional fusion* that occurs in emotionally significant relationships. *Fusion* is a term in Bowen theory that is borrowed from biology. Under certain conditions, for example, two cells fuse to become one cell. Fusion in human relationships is a consequence of the togetherness force, composed of the emotions and associated physiological processes that drive two people to merge into one. In the extreme, it is people living, acting, and being for each other. This occurs to varying degrees, depending on the degree of counterbalancing by the life force for differentiation of self.

The togetherness force pushes all the members of a family to merge into a oneness and function as an emotional unit to one degree or another. This is not a bad thing per se, but when inadequately balanced by solid self and in the presence of high anxiety, the system preserves its stability at the expense of one or more of its members. When family members are strongly fused with one another, they react so automatically and predictably to one another that the family functions like it is a single organism. Most of the pioneering family researchers observed the family as an organism phenomenon, but Bowen was unique in seeing the emotional system as the fundamental basis of it.

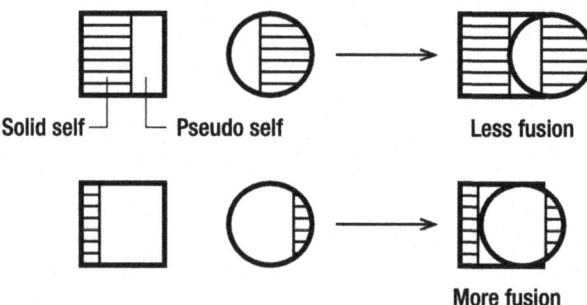

Figure 5.1 *The series of parallel lines in a part of each male and female symbolize solid self. The absence of lines symbolizes pseudo-self. The male and female in the top row function with more solid than pseudo-self and have less emotional fusion in their relationship. The opposite is true for the male and female in the bottom row.*

Figure 5.1 illustrates how people can differ in the proportions of solid self versus pseudo-self in their makeup. The symbols for the relationship at the top depict a male and female with proportionately fairly high levels of solid self and fairly low levels of pseudo-self. (Solid self is depicted by the series of horizontal lines; pseudo-self is depicted by no lines.) The symbols in the upper right depict a moderate to low level of emotional fusion in their relationship. The relationship at the bottom is depicted as low levels of solid self, high levels of pseudo-self, and a large degree of fusion in their relationship. These two relationships demonstrate a difference in the *basic level of differentiation*, comprising the proportionate combination of solid self and pseudo-self. Paradoxically, it is emotional boundaries that enable people to stay connected even when the circumstances are highly stressful.

Differentiation of Self

Bowen theory holds that people's spouses or emotionally significant others each have the same basic level (as indicated in Figure 5.1). A relationship becomes progressively unstable as emotional fusion increases. The instability arises from people being more focused on each other and more reactive to each other's moods and actions. Emotional reactivity and chronic anxiety more easily escalate in a vicious-circle feedback loop. Basic level of differentiation of self is not the only factor that renders a relationship vulnerable to escalations of chronic anxiety. Two other factors are the degree of stress in people's lives and how isolated or cut off a relationship system is from other potentially supportive relationship systems.

Patterns of emotional functioning become active to bind the anxiety. Given that the top relationship in Figure 5.1 is more stable than the bottom relationship, the average higher level of chronic anxiety in the bottom relationship exaggerates the particular pattern in play. Figure 5.2 shows the pattern playing out as a female dominant-male adaptive interaction that is commonly accompanied by an overfunctioning (arrow up)-underfunctioning (arrow down) reciprocity in the relationship. The reciprocity is more exaggerated in the more fused relationship, as indicated by the larger arrows.

Figure 5.2 *The upward and downward arrows on both diagrams indicate that an overfunctioning-underfunctioning tendency is more pronounced (longer arrow) in the relationship on the right that is more fused emotionally than the one on the left.*

Another way Bowen theory describes the dominant-adaptive (deferential) pattern is by a borrowing, trading, and lending of self. It is not solid self but pseudo-self that is being loaned and taken. Solid self is termed *solid* because that is where people draw the line on what they will give up to preserve peace and harmony. One person occupies the functioning position of the "strong, overadequate one" (commonly the overfunctioner) and the other occupies the functioning position of the "weak, inadequate one" (commonly the underfunctioner). Each spouse has the same basic level of differentiation, so these are pretend, barely conscious postures that each spouse assumes to deal with the chronic anxiety generated by the instability of the relationship. Both people pretend to be something they are not, which covers up their mutual difficulty in being a "self" and makes for a more comfortable fit.

If the anxiety in the relationship is not too high, a dominant-adaptive (deferential) pattern can be stable and even preferred by both partners. If the interaction becomes too intense and exaggerated, however, one spouse becomes vulnerable to clinical problems. This is an emotional process, not just a psychological one. The threat level experienced by the person making the most internal adjustments to preserve harmony can reach a point that it significantly disturbs bodily homeostasis, rendering the person more vulnerable to clinical symptoms. People in my clinical practice commonly express the threat they experience in ways such as "dissolving in the relationship, getting lost in it, or feeling overwhelmed and out of control." The spouse making fewer accommodations to preserve harmony may be oblivious to what is playing out between them until the other spouse develops clinical symptoms or wants a divorce.

Pseudo-self can be the basis of increasing a person's *functional level of differentiation* and reduce chronic anxiety. An easily observed example of this is a young man who is functioning in an aimless and purposeless way. He meets a woman and they fall in love. He then decides to jump-start his life and goes back to finish college, develops a professional career, and starts living in a more responsible way. He has borrowed pseudo-self from his romantic partner. People may call this love, but it is love mixed with considerable emotional immaturity in both partners.

Everyone borrows and lends self to some degree. People who join cults and adopt cult beliefs often experience similar improvements in their functional level of differentiation. The myriad forms of tribalism that permeate human societies all lend pseudo-self to their members, and their members borrow it and function more securely because of it. People can draw strength from the perception that those around them agree with them and accept them. Human beings are so profoundly interdependent emotionally that no one is immune from drawing strengths from their association with others. We all depend heavily on that, but some people more than others. This is not a bad thing, but having more understanding of the distinction between solid self and pseudo-self can make an important difference in navigating through life.

The emotional functioning of people at different basic levels of differentiation is significantly different. People with moderate to good levels of differentiation have enough basic differentiation between the intellectual and emotional systems for the two systems to function as a cooperative team. For example, the intellectual system can allow the person to act on feelings if that is what makes the most sense to do but to ride herd on the feelings in other situations. It is an integrated response in that both streams of information are considered. The intellectual system is sufficiently developed to acquire a good level of solid self and correspondingly less pseudo-self, allowing it to function autonomously without being dominated by the emotional system when anxiety increases.

In people with less than the moderate to good range of basic levels, the emotional system has much more influence on the intellectual system. With the intellectual system less developed, the proportion of pseudo-self to solid self is greater than in people at moderate to good basic levels. The pretend intellect of the emotionally dominated pseudo-self interferes with the autonomy of the intellectual system. In people in this range of levels, the intellectual system functions best in noncritical situations, such as thinking through an engineering problem, but in critical situations that are infected with anxiety, the intellectual system lacks the strength to restrain automatic emotional decisions that can complicate a person's life course.

People in the lower range of this intermediate segment below the moderate to good range can frequently describe how automatic emotional reactions can dominate their response to situations in a destructive way but still react to situations as if that insight was of no value whatsoever. What I have just described qualifies under Einstein's definition of insanity: doing the same thing over and over again and expecting different results. This process becomes even more intense at the lowest levels of this intermediate range, where the levels of solid self are very low or nonexistent.

People with the lowest levels of differentiation of self have the greatest degrees of emotional fusion with others. They live in a feeling-dominated world and cannot distinguish between feeling and fact. Having developed in very intense fusions with their parents, they enter the adult world as extremely relationship oriented. The term *relationship oriented* in Bowen theory does not mean being interested in people; it means having hair-trigger automatic emotional reactions to others. This sensitivity makes it very difficult for them to engage comfortably with the larger society, with their moods and behaviors so affected by the experience. Paranoia is always waiting in the wings. With a dysfunctional intellectual system, they have little capacity for self-regulation. Life energy goes into seeking love and approval, leaving little energy of goal-directed pursuits.

This lower group contains the least functional of the people who are diagnosed with schizophrenia, sometimes characterized as the "hard-core" group, and also the most severe of the character disorders, such as the psychopaths that end up cycling in and out of prisons. The lower group also tends to have a higher incidence of severe chronic physical illnesses. They have practically no energy for life goals, such as taking care of themselves and keeping a job. They depend deeply on relationship harmony to manage their own anxiety. Symptoms are an incredibly frequent part of their lives. They are frequently living in institutions. Many are cut off from their families, largely because the family is so reactive to them, which renders them dependent on public institutions to sustain them. People at the upper range of this low group may escape serious dysfunction if life circumstances are unusually favorable.

Hinkle (1974) studied thirteen hundred telephone operators over a twenty-year period and found that one segment of the group had a disproportionate number of health problems and another segment had remarkably few. The healthy group could endure social change and personal deprivation without undue emotional response. The concept of varying basic levels of differentiation of self predicts this type of variation in a population.

Bowen originally used numbers from 0 to 100 to indicate variation on what he early on called the *differentiation of self scale* (Bowen, 1971). Many people interpreted the word *scale* to mean a psychological instrument that could be used to assess basic level of differentiation—this is not the case. The scale idea was intended to be of theoretical importance, a way of presenting or calling attention to the fact of variation in human emotional functioning and a basis for it. It is not a measurement tool. Bowen subsequently dropped the term *scale*. Furthermore, he no longer described people as existing in the very highest range of such a scale, for example, in the 90–95 range, as he did in his original presentation of the idea (Bowen, 1966). He later described his estimate of the highest levels of differentiation in human societies as no higher than 60. Later still, he raised that figure by describing a few people being as high as 75 on this 100-point continuum (Bowen, 1976).

Based on observations to date, it appears as if the distribution of basic levels of differentiation throughout the human population follows the well-known bell-shaped curve, as shown in Figure 5.3. People in the 50–75 range on the continuum, which is estimated at 10 percent of the population, are the ones with the moderate to good levels of differentiation. This means that about 90 percent of the population is below 50 on the 100-point continuum. The group of people with the lowest levels, designated as 25 or below on the continuum, is about 20 percent.

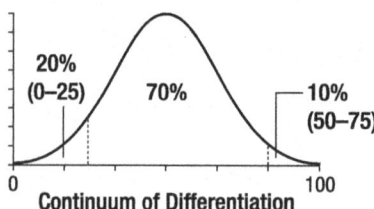

Figure 5.3 This diagram depicts an estimate of the number of human beings at each point on the continuum of differentiation of self. The principal point that the diagram conveys is that the bell curve is shifted considerably to the left.

Key to understand about this lowest group is that their feeling system so floods their thinking that they lack the flexibility to make basic change, meaning to increase basic level of differentiation. An example of inflexibility is being chronically unable to act on a long-term view rather than opt for instant gratification. They lack the discipline that a reasonably well-developed intellectual system can provide in a long-term effort to make progress. Their functional levels of differentiation can change as the level of chronic anxiety fluctuates in the family system over time. A therapist who understands their dilemma and provides the support that objectivity and emotional neutrality foster can help the family raise its functional level and reduce the severity of symptoms. People above 25 on the continuum can make basic changes in differentiation. The higher a person's basic level of differentiation, the more potential that person has to increase the basic level, which takes motivation, hard work, and time. A person's starting-point basic level is not the only factor in sustaining the motivation to progress. One woman said, "My family has always been very important to me, and I yearned to do what I could to improve my relationships with them." Others offer different reasons.

Bowen's change in thinking about the highest levels of differentiation of self in human society was shaped by the accumulation of observations in his own personal and professional lives, as well as of society as a whole. Jonathan Haidt (2012) does not describe a continuum of emotional functioning in society but uses a metaphor that seems to match with Bowen's shift to increasing the chasm between how differentiated any human being is currently capable of being and what humankind could theoretically evolve to be. Haidt's metaphor is that of the *rider* (cognitive processes that support solid self and pseudo-self) and the *elephant* (automatic processes including emotion) to emphasize that the higher brain is capable of guiding things, but its strength pales in comparison to the power of the evolutionary older automatic processes. Quoting Haidt:

> The rider can do several useful things. It can see further into the future (because we can examine alternative scenarios in our heads) and therefore it can help the elephant make better decisions in the present. It can learn new skills and master new technologies, which can be employed to help the elephant reach it goals and sidestep disasters. The rider is skilled at fabricating post hoc explanations for whatever the elephant has done, and it is good at finding reasons to justify whatever the elephant wants to do next. (p. 46)

The higher their basic level of differentiation, the more consistent are people's emotional functioning. Anxious emotional fields buffet them less. As basic levels drop, functional levels of differentiation can rise and fall, sometimes dramatically. The people are much more dependent on the state of their emotional environment and thus more vulnerable to an up-and-down life course. Ups and downs are part of life, but vulnerabilities in that regard vary. A broad generalization is that people in the low range tend to have difficulties in both their work and personal lives; people in the moderate or intermediate range often do well in their work lives but run into problems in their personal lives; people in the moderate to good range are more likely to do well in both areas.

The emotional system can do a good job of guiding people through life. It seems to do a decent job in most areas of people's lives, as it does with dogs, cats, and other flora and fauna, but does less well in critical situations. This can explain why a person can have a fairly high level of functional differentiation at work but much lower in the family, where the emotional intensity is typically higher than at work. The pseudo-self is operating in the service of the emotional system, its subjectively based attitudes reinforcing the feeling process. For example, a person not only can be feeling angry but also can be stuck in obsessing about the "unfairness" of it all.

In developing a continuum of emotional functioning that theoretically has a hundred different basic levels of functioning on it, Bowen theory leaves room for further research to discover the many subtle but significant differences in lifestyles at each level. The differences between lifestyles and life courses are quite obvious between the people with the lowest and the highest levels. People at the higher levels tend to lead responsible and productive lives with stable relationships; people at the lower levels struggle in many areas. It remains to be seen if it will be possible to pinpoint smaller differences, such as between 39 and 40.

Some people will say, "What does it matter what your basic level of differentiation is? All of us still have to play the hand we are dealt." It is a valid point. However, being able to specify the differences in functioning that account for a moderate difference between two siblings and how that difference developed has opened the door to understanding what people need to do to increase their basic level of differentiation. Increasing basic level even a little bit can make a valuable difference in someone's life course.

One example of how levels of differentiation can create significant variation in their emotional function is illustrated by focusing on a unique capacity of the human brain, at least to the degree it is has developed in our species: the capacity to remember the past and to contemplate possible scenarios for the future. This is a very strong asset for people at higher levels differentiation in helping them make adaptive decisions about matters that carry even a high emotional valence. In contrast, it is a liability for people at lower levels who are easily paralyzed by obsessions over past mistakes and fears of what can go wrong in the future. The case with people at lower levels is an example of the emotional system riding roughshod over the poorly developed intellectual system. Again, this does not reflect a lack of intelligence but is an emotionally driven process. Everyone can succumb to it, but it envelopes the lives and decision making of less differentiated people.

To conclude this chapter I make a few other points about differentiation. First of all, some students of Bowen theory mishear the idea of a continuum of differentiation of self as a judgment of people. Bowen theory is an attempt to move toward a science of human behavior. It describes what is, not what should be. Poorly differentiated people are not wrong or bad; well-differentiated people are not right or good. The theory predicts that people with low levels of differentiation are more vulnerable than people with higher levels to behavior that society judges as bad or wrong. But it also predicts that poorly differentiated people are more vulnerable to the opposite types of behavior, such as scrupulous religious practices. People have to take responsibility for their decisions to maintain an orderly society, but it is important not to lose sight of the power of the emotional forces that drive maladaptive decisions. The concept of differentiation has shown that differences in emotional functioning among people are quantitative, not qualitative. All families have much in common, as do all human beings.

A second point is that people do not choose their basic level of differentiation. As I discuss in Chapter 11, all multigenerational families produce well-differentiated people, poorly differentiated people, and the full range in between. No one is in control of the emotionally driven processes that create individual variation, but every family member participates in those processes. It is a natural process related to the counterbalancing life forces of differentiation and togetherness. Every human being acts in ways that promote differentiation in others, and every human being acts in ways that undermine differentiation in others. The important thing is that when people begin to recognize how this process works, they can do something about it.

A related point is that people often ask, Is there such a thing as too much differentiation? The question implies that differentiation is equivalent to people distancing from one another. One way I like to answer this question is with another question: Can people ever have too much mutual respect? People who have good levels of solid self are as interested in the welfare of others as much as in their own welfare. They are not competing with one another and are not trying to change one another. They are present and accounted for even when system anxiety is high. They do not have to distance to calm themselves and do not have to get others to be calm for themselves to be calm. They truly understand that calming themselves helps to calm others.

I once treated a couple in which the wife had had a series of psychiatric hospitalizations for psychotic episodes. She had finally succeeded in getting her husband to try family therapy. In the first session, she said that the problem in marriages is that people have a perfectly good relationship when they get married but then start trying to change each other. I thought it was wonderful insight. She was the talkative one in that first session, and the husband was quiet and looked nervous. In discussing her psychiatric hospitalizations, she sounded and acted a little more distressed than she had earlier in the session. Her emotional level seemed quite appropriate for the matters she was talking about. I looked at the husband and saw that he was getting pale and perspiring. I asked, "What is the matter with you?" He said, "Her! See how upset she gets? See what I am dealing with?" I thought, "How can this woman stay sane living with such an anxious man?" The answer was that she could not. He misperceived the degree of her distress level and could not stay calm in face of it. That was his lack of "self." On her part, she had become far too dependent on someone from whom she often felt isolated. It is the lack of differentiation that promotes boundary violations and distancing. That is the opposite of mutual respect.

In Chapter 4 I quoted Jonathan Haidt on how automatic processes run the human mind just as successfully as they have been running animal minds for 500 million years. So too can the human emotional system and pseudo-self contribute to a productive and useful life course in many instances. However, pseudo-self can land us in a lot of trouble and misery if solid self is not available at critical junctures. Solid self endows our species with a flexibility that enhances successful adaptation. As Murray Bowen said, "The world will always need differentiation of self" (personal communication on repeated occasions).

CHAPTER SIX

Emotional Regression

This and the next three chapters address what I refer to as the *three Es* of Bowen theory: emotional regression, emotional objectivity, and emotional programming. I like to group these three phenomena because each concept is unique to Bowen theory. No other theory in psychology or biology has anything comparable. The terms *regression*, *objectivity*, and *programming* are used in other bodies of knowledge, but not in the same way Bowen theory uses them. Placing the term *emotional* in front of each term anchors them to the bridge—the emotional system—that Bowen theory constructs to link human behavior to evolution and the behavior of other species.

One dictionary definition of *regression* is "a return to a former or less developed state" (Oxforddictionaries.com). This definition gets at emotional regression in a general way. I define *emotional regression* in Bowen theory in a specific way: If chronic anxiety escalates in a relationship system, the system becomes dominated by less thoughtful and more reactive ways of interacting that are older in an evolutionary sense than the advanced complex behaviors of a well-functioning relationship system.

A simple example of regression in a human relationship system is the following. Two people are working cooperatively, with neither one dictating to the other and both pitching in with their particular skills. Related to time pressure or other stressors, chronic anxiety builds in their relationship. As it builds, one person may anxiously try to control the other, and the other may anxiously defer to avoid criticism and conflict. It is a reciprocal interaction: both people play a part in the emergence and perpetuation of the new pattern. This is similar to the dominant-subordinate (deferential) interactions observed in many species. Cooperation is a complex behavior in human beings that requires the intellectual and emotional systems to function as a working team. Dominant-adaptive (deferential) interactions are older evolutionarily, more primitive. When this more primitive pattern surfaces in human relationships, it indicates that the emotional system is inadequately counterbalanced by the intellectual system. Another example of system regression is emotionally driven conflict interfering with cooperation in a relationship. In both of these examples, the pressure of heightened anxiety drives system functioning toward less complex behaviors.

Raghavendra Gadagkar and Niranjan Joshi (1985) observed what Bowen theory would label an emotional regression in an Old World species of paper wasp. The social structure of this species is typically one reproductive female or queen on a group nest and other females working to assist her. Fewer males than females are produced in this species, and the males remain on the nest only a very short time. The workers forage for food and building material, feed the queen's larvae, and build cells for her to lay eggs. If a queen dies, a worker usually replaces her, and the other workers help the new queen.

The researchers observed a colony of this species undergo a steep decline over a two-month period in the number of adults present on the colony and the number of brood being reared. After the colony's size had shrunk to eleven adult females (a queen and ten workers), something unusual happened: five workers disappeared from the nest overnight. It was very unusual for such a large group of workers to leave all at once. The researchers soon discovered that the wasps that left had founded a new nest not far from the original nest. The individual who had been the most aggressive of the five workers when they inhabited the original nest became the queen on the new nest. This fission of the original colony was good for both the "Rebels" and the "Loyalists," as the researchers labeled them. The newly established Rebel colony grew rapidly as the queen laid eggs and the group cooperated to rear the brood successfully. The Loyalist colony, still under the prefission queen, recovered from its long decline and began rearing a brood quite successfully as well.

Observing that the level of aggression in the original colony during the two months before the fission was much higher than the aggression in either colony after the fission, the researchers concluded that it was the high rate of aggression that reduced the efficiency of brood rearing before fission and the low rate of aggression after fission that permitted efficient brood rearing. They also discovered that the high rate of aggression resulted from the members of the original colony having divided into two groups long before the fission, with one subgroup behaving highly aggressively toward the other subgroup. Having color-marked each wasp individually, they could see that one subgroup consisted of the future Loyalists and the other subgroup of the future Rebels. They also discovered that prefission the members of each subgroup had associated primarily with one another, coordinated their activities, and actively tried to avoid members of the other group. The aggression before the fission resulted largely from members of the Loyalist group attacking members of the

Rebel group whenever they encountered them. The slow decline in colony size leading up to the fission probably resulted from the Loyalists' highly aggressive behaviors driving individuals off the nest.

The parallels in this wasp species to what often happens in human groups as large as whole societies are uncanny. These wasp researchers described the phenomenon they observed as colony fission. Viewed through the lens of Bowen theory, the colony fission resulted from the original wasp colony experiencing a decline in emotional functioning, an emotional regression. It does not seem too far a reach to suggest that the aggression reflected a rising tension level in the colony. The reason for that rise is unknown. The fission permitted a decrease in tension and a consequent rise in functional level for both groups, a reversal of the regression.

Periods of regression, as the term is used in Bowen theory, may occur throughout the natural world under tense conditions that disturb relationships between group members. The following quote by E. O. Wilson points to parallels between emotional processes in less complex organisms and those that occur in human beings: "All things being equal . . . people prefer to be with others who look like them, speak the same dialect, and hold the same beliefs. An amplification of this evidently inborn predisposition leads with frightening ease to racism and religious bigotry. Then, also with frightening ease, good people do bad things" (2014, p. 31).

The paper wasps changed from a cooperative relationship system to two subgroups; the conflict that then emerged between them undercut cooperation. An interpretation of what Wilson describes as an "inborn predisposition" suggests that what is commonly described as tribalism in human beings may have ancient instinctual roots. People commonly think of tribalism as people uniting based on common beliefs, often viewing the beliefs and behaviors of other groups as inferior. At its best, tribalism fosters working together in a way that can benefit society as a whole—witness the good works religious groups perform in the larger society. However, at its worst, tribalism fosters escalating violence between groups.

Understanding tribalism as having subcortical roots rather than blaming it on, for example, shared common beliefs is a useful perspective. Common beliefs are part of the process but do not cause it. Bowen theory suggests that regressed tribalism in human groups, including the family, likely has deep phylogenetic roots. The mechanisms of communication that support this sort of group behavior are typically different among species, but regression could be considered a principle that may play out at many levels, from cellular relationships in multicellular organisms to simple and more complex social organisms.

I have already mentioned anxiety as a process that drives system regression, but the next question is, What processes lead to the escalation of anxiety? The answer to this question begins with a discussion of the *individuality* and *togetherness* life forces. Relationships function as if these two counterbalancing life forces govern them. Both forces are conceptualized as being anchored in the emotional system; both forces also have feeling and cognitive components, all of which interact as a whole. A disturbance in the balance of these life forces can increase chronic anxiety in a system, and an increase in anxiety can further disturb the balance of life forces. A vicious circle of increasing anxiety and emotional reactivity propels a relationship system into an emotional regression.

Bowen theory does not assume that one life force is better or more important than the other. Good basic levels of differentiation allow people to choose to act based on individuality or on togetherness depending on the realities of the existing life situation. Individuality manifests in autonomy for self, goal-directed behaviors, productivity, and being governed by principle versus feelings of the moment. Togetherness manifests in pressuring for oneness, sameness, and agreement; seeking love, approval, closeness, and assigning positive value to thinking about the other before self; and holding others responsible for one's own happiness and/or holding self responsible for the happiness of others.

Threats to adequate emotional contact (such as rejection) and to sufficient emotional distance (such as excessive expectations) between people in an emotionally significant relationship system appear to be the fundamental triggers of anxiety that drives emotional regressions and ultimately fuel symptom development in a family. This interplay in human beings may be related evolutionarily to the approach-avoid responses that are fundamental to all living organisms. Organisms automatically approach what they perceive as benefiting them and automatically avoid what they perceive as being bad for them. These ancient instinctive tendencies are perhaps the major obstacles to human beings maintaining emotional autonomy in intimate relationships. Most of us are barely conscious of how subtle the reactivity that drives these behaviors can often be. Verbal and nonverbal signals trigger the reactions.

As anxiety rises in an anxious emotional field, automatic intensification of the togetherness force is the default mode. This makes it more difficult for people to balance contact and distance. As the togetherness pressure intensifies and relationship fusion increases, people experience strongly conflicting urges. For example, one person might experience a heightened sense of responsibility for the other person's distress, which inclines the person to move toward the other. However, this may be coupled with a compelling urge to avoid getting entangled in the other's person's expectations, which inclines the person to withdraw. The other person experiences conflicting urges as well, such as wanting the person to soothe the other's distress and take responsibility for solving whatever the problem is, which inclines the other to move toward the person. However, this may be coupled with guilt about acting helpless and expecting too much from the person, which inclines the other to withdraw. The conflicting urges raise each person's anxiety, which further infects their interactions.

People with moderate to good levels of differentiation are best at managing threats to contact and distance. They do not act out their anxiety in ways that increase the threat level in the system as a whole, such as by distancing or becoming overly controlling. Their intellectual systems can perceive and reign in the feeling-driven togetherness pressure within themselves, and that allows them to be in supportive contact without feeling they have to fix the other person's problem.

Reigning in feeling states generated by increased togetherness pressure does not mean suppressing the feelings. The feelings subside based on having an objective perspective on the reciprocal relationship process at work, which can make the interaction less threatening. The objective system knowledge is available to process information about the interaction, and that renders the cause-and-effect driven feelings and subjectivity less overwhelming and compelling. This counterbalancing of the feeling state can also result from adhering to a solid self-based principle, such as understanding that jumping in to help can undermine another person's capabilities.

One phrase to describe this ability to be present and accounted for in a relationship system and not overcome by feelings is *being in contact with, but outside of, an emotional system*. One system member being calmer and more thoughtful is helpful, but often that is not enough for moderating the system's anxiety spiral. It may also require an I-position, such as "I am no longer willing to believe and act as if our son's behavior is *the cause* of this family's anxiety. We all have a part in this." Such a person is a powerful resource to an anxious family. This person is not telling others what they should do; just defining what the person is going to do. Emotions such as confidence, courage, and interest accompany effective I-positions and communicate a firmness that others may react to strongly, but well-thought-out positions are ultimately calming and useful to an anxious system. It does not help to tell others to calm down; the key is to live it by calming oneself.

When I was writing *Family Evaluation* in the mid-1980s, I told Murray Bowen that I was planning to title the first chapter "Individuality and Togetherness." He strongly advised me not to do that because people will think it is a philosophy. He suggested anchoring the theory firmly in evolution and the emotional system before introducing individuality and togetherness. I got his point. The first chapter became "Toward a Natural Systems Theory," the second chapter was "The Emotional System," and "Individuality and Togetherness" waited until the third chapter.

A common source of confusion is people equating the concept of individuality in Bowen theory with individualism, a moral, political, philosophical, ideological outlook that elevates the interests of the individual over those of the social group. Haidt (2012) refers to individualistic societies as ones that place individuals at the center and make society a servant of the individual; sociocentric societies place the needs of groups and institutions first and subordinate the needs of individuals. Polarized political and philosophical debates abound as to which type of society is in the best interest of humankind. *Rugged individualism* is also a philosophical/political belief or position. The individuality-togetherness concept in Bowen theory is part of the effort to move toward a science of human behavior. Debating whether individuality is better than togetherness misses the point that both life forces are needed for the smooth functioning of a relationship system.

Many people who have been reared in sociocentric societies—and no culture is entirely homogeneous in this regard—question whether differentiation and individuality apply to or are even possible in their culture. The question arises from confusing individuality with individualism. Both a culture of individualism and one of sociocentrism have their more and less differentiated members. The phenomenon is cross-cultural because the emotions that support differentiation and individuality spring from universal biological roots.

A particular culture might describe the characteristics of a well-differentiated person in its own way, but variation in basic levels of emotional functioning exists in every culture. Culture might be best thought of as the content of a society's beliefs, principles, and values. Differentiation is about how people acquire those ideas, whether thoughtfully or passively, and their flexibility in living them (solid self). For example, principles such as duty, respect for elders, service to the group, and negation of self's desires would play out very differently in a poorly differentiated family system compared to a better differentiated one. In the former, the principles may be regarded as dogma and adhered to rigidly (pseudo-self); in the latter, the principles are open for thoughtful discussion about whether they apply in all circumstances (solid self).

A somewhat tangential example of what I have described above may illustrate the point better. After being involved with Bowen theory for many years and having gained a decent understanding of the emotional process between my mother and myself, I told Mother on a visit home that I was there because I wanted to be there. She reacted with some shock replying, "You should come to see me because it's your duty!" She feared that if I did not consider it a duty,

I would not come. That was her deep insecurity, of course. When I began my efforts to function as a more differentiated person with Mother, I had been using emotional distance to shield myself from her anxieties and expectations. Going to see her was indeed a duty at that point. That changed when I better understood my part in the reciprocity in our relationship. Before I understood the process better, I would anxiously lose self on visits. I would placate and often not say what I thought. Later, I could maintain a "self" on visits and have more genuine interest in Mother. She became a highly valued elder instead of someone I was intensely reactive to despite surface congeniality. Responsibility based on obligation had given way to responsibility based on genuine interest and respect.

The essence of togetherness in Bowen theory is the profound need in all human beings for a feeling of connection. One woman described her part in a very involved relationship with her adult but not very responsible son as wanting to "be there" for him. She derived great pleasure and satisfaction from helping him, even though she recognized that she "probably" undercut him by doing things for him that he should do for himself. Fear that he would do less well if she did not step in also propelled her involvement, but living, acting, and being for him—the essence of the togetherness-propelled fusion process—seemed a stronger influence. The powerful push for oneness, sameness, agreement, and emotional closeness functions to support a feeling of connection.

Differences in the individuality-togetherness balance explain the continuum of variation among relationships just as Bowen's original conceptualization of a differentiation scale explains the continuum of variation in individual emotional functioning. At one extreme of the continuum, the relationship balance tilts heavily toward togetherness; at the other extreme the balance tilts more toward individuality.

Being tilted more toward togetherness than individuality means that people are less flexible, are more emotionally interdependent, and have less resistance to anxiety-driven togetherness pressure in the relationship system than when the balance is tilted in favor of individuality. The reduced flexibility results from, in face of increasing anxiety, people's emotional/feeling systems overriding their less developed intellectual systems and the anxiety-induced greater push for togetherness. This reduces behavioral options to more automatic behaviors, such as anxiously trying to control the other or going along to preserve harmony. Consequently, the more a relationship is tilted toward togetherness, the less resistance it has to being disturbed in face of anxiety. If anxiety goes up, fusion increases. This represents a functional shift in individuality-togetherness balance, not a basic change. The less resistance a relationship has to being disturbed by anxiety, the greater the fluctuations in functional level tend to be.

The term *fusion* confuses many students of Bowen theory because it applies both to interpersonal relationships and to the relationship between the emotional system and the intellectual system within the individual. The degree of fusion in relationships parallels the degree of vulnerability to fusion of the intellectual and emotional systems in the two people. Increased fusion in a relationship means that the togetherness force is having more clout than the individuality force. Increased fusion of the intellectual and feelings systems means that anxiety-driven feeling states are overwhelming the thinking system.

Fusion is an apt term to describe both processes because functional separateness erodes in both cases. Loss of functional separateness results in two becoming one. The togetherness force, with its component emotions/feelings, cognitive components, and associated physiological systems, drives the process of fusion in relationships. The togetherness force also drives fusion of the intellectual and emotional systems within the individual. It manifests in an intense feeling-system-driven interference with objective thinking and pursuit of love and approval.

A logical question to ask is, Where exactly is the togetherness force that exists within a person and plays out in relationship interactions? My speculation is that many components of the "bodymind" (Pert, 1997), which is a term that emphasizes the intricacy of the connections between body and mind, make up the togetherness force. For example, neuroscientist Jaak Panksepp (1998) has discovered at least seven major emotional operating systems in the body that are intricately connected to one another and to the rest of the body. One emotional system, the panic system, seems a fairly obvious component of the togetherness force. This system is involved in distress vocalization and social attachment. Many other components likely exist as well. Both the individuality and togetherness forces are useful conceptualizations of two categories of counterbalancing processes that appear to be playing out in and governing relationships. They are likely best thought of as two distinct but interrelated networks of processes in the bodymind rather than existing at specific anatomical locations.

Another question to address is whether individuality and differentiation convey different ideas. Why two words? My conclusion is that the individuality-togetherness terminology best applies to conceptualizing relationships. Differentiation and individuality are attempting to conceptualize the same idea but in different contexts: one within the individual and the other within the relationship system. The important thing to recognize is that lack of differentiation or fusion between the intellectual and emotional systems within an individual's brain parallels the degree of fusion that plays out in the individual's relationships. The reciprocal relationship togetherness-driven fusion process reinforces the reciprocal brain fusion process and vice versa. When Bowen theorists sometimes talk about the differentiation-togetherness balance in relationships (as opposed to the individuality-togetherness balance), they are describing the same phenomena that the individuality-togetherness balance describes.

Anxiety-related changes in functional level of differentiation can occur within the same individual over time. The changes correlate with the degree the feeling system fuses with and overrides the intellectual system. Anxiety-related functional shifts in the individuality-togetherness balance in relationships also occur. They correlate with the degree the togetherness force increases fusion in the relationship and overrides individuality. Furthermore, just as individuals vary in their basic level of differentiation, relationships vary in their basic level of individuality-togetherness balance. The individual and relationship processes correlate, in that more of one force is associated with less of the other force. Unlike functional shifts in relationship balance, anxiety does not affect basic relationship balance.

Functional level of differentiation is discussed in Chapter 5, but deserves more emphasis in the context of the interplay of individuality and togetherness in relationship processes. Very commonly, people function on a higher level in the relationship system of their workplace than in their family relationship system.

A case in point is the fourth president of the United States, James Madison, and his wife, Dolley. Mr. Madison is often referred to as the Father of the Constitution. Later as president, he adhered to a maxim that "public functionaries never display, much less act, under the influence of passion" (Howard, 2012, p. 226). When faced with considerable anxiety- and passion-driven pressure from colleagues and a multitude of others to surrender to the British in the aftermath of the burning of Washington in 1814, he replied, "It would be dishonorable to send any deputation, and . . . we will defend the city to the very last" (p. 216). It turned out that the War of 1812 turned more in America's favor after that decision. If that is not acting on principle and defining a "self" in face of tremendous pressure from the social/political system, I do not know what is! Mrs. Madison, known for her social graces, defined the role of a First Lady during the eight years of her husband's presidency. James and Dolley Madison were a most impressive team during those years. However, in their nuclear family system it was an entirely different story, similar to ones I have seen many hundreds of times in my career as a family therapist.

James Madison met Dolley Payne Todd in Philadelphia in May 1794. He had moved from his native Virginia to Philadelphia in 1789 to serve in the new House of Representatives. He had served in other prominent political positions by then and had a long list of accomplishments. He was forty-three years old and had never married. She was a twenty-six-year-old widow and mother. She had married a Philadelphia lawyer, John Todd, in 1790. They had two children: John Payne Todd (called Payne), born in February 1792, and William Temple Todd, born in July 1793. In August 1793, a yellow fever epidemic broke out in Philadelphia. Two months later Dolley's husband and second son died of the disease on the same day. Her husband's parents, who were both living in Philadelphia, died of yellow fever not long after. Dolley Todd had been a widow for seven months when she met James. They married in September 1794. Mr. Madison adopted his wife's son Payne. They never had children of their own.

After serving two terms in Congress, Mr. Madison retired from politics in 1797. The family then moved back to James's boyhood home, Montpelier, in Orange County, Virginia. He returned to politics in 1801 to serve as secretary of state during Thomas Jefferson's two presidential terms. He succeeded Jefferson to become the fourth president of the United States in 1809 and served two terms. After leaving office the family moved back to Montpelier. Mr. Madison ran the large tobacco plantation on that property that had been started by his grandfather. Mr. Madison died at Montpelier in 1836, Mrs. Madison died in Philadelphia in 1849, and Payne Todd died in Washington City in 1852.

Despite the highly successful public lives of the Madisons during the two presidential terms, they managed to raise an extremely dysfunctional son. Payne was irresponsible in most areas of his life, had a serious drinking problem, and drained great amounts of money from the family coffers. James's functional level of differentiation in the triangle with Dolley and Payne seems to have been low. Dolley was tremendously overinvolved emotionally with Payne, and she appears to have followed the pattern of "I love you no matter what you do." The permissiveness in this pattern typically fosters sociopathic traits in an offspring. James seems to have completely supported Dolley's focus on Payne, perhaps thinking that she was just being a good mother and possibly also wanting to avoid disharmony. I conclude this because that is a very common way this type of triangle pattern plays out.

James sold off large parcels of the Montpelier property to pay debts that Payne had incurred. Payne landed in debtor's prison twice. Profits from growing tobacco were in decline, but the debt incurred in helping Payne was an equal or even larger factor that eventually forced Dolley to sell Montpelier several years after her husband's death. She moved to Philadelphia and lived out her life in poverty. She did receive a lot of help from her friends.

James had a keen intellect and thrived on learning. His preparation for the Constitutional Convention in 1787 was extraordinarily diligent and disciplined. He read hundreds of books about government in an effort to form his ideas about what would be important in the U.S. Constitution. Not all agreed with his views, but he was capable of compromise and provided important leadership during the Convention. I judge his functional level of differentiation in that context to have been very high. It again would contrast sharply with his functioning in the family triangle. The contrast in functioning in different relationship system contexts as illustrated by the Madisons and many other families has prompted psychologist James E. Jones, an expert Bowen theorist and highly experienced family therapist and one of my Bowen theory colleagues, to conclude that basic level of differentiation of self has little to do with occupational success (January 2018).

Theory suggests that neither James nor Dolley could maintain much of a "self" in the parental triangle and that Payne developed minimal "self" as a consequence. Payne never married or had children. In trying to explain the intensity of Dolley's emotional involvement with Payne, certainly the death of her first husband and younger son when Payne was only twenty months old could have catapulted Dolley into a highly anxious emotional investment and protectiveness of her surviving son, but James's willingness or vulnerability to support the overfunctioning with Payne suggests that both James's and Dolley's basic levels of differentiation were not as high as they appeared to be in their public lives. Two other prominent world leaders, Winston Churchill and Franklin Roosevelt, also had similar well-publicized significant discrepancies in personal and public life functioning. I find this context-dependent contrast in emotional functioning a challenge to understand.

As described in Chapter 5, the intellectual system functions best when largely free of pressure from the feeling system. Mr. Madison's emotional fusion with and dependence on his wife would make him vulnerable to sacrificing intellectually acquired principles in favor of trying to relieve the anxiety of the moment in reference to Dolley's worries and fears about Payne, for example, going along with and even encouraging giving into the demands Payne would have made on his parents. Such parents typically threaten harsh punishments periodically in desperate attempt to effect change in the child but routinely flip back to longer periods of permissiveness. The Paynes of the world, despite good intentions, exploit the parents' unsureness and take the easy way out, opting for instant gratification.

Oddly, many of the Paynes of the world disparage themselves for getting away with so much irresponsibility. They are rarely out to hurt their families but lack the discipline not to take advantage of them. Parents who have been so responsible in many areas of their lives typically puzzle over where their son's or daughter's irresponsibility comes from. They conclude that the problem is in the child, not the family. They try to do more of what they have already been doing to make things change but get the same ineffectual result. The parental triangle in families like the Madisons is a veritable cauldron of feelings.

Mr. Madison would have been in the outside position of the triangle with his wife and adopted son. It is important to keep in mind in treating such families that part of the dynamic is the mother meeting needs for emotional closeness with their son. It is not just about worry and protectiveness. It is also about a special closeness that exists between mother and child that renders her vulnerable to giving in to the child. Another process present in the parental triangle is an undercurrent of tension and distance in the marital relationship. The son functions to stabilize the parental triangle, at least up to the point that symptoms appear and the regression deepens.

As the outsider in the triangle, but with a fundamentally a supportive connection to Dolley, James was likely freed to be all he could be in his political life. No matter how challenging the world outside the family is, it is generally easier for people to deal with than an anxious family. A retired army colonel once told me, "I would rather face a phalanx of enemy tanks than deal with my wife's periods of deep distress. I unravel, I can't think." This is not to blame the wife—part of her distress derives from her mate's inability to engage her on an emotional level.

Finally, a core question that arises from this discussion is, What is the basis for assessing the solid self component of the basic level of differentiation of self? It is clear that James Madison manifested a good functional level of differentiation in his public/political life and a much lower functional level in the parental triangle. A question is how much weight to attach to public/political versus personal life functioning in assessing anyone's level of solid self. In most cases, based on a wide range of clinical observations, it is evident that people are most vulnerable in their personal lives to abandoning principles, beliefs, and values, or to dogmatically adhering to them, to relieve the anxiety of the moment, opting for a short-term versus long-term solution. In terms of solid self, one's personal life is where the rubber meets the road.

An important point to consider in this question is that how people manage themselves in the intimate relationship with their spouses, and not how they manage themselves in their work lives, is the primary determinant of the basic levels of differentiation of their offspring. Consequently, assessing solid self as it manifests in decision making and actions in people's personal lives seems to be the most sensitive measure of solid self and basic level. It is often amazing, however, that when people's intellectual functioning is under little pressure from the feeling system, how much they can accomplish even if their solid self is not all that well developed.

Another reason for assuming that basic level is best assessed by looking at the most intimate relationships is that those relationships best reflect the person's unresolved attachment to the family of origin. The unresolved attachment is replicated most in the adult intimate relationships of one's nuclear family. A spouse is the most likely target as a replacement for one's primary caretaker. It is conjecture, but personal and clinical observations support the idea that all human beings have some level of infantile yearning for oneness with their mother. Can the early symbiotic attachment between mother and infant so powerfully program the child's emotional system? A "yes" answer would explain what often seems to be an exponential increase in emotional fusion when a person falls in love. It is an emotional attraction as well as a sexual one. Most friendships seem to fall far short of that intensity. It is that intensity that makes it difficult for a person to maintain a "self" in intimate relationships. People with good basic levels of differentiation can ride herd on the intense togetherness urge for oneness more successfully than people with moderate and low basic levels. People high on heroin often describe feelings of warmth and safety. Is oneness with mother at the heart of such feelings? I offer this conjecture only as something to think about. Perhaps the safest statement that can be made on this issue of what context is best for assessing basic level is that a good level of differentiation of self predicts that individuals will likely do well in whatever career they pursue but excelling in their occupation is not a reliable measure of their basic level of differentiation.

Conventional psychiatry and psychology, still dominated by individual, cause-and-effect theory, would typically view Payne's alcoholism as the primary cause of his dysfuncton and irresponsible behavior. Alcoholism often runs in families and, consequently, many people assume that it has a genetic basis. The National Institute of Alcohol Abuse and Alcoholism currently concludes that multiple genes may be involved constitute about half the risk in alcoholism (Niaaa.nih.gov., 2018). Environmental factors account for the remainder. The role of epigenetics in the regulation of expression of these genes—in other words, gene-environment interactions—is now considered important as well.

People studying the impact of environmental factors do not appreciate how Bowen theory's concept of the family as an emotional unit aids the study of environmental factors. For example, when it comes to factors that adversely affect psychological development, factors such as child abuse, trauma, and neglect are usually considered. Situations like the Madison family show that those three usual suspects are not necessarily present. Furthermore, child abuse, trauma, and neglect are typically secondary manifestations of a family's basic level of differentiation. The concept of differentiation and its relationship to chronic anxiety are not included in research studies. Granted, it is currently a difficult variable to assess in research studies. Bowen theory offers a more comprehensive picture of all the variables involved. Payne Todd's alcoholism certainly complicated his life course, but it is an inadequate explanation. Bowen theory considers it as much a symptom of a dysfunctional life course as its cause.

CHAPTER SEVEN

Emotional Regression and the Individuality-Togetherness Balance

This chapter describes how emotional regression plays out in terms of the individuality-togetherness balance in relationships. I illustrate this by describing a relationship descending into regression and then emerging from it. These two counterbalancing life forces are often hard to see distinctly in a relationship process because they are both acting simultaneously. Any given behavior may reflect a component of both forces. However, when one member of the relationship manages to increase the ability to maintain a "self" in the relationship, as I describe in a clinical case, the distinctness of the two forces is more easily observed.

Most couples have a fairly comfortable courtship, but most find it difficult to sustain a high level of comfort and closeness over time. A core idea in Bowen theory is that people with the same basic level of differentiation predictably select one another as partners for an intimate relationship. Frans de Waal (1996) writes about the *similarity principle* playing out in many species, including human beings, as a basis for attraction between conspecifics. The similarities that he lists for human beings are age, socioeconomic status, political preference, religion, ethnic background, IQ level, education, physical attractiveness, and height. Basic level of differentiation can be added to this list.

People are usually not surprised to see two fairly immature people form a relationship—birds of a feather flock together. It is harder to accept that this applies to all intimate relationships, regardless of maturity level, but that is Bowen theory's assumption. Basic levels of differentiation also influence the development of close friendships but somewhat less precisely. Exceptions occur rarely in marriages—there are not nearly as many exceptions as marital partners often claim! At this point, it is difficult to research this idea because of the difficulty of being more precise about basic levels of differentiation than just making estimates. This phenomenon is also difficult to study because of the borrowing and trading of pseudo-self that occurs in relationships, often resulting in one member of a relationship appearing more mature and functional than the other.

Two fairly common observations are consistent with the idea that spouses are at the same basic level. One observation comes from the histories of marriages in which one partner is currently fairly dysfunctional and highly dependent on the seemingly high functioning mate. The observation is that usually the partners did not begin their relationship having such a discrepancy in their functioning; the discrepancy developed over time. For example, the partners' emotional functioning is very similar at the beginning of the relationship, but an overfunctioning-underfunctioning pattern unfolds to manage the chronic anxiety generated in their relationship over time; the higher the level of chronic anxiety, the greater the divergence in functioning that occurs.

A second common observation that is consistent with the idea of two partners having the same basic levels is that, if two spouses with significantly discrepant functioning split up, the dysfunctional one often becomes more functional and the previously higher functioning or overfunctioning spouse becomes less functional, occasionally to the point of serious dysfunction. It does not always happen this way, but its occurrence strongly suggests that the spouses' basic levels of "self" were not different. I call this phenomenon a "whisper of nature," meaning that it reveals an underlying process in nature that is often difficult to see if it is less extreme.

The partnering process begins with each person investing an equal amount of emotional/psychic energy in the relationship. The term *emotional/psychic* indicates that there are many psychological components of this investment, but the process is anchored in biological forces that govern emotional attachment.

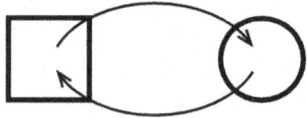 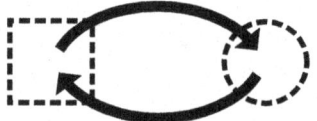

High basic levels DOS   **Low basic levels DOS**

Figure 7.1 *The solid lines around the male and female symbols on the left and the dashed lines around the male and female symbols on the right indicate a moderate to good level of differentiation in the relationship on the left and a low level of differentiation in the relationship on the right. The thinner reciprocal arrows in the relationship on the left compared to the one on the right indicate less emotional or psychic energy invested in the relationship by each partner than on the right.*

This process can be diagrammed as in Figure 7.1. The drawing on the left symbolizes a relationship with each person having equal and good basic levels of differentiation, with associated fairly intact emotional boundaries (solid lines). The drawing on the right symbolizes a relationship with each person having low basic levels of differentiation, with associated highly porous emotional boundaries (dashed lines). The thickness of the arrows between the male (square) and female (circle) indicate that the couple on the right has an equal and much higher investment of emotional/psychic energy in each other than does the couple on the left. The relationship on the right is much more emotionally fused than the one on the left. In the less differentiated relationship, each person's sense of well-being and functioning is more dependent on the amount of attention and acceptance experienced from the other person compared with the relationship on the left. The members of both couples make continuous adjustments to keep the relationship in balance. The members of both couples monitor each other and adjust accordingly, but the monitoring is more intense in more fused couples.

The amount of investment of emotional/psychic energy in the relationship each person makes establishes the individuality-togetherness balance of the relationship. In relationships that are tilted more toward togetherness, each person is investing a greater amount of energy than in relationships that are tilted more toward individuality. In Figure 7.1 the relationship on the right is balanced more toward togetherness than the relationship on the left. It is important to note that the amount of emotional/psychic energy invested in the relationship does not equate with a deep, genuine, unselfish, and respectful interest people can have in each other. In contrast, it equates with the level of dependence each person's sense of well-being has on the other's real and imagined investment in the other; the more energy invested in the relationship, the more people are "completing" themselves by borrowing pseudo-self from the other.

The borrowing and trading of pseudo-self can be equal, resulting in each person's functional level being enhanced and similar. However, an increase in chronic anxiety and accentuation of the togetherness force propel a disparity in functional levels if the predominant pattern of emotional functioning that plays out is dominant-deferential. If the predominant pattern is emotional conflict, the chronic anxiety predominantly plays out in conflict, and each partner's functional level is maintained reasonably well; but, their relationship is full of turmoil. If the pattern is a triangle with focus on a child, the parents overfunction and the child underfunctions. Sometimes with a child-focused pattern the child functions fairly well for a time but eventually dysfunctions. This often happens when the child leaves home. In such cases, the child has been more involved in stabilizing the marital relationship than was apparent.

During a couple's courtship, each partner is typically comfortable with the amount of attention and affection being received, and their communication is quite satisfactory. If either person has suspicions that this may not be the case, this can be the basis of arguments, but the suspicions are often buried in a "love conquers all" attitude.

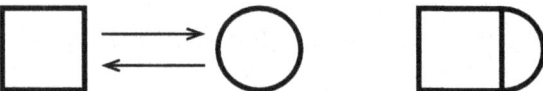

Figure 7.2 *The thick black reciprocal arrows symbolize the strength of the togetherness force in the relationship. The diagram on the right symbolizes the clinically estimated average level of emotional fusion, with the husband being the more dominant partner. It is a stable and low anxiety-generating (no shading in the symbols) at this point in the early history of the relationship.*

Figure 7.2 symbolizes a relationship in the comfortable courtship phase. The diagram on the left symbolizes the individuality-togetherness balance of a relationship in the lower range of moderate basic levels of differentiation on the continuum of differentiation. (If the individuality-togetherness balance is less tilted toward togetherness, as is the case in relationships at good levels of differentiation, it is symbolized by thinner arrows between the people.) The symbols on the right indicate the level of relationship fusion during the courtship period in this example. The clinical vignette I will be describing begins with the Figure 7.2 diagram. The male overlapping the female symbolizes one version of a dominant-deferential pattern of emotional functioning (male vs. female dominated) Early in the courtship period the pattern often contributes to a comfortable fit in that each person may be playing out a functioning position that replicates aspects of that person's particular developmental years, such as when an older brother of a younger sister courts a younger sister of an older brother. It binds any relationship-generated chronic anxiety in that if the female in this case was less deferential and the male is bothered by it, the relationship might not take.

It is a fairly well-recognized phenomenon that when people marry, some increase in relationship tension may occur. Explaining this increase in tension begins with distinguishing between stressors internal to a relationship and ones that are external. Each partner's reactivity to real and imagined verbal and nonverbal cues perceived in the other related to attention, approval, expectations, and distress, a reactivity that varies with basic level of differentiation, are internal stressors. These sensitivities can color their interactions in a way that escalates tensions. External stressors are ones brought into the relationship from sources outside the relationship that affect either partner, such as work issues. Internal and external stressors are interrelated because, for example, one partner's worry and preoccupation with a work issue may result in the other's feeling inadequately attended to, thus setting off an escalating interactive process between the partners that increases chronic anxiety. In the following clinical vignette, the couple's emotional isolation was an important external stressor and their marked reactivity to each other due to low levels of differentiation fueled the internal stressors.

Before proceeding with the case vignette, I want to apologize to the reader for a somewhat complex explanation of relationship process. My goal is to provide clarity, not confusion. In the Bowen theory's defense, once grasped, the explanation above is far simpler than the myriad rationalizations human beings often inflict on one another to "explain" relationship difficulties they are experiencing. That said, I shall continue with the clinical vignette.

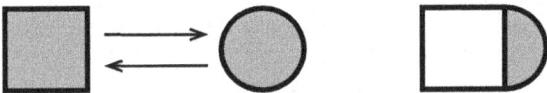

Figure 7.3 *The diagram on the left symbolizes a slight increase in the togetherness force and the light shading of each partner indicates some increase in chronic anxiety that drives the togetherness force. The right hand diagram symbolizes the deferential wife absorbing the slight increase in chronic anxiety that the relationship has generated.*

Figure 7.3 indicates how the relationship in this vignette changed slightly after marriage. The diagram on the left symbolizes some increase in the togetherness force activity (fractionally thicker arrows), which results in a slight functional shift in the individuality-togetherness balance of the relationship toward togetherness. This is not a basic change but an anxiety-driven functional change. The shading in the symbol for each partner indicate some increase in relationship-generated chronic anxiety based on their more reactive reciprocal interactions. The diagram on the right symbolizes a slight increase in the level of emotional fusion between them and, in this case, the female absorbing the chronic anxiety generated by the relationship interaction of a dominant and adaptive pattern of emotional functioning. (She is the one making the most adjustments to preserve relationship harmony.) At this juncture in the relationship, not enough chronic anxiety existed to trigger clinical symptoms. The increased fusion results from the more intense focus each person has on the other; the relationship is tying up more of each person's emotional/psychic energy. This is the first inkling of a regression in relationship functioning.

As months passed for this couple, external stressors accentuated the internal stressors. Prime external stressors were financial pressures the husband worried about and his adult son from his previous marriage distancing from him. The isolation of the couple resulted in part from the husband's possessiveness, which manifested in him pushing his wife to spend less time with her friends. She reluctantly complied, which is her part in the process. Furthermore, neither spouse had extended family members with whom they maintained close contact. The husband obsessed constantly about money, and the wife complained about her husband's unhappiness and her isolation. Both people were stressed, but this was greatly magnified by their intense reactions to each other's distress.

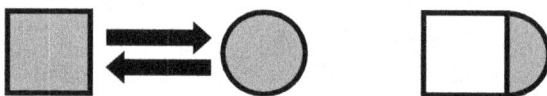

Figure 7.4 The thick black arrows indicate a significant increase in the togetherness force activity related to each person's increase in chronic anxiety level. As the more adaptive (deferential) partner, the diagram on the right symbolizes her chronic anxiety increasing disproportionate to the husband's anxiety (no shading).

Figure 7.4 symbolizes these changes, leading to a more regressed relationship. The diagram symbolizes that each spouse contributes to the relationship tension and the individuality-togetherness balance tilts still further toward togetherness, which is a further functional shift.

The level of emotional fusion increases, and the wife now absorbs even more chronic anxiety from the relationship. The husband is both controlling of the wife and reactively distancing from her upsets. She feels increasingly overwhelmed and out of control. The regression has deepened, and fueled by the anxiety she has absorbed, the wife develops symptoms of depression and irritable bowel syndrome.

As tension continues to escalate, the husband accuses the wife of refusing to meet his emotional needs and threatens to find another woman if she does not change. He aggressively dominates and externalizes even more of his anxiety into the relationship. The wife tries to please and passively submits. She says, "I feel responsible for his happiness and fear his rejection." She internalizes relationship-generated chronic anxiety and her symptoms worsen. Her long-standing type 2 diabetes becomes increasingly difficult to manage as well. Not only is the relationship in a regression, but her bodily homeostasis is so disturbed by her level of chronic anxiety that her body is in a regression too. It is speculative at this point, but it is possible that the regression that can impair the functioning of one member of a fam-

ily may obey the same natural laws that govern the regression in a body that leads to organ and tissue dysfunction.

It is common in these types of situations for the husband's behaviors to be depicted as "selfish" and the wife's as "unselfish." The wife views it that way, and outsiders usually do too. Bowen theory views selfish and unselfish as emotionally based postures people take in relationships in an effort to satisfy togetherness needs. Both postures reflect the inability to maintain "self" in the relationship. In this case, one manifests it by pressuring the other, the husband encroaching on the wife's emotional boundaries, and the other manifests it by trying to please, molding her words and actions to appease him and gain what she wants from him. If the selfish and unselfish terms are thought of as character traits rather than as polar opposite positions produced by a reciprocal process, it is almost impossible not to view the "unselfish" partner as a victim and the "selfish" partner as the culprit.

What happened next in the relationship was fascinating. A first cousin of the husband, with whom he had little contact in recent years, came to town on business and contacted him. They had been close in earlier years. The cousin had had some emotional upheavals in his life and sought the husband out to talk about it. The cousin and husband went out to lunch together several times during the week and talked by phone for long periods on most nights that he was in town.

At the session just after the husband's cousin left town, the wife described a dramatic improvement in her depression and bowel symptoms. Her endocrinologist told her at an appointment that occurred at the end of the week her husband was so involved with his cousin that her blood tests related to the diabetes had also significantly improved. She was alone a lot during that week the husband was involved with his cousin and described lying on her bed and feeling like a great pressure had been lifted. She explained, "I feel free to be my own person, back in control of me."

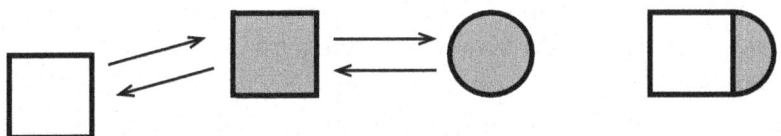

Figure 7.5 A third person has formed a significant attachment with the husband, which reduces the togetherness force and relationship generated chronic anxiety. This results in the relationship being less emotionally fused and reduces the chronic anxiety absorbed by the wife.

This change is symbolized in Figure 7.5. The husband's reactivated relationship with his cousin (symbol on the far left) calmed him and distracted him from focusing so anxiously on his wife. The diagram of the marital relationship symbolizes the couple focusing less on each other during that period and both their levels of anxiety decreasing. The diagram on the right symbolizes less emotional fusion and the wife absorbing less anxiety. Bowen theory assumes that this change helped improve all of her symptoms. The change in the relationship while the cousin was in town reflects a functional shift toward less togetherness, more individuality.

It did not last long after the cousin left town. The regression again deepened, and her symptoms returned. The wife then absolutely insisted that they begin family therapy. They did. It was amazing how quickly the therapy was helpful to them. The wife took the lead. With the lesson of the dramatic improvement in her functioning when her husband was preoccupied with his cousin, the idea that the therapist presented that her symptoms reflected a relationship problem, not a wife problem, made great sense to her. The husband mostly accepted that her symptoms could be linked to their relationship but was not ready to give up the view that the fundamental problem was his wife being unable to meet his needs. He did not comprehend the part his upset and dissatisfaction with her had in making it very difficult for his wife to respond to him in the way he hoped for. He had been unwittingly helping to create her rejection of him.

With the therapist's questioning about the back-and-forth of their interactions, the wife grasped the reciprocity in their relationship. It was that earlier-mentioned "breath of fresh air" experience for her. The new perspective helped her get freer of self-blame and blaming her husband. She felt less responsible for his unhappiness and less frightened by his threats to leave. Most important, she summoned the courage to act on her new perspective. She told her husband, "If you have to leave to seek happiness, I will have to accept it. I don't want that, but I can accept it."

The husband responded in a predictable way when someone effectively defines a "self." He repeatedly said, "You're wrong, change back; if you don't these are the consequences." The consequence was that he would indeed leave. The wife had enough conviction about the fruitlessness of going back to old patterns and in her new way of thinking that she was able to hold the line against her husband's ratcheting up of the togetherness pressure. In an easily observable way, she was reflecting the individuality force, and he the togetherness force. She stood for autonomy; he pressed for oneness.

After nearly a week of the husband's anxiety at its peak and the wife holding her own against the togetherness pressure, the husband blurted out, "You are acting disgustingly mature." He laughed! The individuality-togetherness balance had shifted slightly more toward individuality than was the case early in their relationship. This was a basic change brought about by the wife developing a fraction more solid self; it was not like the previous improvement, a functional shift brought about by the husband's focus on his cousin. The relationship became a bit more emotionally mature, it exhibited a bit more mutual respect.

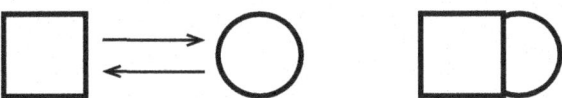

Figure 7.6 *The two diagrams indicate a significant decrease in chronic anxiety, togetherness pressure, and emotional fusion.*

This change is diagrammed in Figure 7.6. The arrows in the diagram on the left side are slightly thinner than shown during their courting period, to symbolize a slight basic shift in the relationship toward more individuality force and less togetherness force operating. The diagram on the right side symbolizes less emotional fusion. The fundamental pattern of the husband in the dominant position and the wife in the deferential position is still present, but overall less chronic anxiety is generated in the relationship and the pattern is less active. She is asymptomatic.

The wife's ability to function with a little more "self" left the husband with no choice but to respect emotional boundaries better than he had been doing. Consequently, anxiety and reactivity became less infectious, resulting in less anxiety-driven togetherness pressure. They now generate less defensiveness and anger in each other, which promotes a more comfortable closeness and associated desire to be helpful to each other.

This case got an excellent result in a relatively short period of time. The wife's brief respite from her husband's pressure and associated decrease in her symptoms made her more receptive to a systems viewpoint than she otherwise might have been. This does not mean that their relationship is quite mature, just that it is more mature than it used to be.

It usually takes longer than six sessions for a family leader to emerge and define a "self," and the process is usually more complicated than in this case. This case is a bit overly simplified to make the points of how anxiety drives regression and the distinction between functional and basic changes in the individuality-togetherness balance. Family therapy based on Bowen theory generally has the reputation of being long term. Indeed, it is usually more long term than in this case. I saw this couple weekly, but therapy can be successful with less frequent sessions as well. The thinking people do between sessions propels much of the progress they make. People are educating themselves to view relationships in system terms, and a family therapist assists such learning. The therapist does not instruct the family on how to change. The therapist primarily helps the family define the problem more factually, which automatically opens up new options.

CHAPTER EIGHT

Emotional Objectivity

The capacity for emotional objectivity is a key ingredient for working toward a science of human relationships. People can learn to describe the emotional process in relationships factually and to recognize the reciprocal interaction between one's internal feeling states and attitudes and what is transpiring in relationships. Bowen theory's highly specific description of emotional process as it plays out in a relationship system has propelled the capacity for emotional objectivity to a new level. The excerpt below from a recorded family therapy session with a person illustrates the development of increased emotional objectivity:

Before I studied anything about Bowen theory, I would have said that I am . . . a perfectionist, wanting to make sure things go a certain way, go well. And now I have identified that I am anxious. And that was a big thing for me to recognize. I would just say I'm anxious—period. And . . . before I would always attach my anxiety to something someone did in relation with me or something I did. And so it was a lot of time spent either blaming someone else or blaming myself when things in a relationship created anxiety and stress. Now I identify myself as being anxious and more aware when I get anxious, when it goes up. . . .
What made it possible to think differently was understanding that emotions are part of a system and that they are going back and forth; and trying to really understand my part in that and take responsibility for my part; and then respect her [adult daughter's] emotions and, I guess, allow her to have them. And also I have learned to lighten up a little. . . . I can find a way to go from catastrophe thinking to seeing what that catastrophizing does in my response to people, and lightening up, and then responding from there, from a calmer place.

What this mother describes is a very common sequence for people trying to gain more objectivity and function with more "self" in their relationships.

The first part in the sequence is recognizing one's own anxiety as just that: one's own anxiety. The second part is recognizing the verbal and nonverbal cues in others that trigger the anxiety and the impact that an anxious response has on others. When the coach (an alternative term to therapist to highlight that the learning tasks place in real world relationships more than in the relationship with the therapist) asked this person if she could explain how she got from there (before family therapy) to here after about ten coaching sessions spaced over nearly a year, she replied that she had heard a few lectures about Bowen theory in the past and that the ideas resonated with her. "I have always been interested in theories," she said—her profession is teaching—"but until Bowen theory, I never found a theory I could really apply."

Two key terms that have already been mentioned briefly are central to understand for developing more emotional objectivity: *functional facts* and *functioning position*. The person quoted above is describing functional facts that she has been able to observe in her relationships, with her daughter, with other family members, and even in her classroom. She had no doubts about her daughter's love for her, but she compared their relationship to the sparks that fly when two bare wires touch. She recognized that when she had not heard from her daughter after a certain length of time, she would begin catastrophizing about what could be wrong. This is a functional fact, a predictable change in her emotional functioning in response to a predictable social cue. As she reflected on this fact, she also realized that it was another functional fact that she would then call her daughter and leave a message like, "I haven't heard from you for a while. Are you all right?" She realized that the anxiety in her voice and her message amounted to an expectation that the daughter call her—and soon—to reassure her that she was okay. The daughter never responded to such messages, which is another functional fact. This predictably further increased the mother's anxiety and frustration.

The mother began to see this as a pattern. Looking at functional facts gets beyond blame and self-blame to reveal a pattern that includes, in this case, two participants, each highly tuned to the other's emotional state. The next time the mother had not heard from her daughter for a long period, she left a message on her daughter's phone, "Hi. It's Mom. Haven't spoken with you for a while, and I just wanted you to know that I'm all right."

Some react to Bowen theory and the above sort of exchange as being manipulative. Some might say the mother was trying to guilt-trip her daughter. Someone might say what the mother said was an attempt to make the other person feel guilty, but recognition of a reciprocal pattern of interaction propelled this mother well beyond blame. Her tone of voice in the phone message was lighthearted, not a guilt-inflicting tone. When Bowen (1978) was developing his ideas about differentiation of self in one's family of origin, he hit on the idea of the logic of an emotional system. It is not a rational logic; it is an emotional logic. The mother's phone message, unlike previous messages too numerous to count, was devoid of any expectation that the daughter respond.

The mother was able to shift from diagnosing herself and others to seeing patterns in relationships and how the pattern affects the functioning of both people. There is no question that the major obstacle to observing these phenomena is intense feeling reactions, of others to self and of self to others. As she said, she knew that emotions were important but was stuck in a cause-and-effect way of thinking about them, blame and self-blame. The content of her message and lighthearted delivery had erased a decades-old emotional cue from the system. It disrupted the emotional logic of the system. People immediately take notice when that happens because the expected sequence is not playing out. The impact that the mother's change had by virtue of being based on a new way of thinking and not on a technique was powerful. The daughter was able to hold onto her "self" better when less burdened by her mother's anxiety-driven expectations. She began reaching out to her mother more. If the mother had not developed emotional neutrality about how things had played out with the daughter in recent years, the daughter could have easily heard her comment as sarcastic. People sense the difference between neutrality and same-old same-old. The mother had truly lightened up, and she did it on the basis of gaining a better understanding of what was going on. It became more interesting than tragic. When such a shift occurs, the prognosis is excellent.

The term *functioning position* refers to how a person's position in a relationship system regulates that person's functioning and contributes to a system process. An example from my own family illustrates this idea. My early efforts on trying to increase my basic level of differentiation by increasing solid self involved several different areas of focus, and the relationship with my mother was one of the major ones. I was thirty years old, in my psychiatric training at Georgetown Department of Psychiatry, married, and father of a two-year-old daughter. I had been studying and trying to apply Bowen theory for seven or eight months at a point that my mother had agreed to come to Washington, D.C., for a visit.

I had begun to recognize that I was much more anxious in relating to Mother than I had realized. My wife had to point that out to me from listening to me talk with my mother on the phone. I denied it initially, but her critique soon helped me observe what she had been observing. It was not until after this visit that I recognized my increase in anxiety prior to contacts with Mother. I loved Mother, wanted her to come, and was very glad to see her, but there was anxiety afoot that I did not recognize as such.

Something important happened about two days into the visit. I was standing at the bottom of the stairs of our two-story townhouse and was about to climb them. At that moment, Mother appeared on the upstairs landing. I watched her place the back of her hand on her forehead and saw that her posture slumped a bit. In retrospect, I had seen this change in her many hundreds of times before. My stomach immediately tightened, and I experienced an associated attitude that I needed to do something to relieve Mother's distress. I also felt the urge to move toward her, to say or do something that would make her feel better. I even started to move slightly, but I caught myself and stopped.

I think because I had been exposed to systems thinking for many months and had also come to recognize my anxiety better, this somehow helped my intellectual system to kick in at a critical juncture. I could suddenly observe a process I had not been able to observe before. The image of Mother's facial expression and body posture traveled down the stairs at 186,000 miles per second, entered my eyes, and traveled swiftly to my stomach and brain. I also realized the instant compulsion I felt to fix the problem. I realized this was a dance that Mother and I had been doing since I was a child. I was incredibly tuned to her and her distress. The impact of seeing the process as between us rather than as a mother problem resulted immediately in my feeling less threatened and amazingly relaxed. I smiled at her and asked if she was coming downstairs, which she did. Smiling at her and feeling compassionate at such a moment had never occurred before. The moment passed. She was fine.

Other thoughts related to that event occurred over the next few days. The guilt I had felt in dealing with Mother disappeared. The pattern was that, if Mother appeared to be slipping into an underfunctioning position, I would move into an overfunctioning position. This happened enough over the years that it was a source of chronic worry for me, especially when we were in each other's presence. We each had a part in this process. I was more aware of how much I had seen Mother as the cause of the problem. Now I saw a two-person emotional process at work for which neither person was to blame. Guilt was the product of a relationship interaction, not a property of me. The objectivity about the process rendered me emotionally neutral about it in my mind.

I realized that the anxiety I experienced prior to seeing Mother physically was related to my lack of confidence in dealing with just this type of experience on the stairs. Having recognized the process and being able to think about it unencumbered by cause-and-effect thinking, I now had the confidence I could manage myself better with her. My anticipatory anxiety evaporated. I did not take any obvious I-position with Mother; I just did not anxiously hover over her. I could see that who Mother was in relationship to me was intricately connected to who I was in relationship to her. It was also clear to me, although I gained more understanding of this as time went on, that the relationship between Mother and me was embedded in the triangle with Dad, and this triangle was interlocked with other family triangles.

I wrote in Chapter 2 that the problem is not in the past; it is in the present. It started out in the past but is continually replicated in the present. This was my first experience of intrapsychic process (guilt and "should" feelings) being significantly modified by functioning with more solid self in a relationship with an emotionally very important person. I modified my functioning position with Mother, and she modified her position as well. It was a dance based on emotional logic.

I provide more details in Chapter 16 about the process of differentiation and use other examples from personal experience to illustrate it. Suffice it to say, that stair experience of many decades ago was just the beginning of trying to gain as much resolution of my unresolved emotional attachment to Mother as I could. The whole of these many experiences got me thinking that, as neutral and nonjudgmental as any psychoanalyst can be, that person is not your mother. The analyst does not place the back of his hand on his forehead and slump a bit. Working things out in the real world of important relationships has distinct advantages over trying to work it out lying on a couch. Bowen opined that more intrapsychic change occurred by developing more of a "self" with one's parents and important others than could occur with psychoanalysis (personal communication in 1970). An important implication of this opinion is that dividing problems into relationship ones and intrapsychic ones, as many therapists do, is a false dichotomy. The relationship process and intrapsychic process are intertwined.

My assessment of what changed for me consequent to this interaction with Mother (and many others) is that I gained a new way of mentally processing potentially anxiety-provoking social cues from Mother that interrupted the automatic reaction of my stress response system. Previously threatening stimuli were no longer threatening. I felt more in control of myself, less helpless in the face of an adverse stimulus, more emotionally neutral about the process. This resulted in less activation of adverse feelings such as guilt and subjective attitudes. I have coached hundreds of other people who have described the identical process. It is a tiny change but a substantive one. A major dividend of the long-term effort was that I became more comfortably available to Mother than I had ever been.

Bowen's research on the unresolved symbiotic relationship between a mother and a severely dysfunctional adult offspring at the Menninger Clinic and then at the National Institute of Mental Health (NIMH) led to him and his research team being able to describe an intense emotional process fairly objectively (Bowen, 1978, 2013). Observing repeated interactions between mother and offspring revealed that both people perpetuated the intense attachment. The conclusion was based on the functional facts of their interactions, on what they did, not on what they said they did. These observations opened a door that led to objective relationship process descriptions of all the family relationships and to the idea of the family as an emotional unit. The key obstacle to overcome in those early studies was a commitment to individual, cause-and-effect thinking. All the researchers started with an emotional as well as an intellectual commitment to individual thinking. Bowen led the charge for letting go of one way of thinking, and that made room for another way of thinking.

As I reflect on the obstacles that the researchers faced in shifting from an individual to a systems paradigm in the heavily psychoanalytic climate of the 1940s and 1950s, I compare it with my own difficulty making the paradigm shift in my own family. Powerful emotions can support a groupthink at multiple levels in society. I do not think that I could have pioneered that new way of thinking, but I was extremely receptive to it when I first listened to Murray Bowen. However, I still had to make the theory my own by applying it in my own family and also in other research areas of my own.

CHAPTER NINE

Emotional Programming

The phenomenon of emotional programming occurs through the transmission of information across generations in a family by relationships and learning, not genes. Important to note, however, is that the exploding field of epigenetics, which examines the interplay between the environment and the switching off and on of genes, opens the door to studying the interaction between emotional programming and gene expression. The research in this field is at too early a stage to form firm conclusions about such a process. The programming results from the verbal, nonverbal, and behavioral interactions that occur within and between the generations. The most intense programming occurs in a person's parental triangle during development, but siblings and other family members have an important influence on it as well. People are not conscious of most of the emotional programming that occurs, but it affects myriad automatic behaviors that govern much of people's lives, for better and for worse. For example, the programming can intensify or deintensify fear reactions to social stimuli. Automatic responses have interconnected emotional, feeling, and subjective cognitive components.

Like Murray Bowen, B. F. Skinner (1953) worked toward developing a natural science of human behavior. Skinner studied measurable behaviors and specific triggers that influence them. He did not study the mind because he did not think such study could be objective. For example, he did not think useful research data could come from asking people to think about things and talk about what is in their heads.

Bowen theory does consider people's introspections to be useful in research and clinical work, but only if they are understood in a relationship system context. They are useful because a Bowen theorist can listen to people's explanations for why they do what they do and think about them not in cause-and-effect terms but as just one of many reciprocally interacting elements of a relationship system process.

Bowen theory's road toward a natural science of human behavior is different from Skinner's in that the bedrock of Bowen theory is the study of family relationships and the functional facts that can be observed in them. The interplay between cause-and-effect thinking and the functional facts of relationship process is illustrated by the following clinical vignette:

> *The mother of rebellious adolescent son explains her fiercely protective attitude toward him as resulting from a deep yearning to be able to make him happy. These feeling-driven attitudes manifest in her ongoing efforts to intervene to solve his life dilemmas. She overfunctions with the son. The son reports feeling his mother hassles him, and he fights her on most every issue, even to the point of sometimes aggressively pushing her away physically. The son feels that his mother wants to control him and that she does not trust him to make good decisions. Such interactions have occurred repeatedly in their relationship, especially since he reached adolescence.*

This is the type of interaction that emotionally programs the son, and the mother's actions stem from her own emotional programming. For example, it programs the son to be hypersensitive to criticism and for his first response to be oppositional. The mother's programming relates, in part, to her matching her mother's worry about her younger brother and feeling sorry for him.

It is not a great leap to associate the mother's feeling state with specific actions on her part. Her predictable actions are functional facts, such as observing her son not working on his homework and prodding him to get it done. When the son is moping around the house and parked in front of the television, that functional fact triggers the mother into feeling that he is unhappy and that he needs more support from her. He predictably feels angry at her prodding, feels controlled by her, retreats to his room, but dawdles on starting his homework. Neither person's feelings, attitudes, or actions cause the problem. They are all part of reciprocally interacting functional facts of their relationship.

It is sometimes magical in family therapy when a mother such as this one, through introspection, is able to identify the subjectivity in her attitudes that trigger her actions toward the son and link them with the triggers coming from the son's verbal cues, nonverbal cues, and behaviors that reinforce her attitudes. Furthermore, insights about the reciprocity in the interaction with the son need to be broadened to the parental triangle (and usually other interlocking triangles in the nuclear and extended families) to gain a more complete picture. In this case, the father's often harsh responses to the son's anger and procrastination increased the mother's feelings of needing to protect the boy. Seeing all the relationship reciprocity that is playing out gives her a reason to work at changing herself and to lay off trying to change her son and husband. Part of the husband's harshness is in reaction to viewing his wife as choosing their son over him.

Backing off from anxiously prodding the son is not about giving up but about the mother taking more responsibility for the impact of her own attitudes and actions on the triangle and how it programs the son's hypersensitivity to his parents' approval, expectations, and upset. The dividend of such a change on the mother's part is that it markedly reduces the chronic anxiety generated in the triangle. This allows the mother to become more available to her son in a calmer way, reduces the father being in the outside position, and helps him to be less critical of the son. In response, the son is calmer and less defensive and procrastinates less. The mother's leadership in seeing the triangle enables her to function with more "self" in it.

If a person's attitudes, feelings, and actions are not studied in the specific relationship context in which they occur, it is easy for the researcher to drift into the subjectivity that Skinner wanted to overcome. Skinner's research was solid, but he lacked a theoretical frame for studying conditioning or programming in a family relationship context (a weakness of cognitive behavioral therapy as well). Ignoring the mind and people's perceptions of a situation leaves out a key component of what sustains troublesome human interactions; ignoring the relationship process leaves out the context in which the mind is functioning. It is difficult to think about the individual and the relationship system simultaneously, but people can learn to do just that.

The child triggers emotionally programmed reactions in the parent simultaneously with the parent triggering emotional programming in the child. As I describe in detail in Chapter 11, the specific processes that are playing out between parents and an offspring require a multigenerational relationship system perspective to adequately explain them. I touch on this in the epilogue, where I describe how the triangle involving Mother, her brother, and their mother influenced the triangle of Mother, Father, and my schizophrenic brother. The degree of fusion in a parental triangle cannot be explained adequately by looking at just two generations. Emotional programming comes down through the generations in myriad forms that with research can be defined objectively. Seeing the multigenerational process provides a much-needed broad perspective for what is unfolding in the here and now.

Emotional programming occurs in the context of the interplay between the counterbalancing life forces of individuality and togetherness in parent-offspring relationships. Variations in the particular balance of these forces can explain variation in the intensity of the emotional programming that occurs, as well as variation in the capacity for self-regulation.

Bowen theory describes a unique understanding of human emotional development. The fundamental idea is that a biologically anchored growth force for individuality and the gradual differentiation of "self" counterbalances the biologically driven force for togetherness in parent-offspring relationships. The forces operate within both parent and child and play out between them. The togetherness force is dominant early in the development of a helpless infant, but as the child matures physically and emotionally the balance normally shifts away from togetherness. Similar processes are easily observed in other mammals and birds.

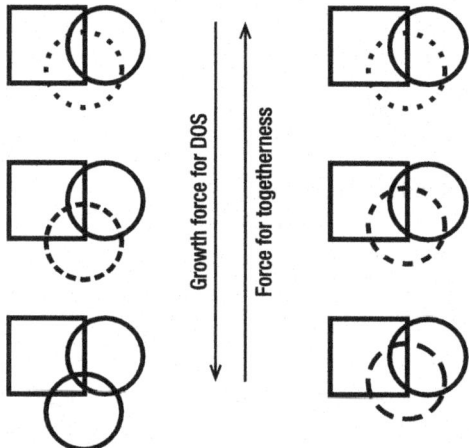

Figure 9.1 *The columns on each side of the diagram symbolize differences in the degree of resolution of parent-offspring emotional attachment during the course of the child maturing biologically.* On the left, significant resolution is occurring as the child matures biologically and psychologically and the parents separate from her based on the realities of her capabilities, and very limited resolution occurs on the right. At the top of each column, the dotted circle symbolizes a newborn baby girl embedded between her two parents. A parent child symbiosis is normal at this time. At the second level down of the diagram, the column on the left shows the daughter having dashed lines around her as she approaches puberty, indicating the development of some "self". The parent-child relationship is partially resolved. On the right, the preadolescent daughter has developed little "self", as symbolized by the slightly heavier dots of her circle. Little resolution of the parents-daughter attachment has occurred. At the bottom of the two columns, the solid line around the daughter on the left and near complete resolution of the attachment to parents (less overlapping) symbolize a significant development of "self" during the child's development. On the right, the dashed circle and little reduction in the overlap of parents and child symbolize little resolution of their emotional attachment and little development of "self." The arrows between the two columns symbolize a growth force for individuality and the development of a separate "self," which promotes emotional separateness between parents and child, and a togetherness force, both in parents and child, that retards resolution of the early symbiotic attachment.

Figure 9.1 diagrams the process. The individuality force propels child and parent toward emotional autonomy in their relationship, and the togetherness force propels parent and child to remain as one. The left diagrams show an infant daughter born in a fairly undifferentiated state (symbolized by the lightly dotted circle embedded between the parents) and strongly fused with her parents. This is a normal symbiotic attachment that favors the survival of the helpless infant. Mother and offspring are like one person, in a near complete state of emotional fusion—recall the quote from Diane Ackerman (2012) in Chapter 4: "A fusion in which the self feels so permeable it doesn't matter whose body is whose." Besides the baby's isolation or distress call, which triggers the mother's response, the child has the instinctive urge to grow away from the parents, to become a separate, distinct, and independent adult. The caretaker has instinctual urges to protect, comfort, and nourish the baby, but also an instinct to separate gradually from the child.

The left diagrams symbolize the daughter maturing psychologically as she matures biologically. The circle of the daughter becoming better defined and less embedded in the parental relationship symbolizes her being age-appropriately more separate emotionally and physically from the parents. The diagrams show that, by the time she has reached her late teens, she has a reasonably well-developed "self" that parallels a reasonably resolved emotional attachment to her parents. Ideally, parents and child can be comfortably close, with each respecting the other's emotional boundaries. This reasonably differentiated relationship facilitates parents and nearly young adult daughter having a reasonably open and close relationship as she prepares to move into the adult world.

Thinking in terms of developmental stages is not a useful way of characterizing the separation process that Bowen theory describes. Critical periods may exist for other aspects of development, but that concept does not seem to apply to the emotional separation process. It is a gradual process of parents separating appropriately from the child, which fosters the child separating appropriately from them. One might argue that, given the onset of puberty, adolescence is a stage. The important point from Bowen theory is that adolescence varies significantly depending on the degree of emotional separation existing in the parent-offspring relationship. The separation slowly developed prior to the child reaching adolescence and continues into adolescence. As described in Chapter 4, significant adolescent rebellion (or its mirror image, overcompliance) is more likely to occur in relationships that have the least emotional separation between parents and teenager. The rebellious adolescents tearing themselves away from their family, a process that the parents' high level of emotional reactivity contributes to equally; the adolescent is not growing or maturing away.

Parents have the task of appropriately toning down anxiety-driven togetherness urges as the child matures. Failure to tone down such urges can undermine the child's ability to separate from the parents emotionally, promoting excessive and prolonged dependency of the child on the parents (or on later substitutes for the parents). The parents' difficulty toning down togetherness urges commonly manifests in being obviously anxious and overly involved in managing the child. It can also manifest in being unduly idealistic about the child and, consequently, often blind to some of the child's vulnerabilities. The right side of Figure 9.1 symbolizes this lack of emotional differentiation between parents and child. The dashed lines around the late adolescent daughter symbolize that she has developed less of a "self" than the daughter in the left diagrams and has less resolution of the emotional attachment to her parents at the point she is preparing to move into the adult world. The child has a built-in instinct to separate emotionally from the parents, but it can all too easily be overridden by the seduction of togetherness. Quite commonly, the degree of unresolved interdependence in the parental triangle has not been obvious to parents or child, even if the child has had symptoms of some type during childhood or adolescence. The parents may recognize that they have been anxious but see their child as causing and justifying that anxiety.

Another somewhat common variation of emotional fusion and its associated emotional programming is when a mother is dysfunctional, perhaps chronically depressed or abusing substances, and the fusion takes the form of her son or daughter being highly tuned into the mother's moods and feeling a lot of responsibility for making her happy. It is sort of like a parent-focused child. The intensity of that fusion programs the child into a strong interdependence with the mother, showing itself in strong need for her attention and later in romantic relationships. Such a person often feels like the giving one in the relationship, not getting enough in return. The mother is fundamentally very involved with that child but may go through periods of withdrawal, to which the child is highly sensitized.

Recalling the discussion of Paul MacLean's (1990) triad of family behaviors in Chapter 4, one of the triad was nursing in conjunction with maternal care, which renders child and mother more important to each other. Nursing is a process that evolution designed to promote the survival of the young, but it can get co-opted very easily by anxiety generated in the family relationship system in which a mother-child relationship is embedded. The anxiety comes to rest in the primary caretaker-offspring attachment and retards the child's development. The child weans from nursing, but the intensity of the emotional connection persists. The mother's ongoing need and anxiety-driven preoccupation with the child and the child reciprocating it can function to help stabilize the family system. For example, the triangle with the child can reduce potential tensions between the parents. All family members have some part in promoting this. One aspect of my part in my family-of-origin process was siding with Mother in viewing the cause of family anxiety as my brother. This played out long before he was ever given a psychiatric diagnosis.

In the right column of Figure 9.1, the anxiety-driven togetherness processes in the parents and the child's complicity in the process have unwittingly fostered togetherness and dependence over differentiation, self-determination, and self-regulation in their child. The needs and anxieties of the parents inhibit their appropriate separation from their daughter, and the daughter acts on her own togetherness urges to remain fused to the parents, taken care of by the parents. She has developed little "self" by late adolescence and, consequently, is poorly equipped to move into the adult world. Her original normal emotional attachment to the parents in infancy remains significantly unresolved.

The above description vastly oversimplifies the developmental process, leaving out countless important details. It is intended to capture the big picture, punching up Bowen theory's distinctness from contemporary psychological theories of development, for example, attachment theory, which views parents not bonding adequately with their child as producing a child who forms insecure attachments with important others (Bowlby, 1988). This is similar to the idea that maternal deprivation is the core cause of relationship and other life problems.

In Bowen theory terms, people prone to highly insecure attachments as adults have the most unresolved attachments to their parents. The significant emotional distance that sometimes occurs in parent-child relationships is a reaction to a high intensity of unresolved emotional fusion between parents and child. As a twenty-seven-year-old man explained, "Mom and I love each other dearly, but we have a terrible time being around each other. We get on each other's nerves. It works best if we see each other infrequently and for brief periods." The young man chooses to live in decidedly spare conditions rather than live with his parents. He also has difficulty sustaining long-term intimate relationships with young women. Keep in mind he picks females at his same basic level of differentiation, so his functioning does not cause the difficulty with intimate relationships; it is something that he and his partner cocreate.

The resolution of the emotional attachment that parents have with one child may be significantly less than that with another child. This is what occurred in my family of origin. Sometimes the differences are quite striking, as it was in my family, but other times not. This can help explain the very common phenomena of siblings who turn out very differently (Kerr, 2008). Bowen theory does not explain the specific outcomes of siblings. Many variables contribute to a specific outcome. However, Bowen theory can predict that the sibling with the best resolution of the emotional attachment to the family will likely have the most stable relationships and orderly life course of the siblings.

Bowen and his research team observed sibling differences in emotional functioning during the Family Study Project. Parents who had a son or daughter diagnosed with schizophrenia often had another child who functioned fairly normally. Bowen theory conceptualizes the sibling vulnerable to developing schizophrenia as having less "self," as having little resolution of the early symbiotic relationship with the primary caretaker and less resolution than what occurred with the siblings. It should be emphasized that systems theory considers a designation of "normal" as arbitrary. Emotional functioning varies on a continuum. In the case of my family of origin, two of my brothers and I functioned on a somewhat higher level than my brother who was diagnosed with schizophrenia. Categories of "normal" and "abnormal" imply qualitative differences between people, whereas Bowen theory conceptualizes the differences as quantitative. These quantitative differences are usually not that much, but enough to make a noticeable difference in life courses.

The fundamental idea in Bowen theory that helps explain sibling variation is that siblings grow up in the same family but in different triangles. The mother of four children explained that she has the most mature relationship with any human being ever with her first child, a fourteen-year-old daughter, and the most immature relationship she has ever had with her second child, a twelve-year-old daughter. She described the relationship with her husband and other two children as between those two extremes. The twelve-year-old was having behavioral and academic problems; the other kids were doing better.

Another mother with two identical-twin four-year-old daughters explained that she and one of the twins focus intensely on each other's moods, tones of voice, and facial expressions. Emotions dominate their interactions. "We seem almost addicted to interacting that way," she explained. The mother was not complaining about the relationship but considered it special. It is completely different with the other daughter. They are much less reactive to each other. The father in another family said that he and his wife had raised three sons: two were "rational" and the third was "irrational." He added that he sees this pattern in almost every family he knows. "Why is that?" he pondered. Bowen theory describes one key process that contributes to this common phenomenon.

Figure 9.2 diagrams this phenomenon of same family but different triangles. In the diagram, the triangle involving the two parents and the older son is marked with dots to symbolize that it generates less chronic anxiety than the triangle involving the two parents and the younger son, which is drawn with heavy lines to symbolize that it generates more chronic anxiety. The

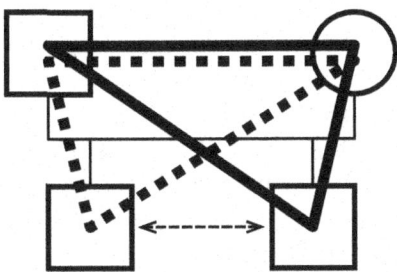

Figure 9.2 *The dotted lines between the parents and older son symbolize a parental triangle with reality based, low anxiety, and mature interactions in the triangle. The heavy black lines between the parents and between the parents and younger sibling indicate feeling based, high anxiety, and immature interactions in the triangle. The dashed arrow between the siblings indicates that their interactions affect each one's development.*

dashed arrow between the two siblings indicates that their interaction affects the overall family emotional process. For example, the older son, not recognizing the overfunctioning-underfunctioning reciprocity between his brother and their parents, may take sides with his parents and criticize the brother for acting irresponsibly and causing his parents so much distress. The sibling relationship is generally less of a factor in the emotional programming of a child than is the parental triangle, but it is not inconsequential.

TABLE 9.1

MORE DIFFERENTIATED TRIANGLE	LESS DIFFERENTIATED TRIANGLE
Less anxious investment	More anxious investment
More mature interactions	Less mature interactions
More goal-directed	More relationship-oriented
More "self"	Less "self"

Table 9.1 lists the differences between the two triangles. First of all, less anxious investment in the child plays out with the older son. Parental investment in a child is obviously a good thing, but if it is chronically laced with anxiety it ratchets up the emotional programming of the child in areas such as needing attention, sensitivity to approval, sensitivity to expectations, and high reactivity to upset in the parents. These are the social cues mentioned earlier. It is not a complete list, but I emphasize these sensitivities because these are the ones that people most commonly identify as needing to work on to try to function with more "self" in their families and other arenas.

As emphasized earlier, the subjective attitudes that get linked to this reactivity, such as being treated unfairly or that the self is the center of the universe, are hugely important to recognize as well. The more intense the emotional programming, the more influence bias and other subjective attitudes have on a person's actions and decisions.

It appears that when children develop in a chronically intense emotional environment—triangles involving other family members and people outside the family are important as well—this makes it very difficult for them to learn to think for themselves because they are functioning so much in automatic reaction to others. Furthermore, the parents may be constantly interpreting the world to the children. This seems to blunt the development of their intellectual system and its associated capacity for self-regulation. It amounts to a double whammy: heightened emotional reactivity to the social environment and impaired cognitive capacities to self-regulate. The combination makes it very difficult for a person to function calmly, except under ideal circumstances. At the extreme it can be markedly impairing and ultimately express itself as clinical symptoms, such as highly unstable relationships, severe acting out when the anxiety is externalized into the system, or the full range of clinical problems that result from the adverse effects of internalized chronic anxiety on body and mind, in the here and now, and the toll that anxiety takes over time.

The second process listed in Table 9.1 is maturity, or lack thereof, in the triangle. Immaturity is reflected, among other ways, in being so reactive to others that it impairs people's abilities to remain in consistent emotional contact with one another or makes it difficult not to be overly intrusive into others' emotional space, particularly when stress levels are high. Distancing emotionally or being overly intrusive changes a relationship from being a potential resource to being an additional stressor.

It is important to keep in mind that this all exists on a continuum of basic level of differentiation of self. People differ in degree and not kind. These processes are easiest to see when they are extreme, but they are always present to some degree in all families, particularly when stress levels are higher than usual.

The third process listed in Table 9.1 refers to where people exist on a continuum of the capacity to be goal directed versus relationship oriented. The more intense the emotional environment one develops in, the more life energy gets consumed by relationship interactions and the less energy is available for goal-directed pursuits. *Relationship oriented* does not refer to a constructive interest in other people but, rather, to an automatic, obligatory strong response to social cues and a lack of self-regulation. All human beings have an instinctively based interest in others, but the emotional status of relationships rules less differentiated people. People can be in denial about this dependence or painfully aware of it. Being goal-directed can be tricky to assess because people can deal with emotions by an intense focus on goals. Emotions and anxiety drive type A personalities along with their functioning positions in their important social contexts. A caveat here is that people who fit the type B personality description do not necessarily have a good basic level of differentiation. People can stay calm by avoiding defining a self when that would be important to do. A related common process occurs in marriages when one partner appears rational and calmer than the other partner, who appears more emotionally intense. It is fairly easy to observe such relationships and see that both are very reactive to the other person, but the "rational one" has a hard time seeing it.

The last item in Table 9.1 has been discussed already. The person developing in a more mature or better differentiated set of interactions over time predictably develops more "self." According to Bowen theory, that is one very important component of why siblings turn out differently.

The *family projection process* is one of the eight concepts in Bowen theory that I discussed in Chapter 4. I mention it again in this chapter because the projection process is embedded in the phenomena of emotional fusion and associated emotional programming. The concept describes a mechanism for how anxiety gets transmitted from a parent to a developing child. It is important to remember here that the level of chronic anxiety in a mother is not simply a property of the mother. Her level of anxiety reflects the level of anxiety in the family system of which she is a part and the larger network of relationships in which the family system exists, such as extended family and community. Her anxiety also reflects her functioning position in the family system. For example, her husband may calm himself by focusing on his work, and his wife, feeling anxious and isolated in reaction to his distance, anxiously overfocuses on one or more of their children. Another example is a wife who loses functional self (a lending and borrowing of pseudo-self) in her marriage regaining pseudo-self through being overly involved with a child.

The family projection process fits sociologist Robert Merton's (1948) description of the self-fulfilling prophecy. He applied the concept to social phenomena, not to the family. In Merton's view, the process begins with a false definition of a situation that evokes a new behavior, which makes the false conception come true.

The mother can focus on an existing minor defect in the child and, as a consequence, exaggerate it over time. The defect may also be a total product of the mother's imagination. In my family of origin, my mother perceived my brother, the one who years later was diagnosed to have schizophrenia, when he was an infant to be "a fragile china doll." Review of home movies from my brother's early years and later discussions with Mother strongly suggest that this was a completely false or imagined definition of the situation. This is an important point because many parents readily acknowledge that they have been anxious about something being wrong with the child since the early period of the child's development but are convinced that the child was born that way. They have great difficulty entertaining the idea that the child's current problems may relate to a faulty perception of the child and their anxiety-driven reactions to that perception.

In the case of Mother and her firstborn son from the second marriage, it was not just her fears that drove her perceptions of him and behaviors toward him but also her need to be needed. Anxiety that was managed by emotional distance in the marriage shifted to an anxious focus on my brother and projection of that anxiety into him. Dad fully supported this process with, obviously, no awareness of its potential fallout down the road. Mother gave Billy highly protective special handling throughout his life. She loved each of her four sons dearly, but her most anxious investment played out with Billy. His mostly no-self makeup crippled him for life. He could not move forward into the adult world. Mother was a kind and loving human being and had the best of intentions. She, of course, felt that her efforts on Billy's behalf were addressing and fixing problems.

I described the family projection process as embedded in emotional fusion because the intense emotional programming that accompanies the fusion interferes as much with the development of "self" as does the particular content of the mother's worry system. Early in my supervision with Murray Bowen he asked me the following question: "If a schizophrenic person sits down in front of you for a therapy session, what are the three most important questions in his mind?" Bowen's answer was, "What do you think of me? Do you accept me? What do you want me to do?" (personal communication, May 1969). I came to understand that these questions are not peculiar to people diagnosed to have schizophrenia but are characteristic of all human beings. The problem is that, at the level of no-self where a schizophrenic person exists, these questions dominate existence. The perceived answers can trigger anxiety or calm it. The schizophrenic person is at the mercy of his or her emotional environment. People with more "self" have less intense reactions, more accurate perceptions of the answers to these questions, and more ability to self-regulate the behaviors that those reactions can evoke.

For reasons largely unknown, when disturbances occur in the most important relationship context of people who are called schizophrenic, their consequent severe emotional disequilibrium manifests in anxiety-driven psychotic symptoms. Psychosis is a place to withdraw to in face of an anxious environment. Psychosis solves a problem, but it also creates a problem.

I describe in the epilogue that Mother's most intense focus on her firstborn son of the second marriage as, by her own statement, that she was simply ready to have a baby when he was conceived. In working with thousands of families over time, I have heard a wide range of explanations from mothers of how they got anxiously focused on a particular child in a sibling group. Bowen theory currently lists five situations that can foster a more intense focus on a particular child: the firstborn child; the firstborn of a certain sex; a child born with a reality defect; a child born at a time of high stress in the family, nuclear or extended; and the last-born child.

It is valuable for parents to think through why the anxious family focus may land on one child versus another, and even why more than one child may be a focus. In my family of origin, Billy being the firstborn of my parents' marriage was a factor, but that has to be understood in the context of the different circumstance that prevailed when Mother's son of her first marriage was born. Billy was conceived at a time Dad's dying father, his wife, and her sister were living with this new nuclear family. It is useful for parents to try to sort out the context in which the intense focus developed because it can help them be more objective about how the process occurred. We are fortunate to now have a theory that can help explain how bad things can happen to good people. It is all too easy to blame parents rather than exercise the discipline to comprehend the many variables that go into the explanation of a human emotional problem.

CHAPTER TEN

Chronic Anxiety

Bowen theory does not view anxiety as a psychiatric disorder. Anxiety exists in all people and, in some form, probably exists in all living things, flora as well as fauna. Neuropsychiatrist Eric Kandel (1983) has studied anxiety in an organism whose evolution dates back to the early Cambrian period of 500 million years ago, the California sea snail *Aplysia californica*. This organism has central ganglia and peripheral motor neurons, but none of the more complex brain structures and physiology that mediate anxiety in human beings. Kandel discovered processes in this mollusk that, despite its not having a complex nervous system, have remarkable parallels to chronic and anticipatory anxiety in human beings. Stress researcher Bruce McEwen (2002) noted that the particular mechanisms that mediate the physiology of anxiety in human beings—the stress response system—first became fully operational in salmon about 400 million years ago. While salmon are on a different evolutionary branch than human beings, evidence for a stress response in organisms on a range of evolutionary branches emphasizes its importance for sustaining life. Anxiety is a natural process. What psychiatry textbooks term *anxiety disorders* are but one of myriad symptomatic manifestations of overly active evolutionarily ancient anxiety systems.

Anxiety is one of two main variables in Bowen theory. The other variable is the degree of integration of self, explained in detail in Chapter 5 as differentiation of self. The two variables are distinct but interlocking. They are referred to as variables because they significantly affect all the other processes that Bowen theory describes, such as the activity level of the patterns of emotional functioning. The concept of differentiation of self describes the existence of a continuum of emotional functioning. The variable of integration of self refers to the phenomenon of thoughts and feelings operating as a working team. People with moderate to good basic levels of differentiation have the most ability for thoughts and feelings to operate as a working team; the feeling system dominates thinking in people with low basic levels of differentiation.

Bowen theory defines anxiety as the reaction of an organism to a real or imagined threat. This is consistent with Kandel's (1983) definition of both chronic and anticipatory anxiety representing a motivational (defensive) state in preparation for expected danger, a preparation that is not necessarily expressed in motor activity. Acute anxiety is typically in reaction to real threats, and chronic anxiety occurs more in reaction to imagined threats. The response to real threats is generally experienced as time limited. The response to imagined threats is not experienced as time limited because such threats are accompanied by more uncertainty about when they will end. Bowen theory distinguishes between *internalized* anxiety, which manifests in one or more locations of the body (inflamed bowel) or mind (hallucination) of an individual, and *externalized* anxiety, which an individual acts out in one way or another in the relationship system. It is important to note that an imagined threat can become real. For example, when an anxious response to a perception that an important other person has become emotionally distant triggers pursuing behavior to reestablish closeness, and the pursuing behavior triggers anxiety-driven emotional distancing by the other—it is a self-fulfilling prophecy.

A way to understand the interlocking nature of the two variables is from the perspective of adaptation. One definition of adaptation in Bowen theory is that it is the ability to respond to life challenges without participating in an escalation of chronic anxiety in a relationship system (*adapt* here refers to a different phenomenon than in the dominant-adaptive pattern of emotional functioning). The capacity to adapt parallels a person's capacity for an integrated response. For example, a triangle that includes three poorly differentiated people is more vulnerable to escalations of chronic anxiety than a triangle composed of three people with good basic levels of differentiation—although no one is sufficiently differentiated to be immune to participation in triangles if the stressors are great enough. Two reasons explain this difference in vulnerability. The first is that if one member of a reasonably well-differentiated relationship system experiences a significant stressor or series of stressors, that person can usually self-manage without acting in ways that make other members of the system anxious, for example, by not withdrawing, acting frustrated and angry, or acting helpless. The second reason a better-differentiated triangle is less vulnerable is that the other members of the system have enough "self" not to become unduly anxious about the stressed person's anxiety. They can remain present and accounted for without invading the emotional boundaries of the somewhat anxious system member.

Examining anxiety in this way illustrates that, even though it is individuals that experience anxiety, chronic anxiety is a consequence of various types of social interaction and, consequently, is most usefully conceptualized as a property of the emotional field (Henry, 1992). One individual in a relationship system may most intensely manifest subjective and objective manifestations of anxiety, but the degree of anxiety that this person manifests is not solely an individual property. This is an important distinction because commonly the most anxious person in a system is seen as causing the others' anxiety, rather than seeing the most anxious person's anxiety as a reflection of system-generated anxiety as well. Thus, in assessing a person's adaptive capacity, it is important to consider the degree of chronic anxiety in the emotional field, as well as an individual's capacity for an integrated response in the context of that emotional field.

To summarize, an individual's level of chronic anxiety is related to two processes that are not under individual control: (1) poorly differentiated relationship interactions in the relationship system in response to a stress or stressors on one or more members that raise system chronic anxiety, and (2) the person's functioning position in the system. In the case of a triangle, for example, whether a person occupies an inside or outside position (see Chapter 3) governs how much system-generated anxiety that person absorbs.

It is important to recognize that the member who is distressed initially by a real or imagined stressor is not necessarily the one who absorbs the system-generated chronic anxiety. The one who absorbs the anxiety depends on the particular patterns of emotional functioning that come into play to manage the anxiety. For example, a mother reacts to her husband's distance, distance that has been triggered in reaction to anxiety generated by problems at his work, and manifests her reactivity by anxiously focusing on their six-year-old child. That night the child "inexplicably" wets the bed. The father, whose anxiety initially tweaked the system, slept peacefully that night. A metaphor for this process is people quickly passing a hot potato to avoid getting burned themselves. It is not usually a conscious process, but people can use the lens of theory to help them become aware of it as a phenomenon and can then learn to control their part in the process.

Viewing chronic anxiety as primarily related to relationship system disturbances does not discount the fact that a person's attitudes often trigger chronic anxiety; for example, a person who perpetually feels that life treats him unfairly is chronically vulnerable to anxiously reacting to a wide array of life situations. McEwen notes that "if we torture ourselves with worst-case scenarios, voluntarily simmering in a toxic broth of dread, we can exhaust our bodies' allostatic systems without ever coming into contact with a predator or adversary, without even leaving home" (2002, p. 10). (*Allostasis* describes the bodily processes that enable the body to keep stable in the face of change, a concept described in more detail in Chapter 23.) A person harboring such an attitude has experienced the programming for it in interaction with other people in the past and acts out that programming with the same or other people in the present. A man I coached in dealing with his family was highly vulnerable to considerable self-criticism. Fortuitously, during the coaching his wife had a rare out-of-town business trip. While she was gone he experienced a marked decline in his self-critical obsessions, but the obsessions came roaring back when she returned. He had not realized how much of his self-criticism, his "toxic dread," was linked to worry about what his wife thought of him. His obsessions were much more intense in the context of the marital emotional field than in his work emotional field.

Conceptualizing chronic anxiety as a relationship problem is useful. By seeing an aspect of the marital relationship process more clearly, including recognizing how reactive he was to his wife's facial expressions that he perceived as critical, the time spent by the husband in a state of toxic dread declined. He realized that his fears and sensitivities to her played a part in her disapproval. This gave him the courage and confidence not to be so reactive to her. The man also realized that key aspects of the relationship with his mother contained a similar dynamic. Murray Bowen liked to say, "That which was created in a relationship [emotional programming in the relationship with his mother] can be fixed in a relationship [in the relationship with his wife]" (personal communication on many occasions,). The success of psychoanalysis was based on resolution of the transference with the analyst. The success of a Bowen-theory-based approach depends being able to change in relationship to important others in the real world. This man's mother had died before this insight about his marriage. Had she still been alive, he could have made changes with her as well.

Two perspectives are particularly important for understanding how chronic anxiety develops in relationships. One is a microscopic view of relationship interactions to reveal the specific details of the interactions. The other is a macroscopic view that examines the total network of relationships in which a given relationship is embedded. Gaining both perspectives is important for gaining objectivity when people are trying to improve their emotional functioning.

The microscopic view examines what transpires in a two-person system. (It is important to keep in mind always that what transpires in a dyadic relationship is intricately connected to the triangles and interlocking triangles in which it is embedded.) One of the important elements in viewing dyadic interactions is the social cues that have been mentioned in Chapter 1.

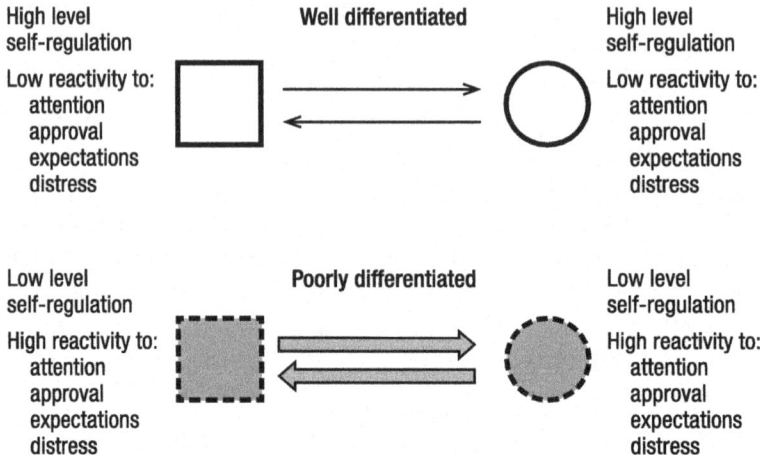

Figure 10.1 Summary of the processes that render a less differentiated relationship more vulnerable to escalations of chronic anxiety and associated instability than a more differentiated relationship. The shading of the male and female symbols in the lower diagram and in the reciprocal arrows between the two people symbolize anxiety.

Figure 10.1 diagrams the basic elements in this process. The symbols in the bottom half of the figure indicate a poorly differentiated relationship, with anxiety-infused interactions (represented by shading in the arrows) between the two people and buildups of chronic anxiety (shading) in the male and the female. The chronic anxiety in each person and the anxious interactions between the two people are intertwined. The principal point that the figure is intended to convey is that the chronic anxiety in each person is connected to a relationship process, which can convert manageable anxiety in individuals into difficult-to-manage anxiety. The dashed lines around each person symbolize porous emotional boundaries related to low basic levels of "self." Porous boundaries foster a high level of reactivity to fundamental social cues.

Beside each person in the figure are that person's most basic reactions that can stabilize or destabilize the relationship. Antonio Damasio calls the triggers for such reactions "emotionally competent stimuli" (Damasio & Brooks, 2009). The triggers are a wide variety of verbal and nonverbal communications, such as conveying disapproval and disappointment that threaten the other person. Repeated clinical observations suggest that the most common threats people experience are to approval, attention, expectations, and distress. The two people in this relationship diagram were emotionally programmed equally during their development to react intensely to these threats. Such reactions set off a range of emotions in each person, depending on, for example, whether the emotionally competent stimuli are perceived as approval or disapproval, attention or lack thereof, expectations met or unmet, and upset or equanimity in the other. Furthermore, uncertainty about if and when such stimuli will occur intensifies the process.

Approval enhances emotional well-being, and disapproval provokes anxiety. Approval can be associated with feelings of well-being; disapproval can be associated with feelings of unease and perhaps shame. The perception of adequate attention from the other can activate the calm and connection system and a reciprocal toning down of the fight-or-flight system (Moberg, 2011). The perception of inadequate attention can trigger feelings of rejection, panic, and emotional isolation.

Above the list of reaction triggers in Figure 10.1 is the phrase "low level self-regulation." One manifestation of a low basic level of differentiation is the difficulty self-regulating one's emotional reactivity. It is the coupling of intense reactivity fueled by the four social cues (and certainly other cues as well) with lack of higher brain self-regulation that drives the escalation of chronic anxiety in the relationship and associated relationship instability. It is not about one person upsetting the other but about two people upsetting each other. Repeated clinical observations that disturbances in emotionally significant relationships are the most fundamental triggers of chronic anxiety are consistent with Henry's earlier-referenced conclusion in this chapter about the important role of social interactions in generating chronic anxiety. A poorly differentiated relationship can remain calm and stable in ideal or minimal stress conditions but is highly vulnerable to instability in the face of challenge. That instability occurs consequent to the processes described above.

The upper half of Figure 10.1 symbolizes a well-differentiated relationship. The solid lines around each person symbolize solid emotional boundaries associated with good basic levels of differentiation. The people in this relationship have not been intensely programmed during their development to be highly reactive to threats to the four social cues listed beside them. They respond to such cues to a degree that facilitates smooth interactions between people. They can perceive the other to be disapproving based on verbal and nonverbal cues, but their perceptions tend to be more accurate and reactions less intense. This is a quantitative and not qualitative difference from less differentiated people. Many degrees of difference exist between the highest and lowest levels of emotional functioning. They are also better able to reflect on whatever reactions they might have, question the accuracy of those perceptions of the emotionally competent stimuli, and respond realistically to them. The diagram shows fewer anxiety-driven interactions and less buildup of chronic anxiety in both people. The relationship is consequently more stable, even in the face of challenging external stressors.

The macroscopic view involves viewing the close-in aspects of one's immediate relationships in the broader context of the extended families and larger social networks. The broader context of relationships can be either stabilizing or destabilizing to the relationships that exist within it. An open relationship is ideal for sustaining the sense of well-being and emotional functioning of the people involved. The problem is that no one is completely differentiated, which means that some degree of emotional distance (associated with less openness) creeps into every human relationship to help manage whatever chronic anxiety develops in it over time. This leaves the members of the twosome with the urge to manage the chronic anxiety that is not resolved with an open relationship through other relationships or activities that can bind anxiety.

Relationships and anxiety-binding activities can stabilize a system for extended periods of time. The relationship process part of the stability involves interlocking triangles. One example is a couple that had been married for fifteen years and had three adult children. The husband was the oldest of four siblings, and the wife, the younger of two siblings. The husband's parents and all four of their adult children lived in the Washington, D.C., area. The husband's father was the patriarch of the family. The wife was from New England. Her parents had died some years before I saw the family in therapy. This family coped with the deaths of the wife's parents fairly well. However, the wife's parent's deaths increased her emotional dependency on her in-laws.

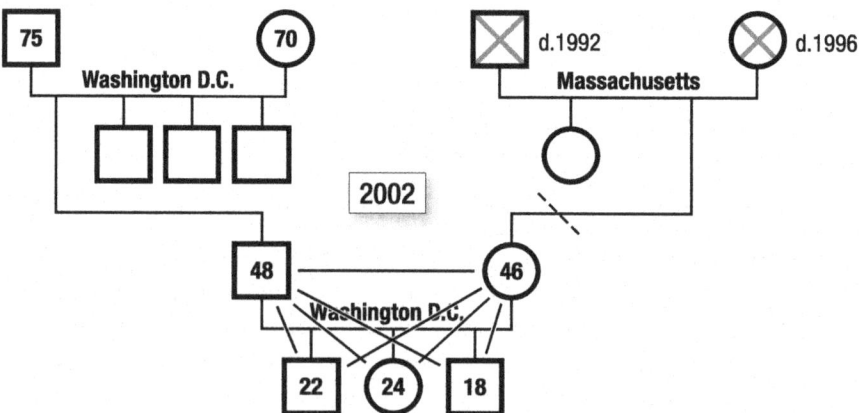

Figure 10.2 *This three generation family diagram depicts the emotional state of the family four years before I began family therapy with them. It is important to note on the diagram that the nuclear family that sought family therapy (at bottom of diagram) lived in the midst of the father's extended family and interacted with family members frequently over many years. The dashed line between the wife in the family I was treating indicates a significant cut-off from her family of origin.*

Figure 10.2 is a bare-bones diagram of this nuclear family and its extended family system four years before the couple sought family therapy with me in 2006. The diagram indicates that the husband's parents were alive in 2002. The lines in the nuclear family of the couple I later saw in family therapy (bottom of diagram) indicate fairly calm and stable relationships as of 2002 and for many years before that. The lines connecting the husband's parents to each of their offspring's families indicate quite involved relationships that were anxiety-reducing and stabilizing for each for the four siblings' nuclear families. The line is heavier with the oldest son's family because the parents poured more time, energy, and money into his family than the families of the other siblings. This is not a very well differentiated family, but one in balance nonetheless as of 2002, not in a regression.

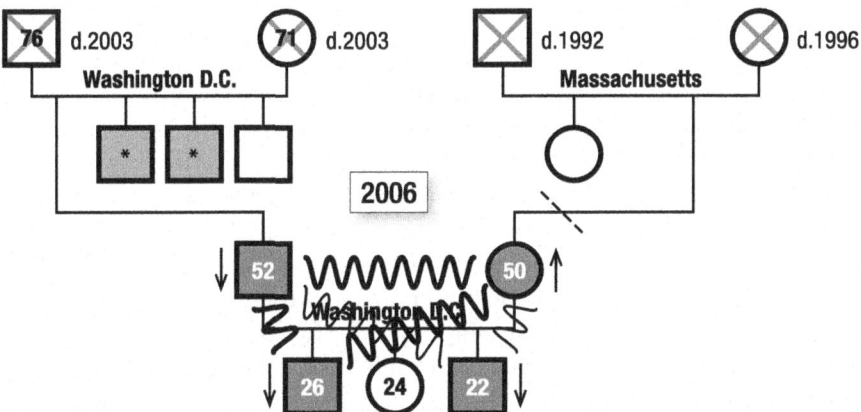

Figure 10.3 This diagram indicates the emotional state of the family when therapy began. The dark shading in the symbol for the father of the family I was treating, in his wife, in his two sons, and in the families of two of the father's younger brothers symbolizes high chronic anxiety in those individuals. The downward arrows next to the father and his two sons symbolize their considerable underfunctioning, and the upward arrow next to the wife of the family I was treating symbolizes her anxiety-driven overfunctioning.

Figure 10.3 symbolizes the changes in the family system in 2006 when the couple sought family therapy. Things had changed dramatically for the couple three years before I met them. The change was associated with the deaths of the husband's parents within six months of each other in 2003. The husband in the family that sought therapy said, "My parents died, and the castle crumbled!" Two of the marriages of the husband's siblings (ones with asterisks) had ended in divorces during the two years following the deaths. The couple that came for help was on the verge of divorce, and two of their three children (the sons) were having significant clinical problems associated with the decline in their functioning (downward arrows). Several of the husband's nieces and nephews were in trouble as well. These were the children of the husband's two brothers marked with asterisks. The functioning of the husband of the family that sought therapy had declined. He was on the verge of being fired from his law firm. The heavy underfunctioning arrow next to the husband symbolizes his major dysfunction. The wife was in an anxious state of overfunctioning. The jagged lines symbolize the high level of chronic anxiety driving those family relationships, which was particularly intense with their oldest son. He had dropped out of college before his grandparents' deaths and had returned home to live with his parents. He had worked at a number of menial jobs but had not worked since his grandparents died. Their daughter, who had been less a focus of family anxiety, completed college, moved to New York City, and had a good job.

The husband explained, "I had not realized how important my parents were to the stability of my family and my siblings' families." The presence of his parents had a calming influence on the whole system. It is reminiscent of the chaos that occurs in many animal social groups if the alpha male dies suddenly. This was a case where much of the potential chronic anxiety of the husband's family of origin was bound by the presence of his parents. The deep emotional dependence of the siblings on the parents was not obvious to them while the parents were alive. The functional levels of differentiation of the siblings were sustained by the presence of their parents. The level of chronic anxiety in the nuclear families of the four siblings spiked after the parents died. The instability that emerged in each nuclear family is related to anxiety-generating interactions mediated by heightened reactivity to attention, approval, expectations, and distress as described earlier in this chapter.

Recognizing the interactive processes in the nuclear family is a microscopic view; recognizing that what is transpiring in a given nuclear family is related to events in the extended family systems is a macroscopic view. The distinction is important because if a member of a nuclear family recognizes this connection, it provides a perspective that may enable that person to bring a calmer and more objective understanding to the immediate situation. The issues family members are reacting to (content) are not the problem; their anxiety-driven level of reactivity related to the larger relationship system (process) is the problem.

Bowen theory refers to what transpired after the parents died as an *emotional shock wave* (Bowen, 1976). The family that I was seeing never recovered. They divorced, the husband lost his job, and his diabetes became very unstable. The husband died a few years later. A poorly differentiated system that had been balanced for more than two decades became imbalanced and descended into an escalating emotional regression.

Another important perspective on chronic anxiety is how it fluctuates over time. I illustrate this with my family of origin in the epilogue, showing how ups and downs in my schizophrenic brother's emotional functioning and symptoms reflected what was occurring in the family a whole. Gaining a perspective on how an increase in the chronic anxiety level of a family system, a process for which no one person is to blame, can help shift people out of blame and self-blame.

One particularly interesting case that illustrates the flow of chronic anxiety through a system involved a couple in which the husband had gotten into an affair about six months after their first child was born. They were living in New York City at the time and began family therapy there after the wife discovered the affair. The counselor the couple was seeing suggested that the wife may have had a part in the affair occurring. She struggled to figure out what her part might have been but could not sort it out. She continued to be in significant distress about the affair despite the counseling. The husband's employer wanted to move him down to their Washington, D.C. office. He and his wife talked it over and agreed to make the move.

After they got to Washington, they sought out a family therapist to help them continue with their efforts to "move on" from the affair. I began seeing them at that point. The husband suggested during the first few sessions that the birth of their child, although wanted by both parents, had adversely affected their marital relationship and that it was probably an important factor in his getting into the affair. The wife tried to understand the husband's point, but it was not helpful to her. After about four or five sessions, in response to questions I asked the wife, she began to realize two important changes in her that occurred after the baby was born. One change was her intense focus on taking care of the baby. The other change was her anxiety about whether her husband would pitch in and help out wherever he could, leading to her critically monitoring his perceived level of involvement. In reflection about that period, she also realized that not only was she devoting less attention to her husband. But, she said, "I think I was hell to live with during that time!"

Her new insight was the first time that she could specifically see how she had played a part in the marital anxiety and emotional distance. She still held her husband responsible for his actions, but she was much calmer than she had been since she found out about the affair. She said, "I am amazed that I can view this objectively: he had a part and I had a part. I see it." She emphasized that up until then she had accepted intellectually that she must have had a part in the affair, but until she comprehended the specifics of that part, it had not helped. She said that my detailed questions to her about that period had helped. This clinical experience reinforced for me that saying someone has an equal part in a process is not especially helpful until that person can comprehend the specifics of it all. People need help with this. Questions based on systems thinking and occasional clinical vignettes to illustrate are the best help people can get to educate themselves about emotional process.

This brief clinical vignette emphasizes the critically important role of chronic anxiety and disturbances in important relationships in the development of clinical symptoms such as an affair. Bowen theory assigns a very important role to heightened and sustained levels of anxiety in the development of clinical symptoms of all types, whether they manifest as mental illness, physical illness, or social illness. Further research will determine if this assertion holds up over time. I hasten to add that heightened chronic anxiety alone does not cause an illness, but it may be one of the most important variables for explaining when clinical symptoms emerge.

One of the key obstacles to recognizing the role of chronic anxiety in symptom development is viewing anxiety as a psychiatric disorder. Many years ago, I asked faculty members in the department of dermatology if I could acquire some slides that illustrate the skin condition psoriasis. One response I received, by a person knowing that I was a psychiatrist, was, "Do you think that people with psoriasis have psychiatric problems?" This response was useful for understanding that I needed to improve my ability to communicate about the subject of chronic anxiety and its manifestation in physical symptoms. I answered the faculty member by saying, "No, they do not have psychiatric problems, but have anxiety manifesting in physical problems. People with psychiatric problems have anxiety that manifests in mental processes." I subsequently published an article on this subject (Kerr, 1992). As stated previously, chronic anxiety does not cause physical and other symptoms; it increases people's vulnerability to develop symptoms. One way to conceptualize this is that chronic anxiety disturbs homeostasis in the body, and this disturbance can render people vulnerable to illness and even death. Referring to anxiety as a psychiatric disorder is a very narrow perspective on a powerful naturally occurring process that affects all human beings.

CHAPTER ELEVEN

The Multigenerational Family Organism

Those who do not remember the past are condemned to repeat it.
—George Santayana

I've got news for Mr. Santayana: we're doomed to repeat the past no matter what. That's what it is to be alive.
—Kurt Vonnegut, Bluebeard

The concept described in this chapter is the multigenerational transmission process. I have titled the chapter "The Multigenerational Family Organism" to emphasize that Bowen theory views the multigenerational human family as a living, evolving organism. Natural systems thinking is essential for conceptualizing multigenerational process. It is not evolution in terms of spawning new species, but one of forces, and patterns that have been shaped by evolution predictably generate increasing variation in the emotional functioning of families over many generations. It is impossible to understand adequately the emotional functioning of any one individual or nuclear family without understanding the multigenerational family emotional system. Current evolutionary theory explains how variation in adaptive functioning evolves among species. Bowen theory explains how individual and family variation in the capacity for adaptation to life challenges evolves within the human species.

The family diagram is used to record data about multigenerational families. When considered as a whole, the data can be used to assess levels of emotional functioning in present and past generations of a family. Many family therapists substitute the term *genogram* for family diagram (McGoldrick, Gerson, & Shellenberger, 1985). Bowen theory has retained the term *family diagram*. The actual terms used are far less important than the theory therapists and researchers use to interpret the data on the diagram. Many family therapists use the term *organism* to convey the idea of the family as an entity in its own right. However, only Bowen theory views the family as not just the outcome of millions of years of evolution that led to our particular species, *Homo sapiens*, but also of the several billion years of phylogenesis that led to the emergence of the genus *Homo*.

Remember that Bowen theory extends the concept of emotion to the earliest forms of life. Consistent with Bowen theory's broad use of the term *emotion*, Damasio (Damasio & Brooks 2009) conceptualizes processes that have an "emotional flavor" developing very early in evolution. Processes such as reward and punishment systems, drives, motivations, and basic life regulation provide a kind of automatic intelligence for triggering action programs that enhance survival and reproduction in primitive creatures. Given the ancient evolutionary origins and fundamental importance of emotions, it makes sense that they are the dominant force in the behavior of our species.

It is important to keep in mind, especially when trying to modulate intense emotional reactivity, that the problems related to too much or too little emotion are not related to the emotions themselves but to the internal and external emotionally competent stimuli to which people have learned to be anxiously overreactive or underreactive (in the sense of automatically constraining emotional expression). Anxiety-driven emotional reactivity is the core problem, not the phenomenon of emotional reactivity itself. The emotional flavor processes sustain the lives of primitive organisms and the emotions they evolved into also sustain the survival of complex organisms.

The multigenerational transmission process could be considered the perspective-promoting concept in Bowen theory. Just as an understanding of billions of years of evolution gives us an understanding of how the fauna and flora that presently inhabit Earth have come to be, knowledge about the emotional functioning of preceding generations of contemporary nuclear families gives us an understanding of their present level of emotional functioning. Gaining such a perspective provides a level of emotional neutrality about the human condition that seems difficult to gain in any other way.

Careful study of multigenerational families provides a factual basis for asserting that families are much more alike than different, but based on varying family and cultural contexts some people develop more emotional maturity than others. Variation in levels of emotional maturity occurs in all cultures. Neutrality is a basis for more tolerance for the nature of the human condition—less judgmental—but also the basis for more ability to stand thoughtfully firm when that is important to do in an anxious world. These two seemingly unrelated abilities both relate to being able to focus on facts and to reason in intense emotional situations. An understanding of evolution adds further perspective by, among other things, showing how much we have in common with other forms of life. It is the antidote for the malignant anthropocentrism that has long dominated the human psyche.

The quotes from Santayana and Vonnegut that introduce this chapter are both important from a Bowen theory standpoint. On the one hand, gaining knowledge about the emotional functioning of previous generations is very important for helping people get beyond blame and self-blame, both of which are anchored in cause-and-effect thinking. Understanding multiple generations increases one's perspective on the present by adding myriad more variables to explain the present and, for example, one's relationship with one's parents, spouse, and children. This knowledge expansion helps people move toward systems thinking. On the other hand, Vonnegut implies that it is extremely difficult to modify automatic emotional processes that have come down through the generations. The effort to consciously control intense emotional reactivity puts free will to the test! However, Bowen theory's ability to help people become more objective about the past helps people shift from how they see the world to how the world really is—within limits, of course.

The study of multigenerational families consistently reveals that every family has high-functioning and dysfunctioning branches. Bowen theory provides an alternative to assuming that this variation occurs randomly. Emotional forces and patterns that come down through the generations create this variation. Variation in emotional functioning among individuals and among families is a predictable outcome of a multigenerational emotional process. The rapidity by which changes in levels of emotional functioning develop varies. There is something about seeing this in one's own family that has a profound effect emotionally. Bowen credits William W. Meissner with helping to document what would become the multigenerational transmission process concept (Kerr & Bowen, 1988). His early 1960s studies included family diagrams and written explanations for each generation of three separate "patient" families that went as far back as three hundred years.

In summary, the development of a wide range of emotional functioning in every multigenerational family is a systems process involving multiple family members, all of whom are embedded in a network of evolving emotional forces that shape their development and adult lives.

The family diagram is a method of recording data that, when considered as a whole, make it possible to draw conclusions about the emotional functioning of nuclear families in present and past generations. The family diagram as used in Bowen theory is a modification of genetic pedigree charts commonly used by geneticists to indicate which members of a multigenerational family have traits or clinical conditions that are transmitted down the generations on a genetic basis. Genes can influence the manifestation of traits or conditions in a family member, but, as related to health issues, they typically do not stand on their own as the cause. Multigenerational family emotional process is composed of myriad more variables than just genes. Recording all the information necessary on a diagram to draw conclusions about emotional process requires more space than the typical pedigree chart provides. Such charts have been modified to allow room for the basic information included on a family diagram.

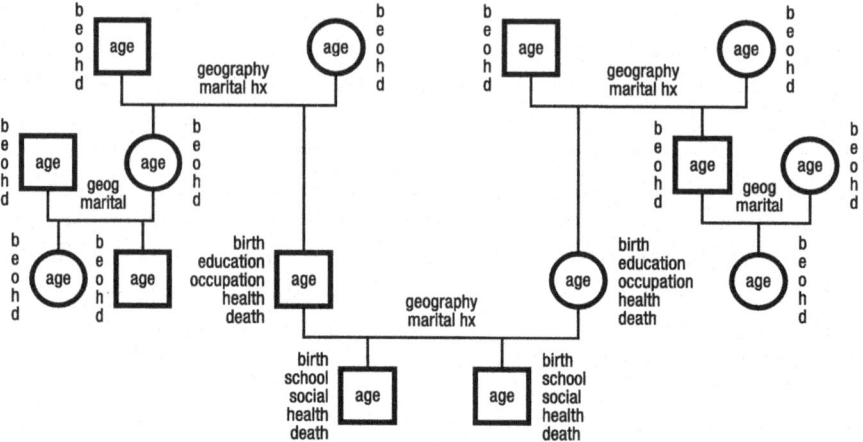

Figure 11.1 This diagram is the basic model for drawing a family diagram and where to place the data collected about a family on the diagram.

An example for a three-generational family diagram is shown in Figure 11.1. Beginning with the nuclear family in the lower center of the diagram (father, mother, and two sons), data are recorded for the father and the mother that include birth date, educational history, occupational history, health history, and date of death. Each parent's age is recorded in the square or circle. Dates of when the parents met, became engaged, and got married are also recorded. Where the parents have lived during their marriage is recorded. Besides indicating a date of death, an X is placed over the square or circle along with the person's age at the time of death. The same data are also recorded for the parents' parents and for the siblings of each parent and their spouses. The data recorded for dependent children and for the parents' siblings' children include birth date, school functioning, social functioning, health, and death date (here abbreviated b s s h d). If an individual has been adopted, that is noted with the letter *a* and the date of the adoption, along with the birth date of the adopted child. There are no hard-and-fast rules for exactly how to record this data; it is most important that it be clear and as factual as possible.

Figure 11.2 shows how to record divorces and remarriages. All the data given in the previous example are recorded for the parents and dependent children. The diagram for Family A indicates that the father had a previous marriage that ended in divorce. He has one son from that marriage. The symbol for the divorce leans toward his ex-wife to indicate that the son lives mostly with his mother. The dates of the separation of the parents and subsequent divorce are recorded above the divorce symbol. This man and his new wife,

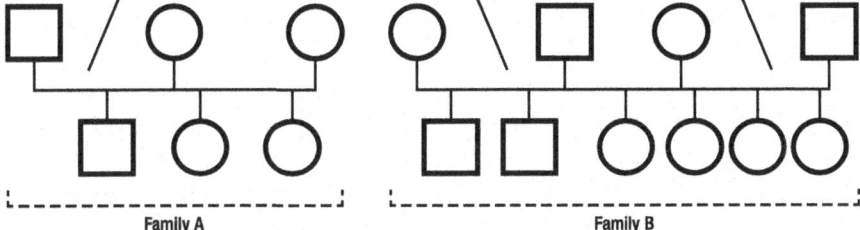

Figure 11.2 *These two diagrams illustrates how to symbolize divorces, multiple marriages, and children from multiple marriages.* The slanted line between a husband and wife indicates a divorce. If the slant is to the right, it indicates that the children lived with their mother post divorce; if it slants the left, the children lived with their father. In family A, the father was married and had one son from that marriage. The son lived with his mother after the divorce. The father later remarried and has two children from that marriage. The family B diagram indicates that the couple in therapy are the male and female near the center of the diagram and that they have one daughter from their union. The father was married before and had two sons from that marriage. The wife was also married before and had three daughters. The slant of the divorce lines indicates that potentially four daughters lived with or did live with the parents seeking family therapy.

who has not been married before, have two daughters from their marriage. The diagram of Family B is a so-called blended family. The current marriage is in the center of the diagram. The husband has two sons from his first marriage, which ended in divorce. The sons live mostly with the ex-wife. She has not remarried or her second husband would be shown to the far left. (These diagrams can get complicated, and people have to improvise a bit to record all the relevant data.) The husband's current wife is divorced and has three daughters from her first marriage, all of which live mostly with her and her new husband. This couple also has one daughter from their marriage.

The family diagram and information recorded on it are usually sufficient for clinical work. Information can be added as the family therapy proceeds if one or both parents research their families more carefully during therapy. The data can be used to assess each individual's functional level of differentiation, and the composite of data from all the individuals can be used to assess the functional level of a nuclear family.

Estimates of basic levels of differentiation necessarily include data for as many generations as possible. Assessing multiple people who are closely connected emotionally to each other to assess basic level is necessary because one family member's functioning can be enhanced or undermined by the reciprocal functioning of other family members. For example, the facts about the functioning of one spouse may be consistent with a person with a good basic level, but the facts of functioning of the other spouse may be consistent with a basic level in the lower range. This discrepancy may be based on an overfunctioning-underfunctioning reciprocity in the marriage, which indicates that both spouses have the same basic level and it is in the moderate range.

The same is true for two parents who have high functional levels but have one or more seriously impaired offspring. Parents can unwittingly enhance their functioning at the expense of a child. Furthermore, a sibling that the data suggest has a fairly high level of functioning compared to another sibling does not necessarily have a different basic level; this can be based on a degree of reciprocal functioning between the siblings. For example, one child may function in reaction to a sibling's acting out by trying to do everything right to win the parents' approval. Both children may be equally relationship oriented and have very similar basic levels of "self." The functioning disparity of the siblings in this case reflects pseudo-self, not solid self. One very successful entrepreneur attributed part of his business success to his twin brother's death at age twenty-one. He described his childhood as living in the shadow of his dominant twin brother and underachieving. He said he was released from the process with his twin brother's death.

The specific data collected for the clinical assessment of a family in therapy or for research purposes is selected on the assumption that the individuals' emotional functioning strongly influences that data. For example, two siblings may each have the opportunity to attend college. One takes full advantage of that opportunity, and the other squanders it. This is one piece of evidence for a difference existing in the basic levels of differentiation of the siblings. However, one piece of data is suggestive but never definitive.

Emotions are not pathological. It is the level of chronic anxiety present in a family system at a given period of time, the person's functioning position in the system, and the person's emotional programming during development that can result in that person being overly reactive emotionally to the relationship context in which that person lives and works. This is when the feeling system, which when operating at an optimum level can improve the efficiency of higher brain processes, overloads higher brain circuits and interferes with judgment, reflective decision making, and other self-regulatory functions. It can also skew moral judgments. Such processes are what undermine the sibling who squanders the opportunity to attend college. This reflects an impaired level of emotional functioning, at least at that point in time. How a person and the family ultimately respond to such a catastrophe can also be an indicator of emotional functioning. It is important to recognize that a person may act calm but inwardly be just as reactive as a person who is obviously highly emotional.

Level of emotional functioning is not a diagnostic category; it transcends all diagnostic categories. The lower the level of emotional functioning at a given period of time, the more the chronic anxiety associated with that lower level accentuates the obsessiveness of a person with a tendency to such traits or the antisocial acts of a person with that tendency. As described in Chapter 5, the lower a person's basic level, the more vulnerable that person is to significant fluctuations in emotional functioning (shifts in functional level of differentiation).

Data about occupational experiences can be misleading. A high level of occupational achievement may indicate a fairly high basic level of differentiation, but not necessarily so. The reverse, however, is predictive: a person with a high level of differentiation, barring glaring unlucky upheavals in life, will very likely have a responsible and productive life course, regardless of the field he/she chosen.

Data on health histories are valuable because Bowen theory assumes that level of emotional functioning has a strong influence on health. It is also important to consider how successfully a person and family adapt to whatever health issues befall them. The ability to adapt responsibly and thoughtfully to health issues suggests a higher level of emotional functioning than the opposite adjustment. For example, there is significant variation in how youngsters and their families adapt to a diagnosis of juvenile diabetes in a child. Clinical observations suggest that a successful adaptation results in a more stable clinical course.

Longevity seems likely affected by level of emotional functioning, but living a long life does not necessarily equate with being a person with a high basic level of differentiation. Two grandparents may live long lives and function well, but their children and/or grandchildren may significantly dysfunction. This discrepancy suggests that a strong projection process played out between the grandparents and their children and an equally strong projection process played out with their children's children.

The data about courtship, marriage, and marital stability helps to assess how differentiation is reflected in the stability of a person's intimate relationships. Very drawn-out courtships and very short courtships may suggest, respectively, people with such limited ability to maintain a "self" that they are leery of the finality of tying the knot and people with a strong need to be stabilized by a marriage and marry very quickly. For example, a divorced mother of two children who was raising them postponed marriage to a man with whom she had been romantically involved for over a decade until her children left home. She said that she was unsure enough of herself that she did not think she could deal with the competing emotional needs of a spouse and children.

No one question or piece of data accurately assesses a person's basic level of differentiation. The variable of differentiation introduces an important understanding for what can render some people more vulnerable than others to problematic life adjustments and clinical dysfunctions and some people more likely to live fairly healthy, stable, and productive lives. A computer program or questionnaire does not yet exist that can estimate a person's basic level with sufficient accuracy. Estimating basic level using a three-, four-, or five-generation family diagram is the most accurate method at this point. John Mulvihill a medical geneticist who was then studying high-incidence cancers in families at the National Cancer Institute, commented that he trusted looking at the pedigree chart as a whole, rather than looking at numbers on chart derived from those data, to understand better the cancer process in those families (personal communication, 1976). I think his comment parallels the value of looking at the multigenerational family diagram to get a glimpse of the emotional flow through the generations. It is commonly something you can see but difficult to put numbers on. A project is currently under way, sponsored Bowen Theory Academy, to computerize all the data from a cohort of people that have collected and verified data from the multigenerational study of their own families (see http://www.bowentheoryacademy.org). Perhaps this project will contribute to developing more accurate ways of assessing basic levels of differentiation.

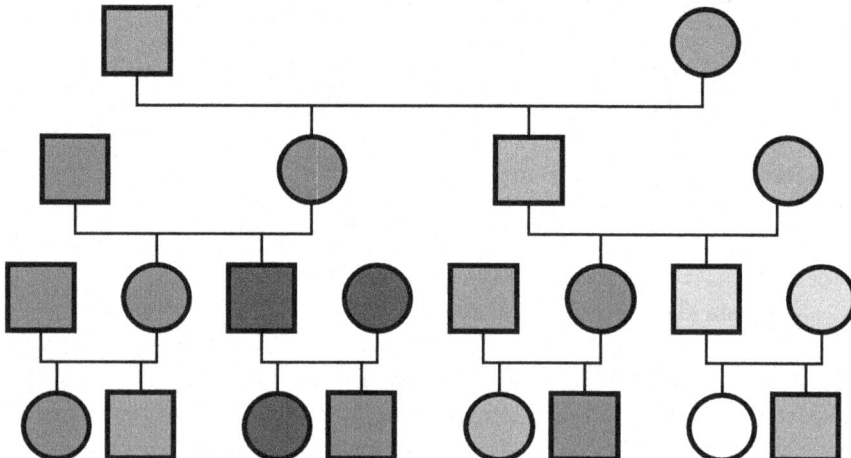

Figure 11.3 *This family diagram is the first of four that illustrate multigenerational family emotional process.* This one illustrates the variation in life functioning of members. The darker the shading, the higher the functioning, the lighter the shading, the lower the functioning.

In Figure 11.3, the variation in the shading of the members of this multigenerational family symbolizes the significant variations in life adjustment that are a consistent fact of all families. Every family has its saints, sinners, and skeletons in the closet. One way to think about what this variation reflects is that family members have different levels of emotional maturity, which has a significant influence on how successfully people adapt to the inevitable stresses, strains, and challenges of life. Most people consider emotional maturity as something people develop as they grow up rather than being genetically based. People mature psychologically as well as biologically.

Sociologist Dalton Conley (2004) studied sibling variation as measured by educational attainment, income, and net worth of individual family members in many different multigenerational families. He commonly found significant variation in members of the same sibling group in whether they moved up or down the socioeconomic scale as adults. Family members described the siblings that did well in their family in the following terms: responsible, disciplined, persevered, motivated, set goals, had a plan. Family members described siblings that did less well in contrasting terms: bad attitude, poor emotional or mental health, lack of determination. These characteristics are closely related to emotional maturity. Most interesting, sibling variation was much more predictive of moving up or down the socioeconomic ladder as adults than the particular socioeconomic status of the family in which the siblings grew up. Having a sibling or siblings that do not adapt well increases one's own chances of doing well threefold! Conley's finding is consistent with a family projection process impairing the functioning of one child more than the siblings. This occurred in my family of origin and occurs to at least some degree in most families.

A high level of intelligence does not necessarily lead to emotional maturity. A person's relationships during development significantly affect emotional maturity, particularly family relationships. Commonly held descriptions of emotional maturity include acceptance of responsibility, ability to make decisions, ability to function as a team member, development of stable and sustaining relationships, and a realistic sense of self-worth. Mature people are able to see the big picture in various situations and to make decisions based on the long-term best interests of themselves and others. The less mature a person is, the greater the tendency to seek immediate gratification and act to relieve the anxiety of the moment.

Bowen (1966) suggested that emotional maturity and basic level of differentiation of self addressed the same phenomenon. However, differentiation is a broader concept for several reasons. First of all, differentiation of self is a life force with deep evolutionary roots. It involves not just psychological maturation but programming of the emotional system and associated physiology as well. Second, the theory describes how differentiation or lack thereof plays out specifically in relationships and broadens thinking about what constitutes emotional immaturity, such as anxiety-driven overfunctioning. A bully is typically regarded as immature, but a parent who is too anxious to stop overly protecting a child is acting immaturely as well. Third, relating basic level of differentiation to the degree of unresolved attachment to the family of origin is an alternative conceptual framework to ideas widely implanted in the public consciousness such as abuse, neglect, and trauma during development as core causes of emotional problems in children and in adults.

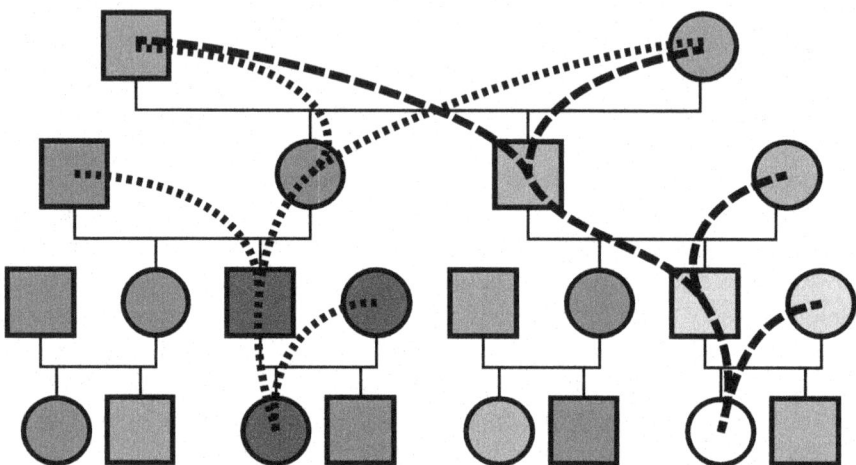

Figure 11.4 *The dotted lines on this diagram track increasing levels of life functioning over the course of four generations. The dashed line tracks decreasing life functioning. Note the slight shading differences between siblings that result from nuclear family emotional process in each family and the fact that people marry who are at the same basic level of differentiation.*

Figure 11.4 symbolizes an important insight from Bowen theory, which views basic levels of differentiation in the members of a multigenerational family as a basis for understanding variation in the life adjustments of those members. Furthermore, the changes that develop across generations are connected and not random. The dashed and dotted lines through members of four generations symbolize two quantitatively different processes. The dashed lines indicate that the intensity of the unresolved emotional attachment between generations I and II, II and III, and III and IV is decreasing gradually. Note that the shading indicating more (darker) or less (lighter) solid self, is changing in four successive generations. The female sibling in the last generation has much less "self" than her great-grandparents. Her brother, on the other hand, was subject to less of the family projection process and has developed more "self" than even his parents. He is back to the level of his grandparents. The dotted lines indicate increasing resolution of the emotional attachment to parents in four successive generations—increasing levels of solid self. Note that the symbols indicate that the parents marry spouses with the same basic levels of differentiation. A parent with a good level of differentiation does not choose a marital partner with a moderate level and then produce offspring somewhere in between. A person with a good level chooses a mate at the same level, and they can produce children with basic levels a little higher, a little lower, or the same as their levels.

The key point here is that it takes more than one generation to go from a very good level of differentiation of self to a very poor level. It could take eight to ten generations or as few as three or four. This occurs because the basic levels of differentiation of offspring are somewhat constrained by the basic levels of their parents—the apple does not fall far from the tree. The emotional maturity of offspring is powerfully affected by the emotional maturity of their parents. However, as Bowen theory describes, some members of a sibling group may be in a more favorable position to mature than others. In my family of origin, my oldest full brother was the subject of an intense family projection process, my parents managed their immaturities with emotional distance, and our nuclear family was moderately isolated from each extended family. This made for a fairly significant decrease in differentiation in my oldest full brother's basic level compared to our parents, but the levels that my other brothers and I developed were not that much higher than my parents' levels.

Some people react to Bowen theory's concept of the multigenerational transmission process as fatalistic. The best way to grapple with this idea is studying it in one's own multigenerational family, either proving or disproving it to oneself. One hypothesis about why it works the way the theory describes is that it is the nature of living systems to compartmentalize tension or anxiety in one part of the system to preserve the stability of the system as a whole. Homeostasis can be maintained in the family organism at the expense of some of its parts. This is obviously an automatic process (with associated psychological elements), not a conscious one. People must be able to grasp the powerful emotional impact people have on one another to wrap their heads around this idea.

Another way to think about this process is that all parents have strengths and weaknesses emotionally. It is inevitable that some children will pick up more of the strengths and others more of the weaknesses. What is important is that when the child that has picked up more of the weaknesses manifests symptoms of that process, the family can approach the problem as a system problem, not an individual problem.

Figure 11.5 symbolizes the multiple interconnections of the members of a multigenerational-family emotional system. Everyone on the diagram, whether dead or alive, contributes or contributed to the evolving multigenerational family organism, emotional field, or system. Deceased family members

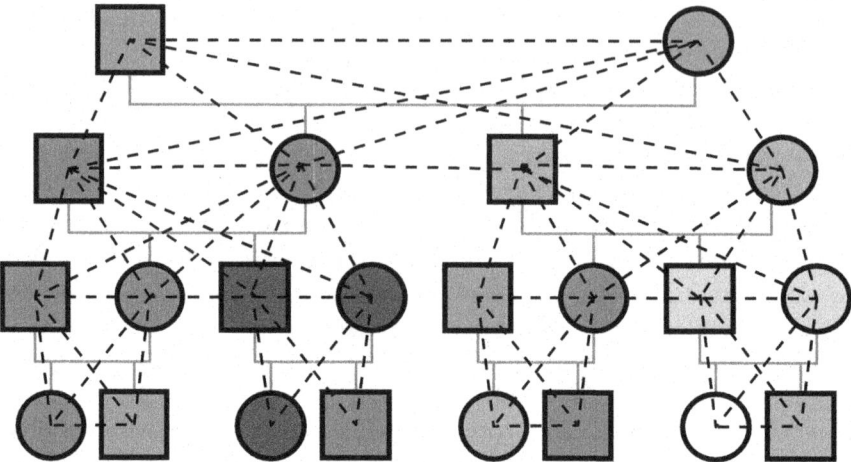

Figure 11.5 *The shower of dots in this diagram is an attempt to help students of Bowen theory think beyond genetic transmission.* The dots symbolize an emotional process or emotional field that flows down the generations. The principal point of this diagram is to emphasize that the particular basic level of differentiation (high or low) of one human being is the culmination of the many generations that preceded him.

contribute through the relationship-transmitted emotional programming of those with whom they interacted. To not clutter up the diagram too much, the interactions between great-grandparents and grandchildren and great-grandchildren are not depicted, but they are important as well. Also not depicted are the interactions between the second-generation members and their siblings' children and grandchildren and third-generation members with their cousins and cousins once or twice removed, which also shape the evolving family organism. This diagram is intended to convey, for example, that the female in generation IV, who is symbolized as having the least "self" of any member of her generation, is not just the product of the unresolved attachment to her parents. Her parents' unresolved attachment to their parents, and on and on, have played a role in the low level of "self" she developed. As has been emphasized already, understanding the multigenerational influences is key to getting beyond blame. Many people played a part, but no one caused it.

I will describe in the epilogue, in more detail, an example of the transmission of emotional process across generations. My mother focused intensely on her mother's tension and distress. Mother wanted to make it better somehow. Mother's mother was also extremely focused on her. In listening to my mother's description of this, I saw that the legacy for Mother of this emotionally intense interactive process was emotional programming of a heightened sensitivity to the feelings of others and feelings of guilt if she could not find ways to relieve the distress of others. Such feelings had a strong impact on all her children, but especially the one with whom she was most fused, my schizophrenic brother. This programmed into my brother a very strong dependency on our mother to help him to manage his feeling states, which is part of what erodes people's "self." This example somewhat oversimplifies the complexity of the emotional programming process down the generations, but does illustrate an aspect of it.

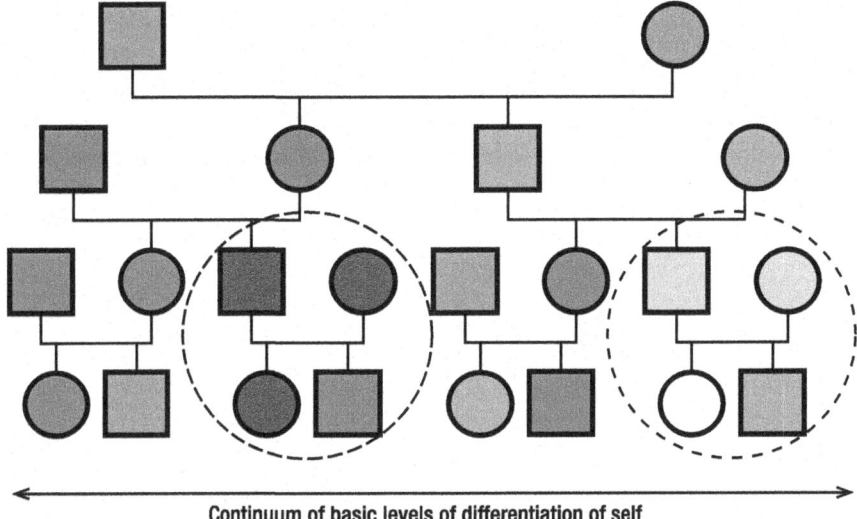

Continuum of basic levels of differentiation of self

Figure 11.6 *This diagram is intended to convey that a continuum of basic levels of differentiation exists in the human population because of a multigenerational transmission process. The darkly shaded individuals of the nuclear family unit surrounded by a dashed circle represents a well differentiated nuclear family and the lightly shaded individuals surrounded by a dotted circle a poorly differentiated family.*

Figure 11.6 is intended to convey two ideas: (1) every multigenerational family gradually produces the full continuum of basic levels of differentiation of self, and (2) families that are commonly described as dysfunctional are the outcome for a branch of a multigenerational family. The more functional branches have unwittingly played a role in fostering the development of the less functional branches. The family with the dotted circle around it is the dysfunctional family in this hypothetical multigenerational family. It contains the most potentially impaired person (no shading, to indicate little "self"), the older sister of a brother. This branch of the family has a quantitative increase in emotional fusion compared to the other nuclear families, and greater emotional interdependence. This means that the same emotional forces and patterns of emotional functioning play out in this branch that operate in other branches, but the processes are more intense. This is due to the need to bind the high chronic anxiety generated by the significant undifferentiation in this particular nuclear family system compared to the nuclear families in other branches.

The horizontal arrow stretching to include the eight members of generation IV indicates a continuum that the multigenerational process has spawned. The marked differences in shading in generation IV indicate a broader span of variation than the degree of variation that occurs between the two siblings in generation II. The essence of the multigenerational transmission process concept is that it describes a natural process that generates variation. The no-self end of the spectrum in some lines may include extinction or severe family fragmentation. At the other end of the continuum the amount of "self" that can develop is limited by what biological and cultural evolution have determined thus far.

CHAPTER TWELVE

Sibling Position

> *He was a systems thinker before his time. Through vision and disciplined research he assembled discrepant and partial facts about family configuration into a precise body of systems knowledge so accurate it was of immediate use in family systems therapy. It could predict the future "all other things being equal" and helped open doors for multigenerational family concepts. In appreciation of his structured approach which helped change the world for all who aspire to a systems view of the human condition.*
> —Plaque presented to Walter Toman by
> Murray Bowen and the Georgetown Family Center

Despite sibling position being a concept in Bowen theory, not much has been written about it by Bowen theorists. Fairly early in his family research, Bowen (1966) saw the need for some type of concept that addressed sibling position. When he read Walter Toman's book *Family Constellation* (1961), he found the profiles of the various sibling positions so amazingly accurate that Bowen soon incorporated them into a concept in his developing theory.

I did not read Toman's book until 1969, when I embarked on a serious study of Bowen theory. At first reading, I reacted to the profile of an older sister of a sister. I felt it was unfair for someone to know so much about my wife, never having met her! He also suggested that a youngest brother of brothers, which is my position, is not the best match for her as a marital partner (compared to a younger brother of a sister), but "he may do."

A faculty member at the Georgetown University Family Center once objected to Bowen including Toman's concept in his theory, stating that it was an individual theory concept. The quote to open this chapter, written by Murray Bowen, conveys his respect for Toman's research and disagreement with the faculty member's opinion that it does not fit into a systems theory. The quote also notes that the concept has useful clinical applications.

Toman described eleven sibling profiles based on observations derived from the study of over three thousand families. Implicit in his thinking is that the predictability of the traits he describes is related to the configuration of the family as a whole. Toman did not know systems theory, but the facts he discovered fit into Bowen's family systems theory. Variations in the functioning of family members are determined as much by the reciprocal functioning of others as by forces within the individual. For example, the functioning of those interacting with a firstborn during that child's development instill and continually reinforce the traits common to most firstborns. If the person marries, those same traits will be strengthened or lessened by how the spouse, children, and others in the extended family systems interact with that firstborn.

Many clinicians and researchers debate the degree of influence sibling position has on a person's development and adult life functioning. Some consider it not particularly important, and others, like Toman, estimate that it accounts for 10–25 percent of a given personality. Bowen theory does not estimate its degree of influence but holds that sibling position is always influencing aspects of how a person functions. The naysayers argue that insufficient research exists to support sibling position being that important.

One reason people who study their own families and do therapy based on Bowen theory readily accept the importance of sibling position is that it is so obvious and useful when observing families. If people grasp the reciprocity in relationships, for example, the interplay in a marriage between an older brother of a sister and a younger sister of a brother, in contrast to the interplay between an older brother of a brother and an older sister of a sister, how the relationship process reinforces the functioning of both spouses is unmistakably obvious.

Toman argues that if an older brother of a sister marries the younger sister of a brother, they have rank and sex complementarity because he grew up with a younger (rank) sister (sex) and she with an older brother. If an older brother of a brother marries an older sister of a sister, they have neither rank nor sex complementarity. If spouses have rank and sex complementarity, it is easier for them to get along than if they lack the complementarity. This does not mean that one marriage is more mature than the other. This is where the phrase in the award plaque, "all other things being equal," comes in. Bowen theory adds basic level of differentiation of self to the list of things that are not equal. For example, the family projection process can so impair the functioning of a firstborn son that his younger brother may function more like an older brother than the firstborn does. In such instances, the younger son becomes a "functional oldest." Alternatively, the younger son may be so babied and protected that he becomes highly vulnerable to helplessness and indecisiveness, which are not characteristic of all youngest children.

Toman and Bowen theory both hold that there is not a best or worst sibling position. Each position has its assets and liabilities. An immature older brother of brothers is likely to be overly controlling and dogmatic, provided his spouse functions in a reciprocal opposite way, such as being passive and indecisive. A mature older brother of brothers can be a very effective and responsible leader and respect the emotional boundaries and integrity of others.

It is valuable to read Toman's book and learn how he describes the sibling profiles to gain a sense of what is fairly constant and what is easily altered by level of emotional maturity. Having spent many hours with Walter Toman on his many trips to Washington, D.C., I realized that he had a knowledge base about family configurations that I cannot come close to matching. Bowen qualified his thoughts about Toman's profiles by saying that they accurately describe people at the midrange on the continuum of differentiation of self.

Tidbits of Toman's eleven sibling profiles follow (Toman, 1961).

Oldest brother of brother(s): He takes charge and leads. He grew up feeling responsible for and leading his younger brother. It is a built-in expectation of his sibling position. He tends to be a good worker, is practical, builds up property, and makes long-range plans for himself and his family's future. A good male friend for him is a youngest brother of brothers. The best match for a marital partner is a youngest sister of brother(s). She grew up looking to and adoring a male. His worst match is an oldest sister of sister(s), a relationship highly prone to battles over being in charge. Murray Bowen and I worked very well together. The fact that he was an oldest brother of brothers and two younger sisters and I am the youngest brother of four brothers played some part in our relationship.

Youngest brother of brother(s): He is not a natural leader but can learn to be one. He reacts off others sometimes to the point of being oppositional and rebellious. He is not careful about money or creating and preserving property. Women like to do things for him and want to take care of him. His best choice for a marital partner is the oldest sister of brothers. The worst match is a youngest sister of sisters. Politically he tends to laissez-faire.

Oldest brother of sister(s): He is very tender and loving of females. He gets along with men but communicates best with females. Female colleagues and coworkers help him be a good and responsible worker. If in a position of authority, he is more causal than the oldest brother of brother(s). He is a decent preserver of property but is not driven to accumulate. His best marriage partner is a youngest sister of brother(s). He is not a "one of the guys" type, unlike the oldest brother of brother(s).

Youngest brother of sister(s): He is loved and doted on by girls. He is less reactive and competitive than the youngest brother of brother(s). He does not build up property well and is even prone to squander it. He is bigger on grand plans than specifics, for him and his children. He does well with women but can lose sight of their needs and interests. His best marital partner is the oldest sister of brother(s). He is not a "man's man." As for politics, he has no or limited opinions.

Oldest sister of sister(s): She is a caretaker who stands on her own feet, even bossing others to some extent. She is not a bully, just good at what she has been trained to do. She likes to be in charge and is a responsible, detail-oriented, and effective worker. People may resent her being in charge but easily flow into her wake. She can be a true and loyal friend. She may appear more strong and independent than she really is. She does best with men who are used to being bossed, and their compliance can bring out her tender and motherly side. Her best marital partner is a youngest brother of sister(s), but he may have trouble with her unwillingness to budge in arguments.

Youngest sister of sister(s): She is the adventurous and colorful type, thriving on entertainment and novelty. She can be charming, capricious, and gullible. She can also be hard to pin down, jumping from thing to thing. She can be quite seductive to men with her submissive qualities. She can range from being a good worker to an erratic one and vulnerable to intensifying the gossip system. She is not a good leader. She does many tasks very well but has difficulty deciding on a direction. Men are attracted to her, but she is prone to histrionics. Her best choice for marriage is the oldest brother of sister(s). If they have children, she is highly prone to getting overwhelmed by them.

Oldest sister of brother(s): She takes care of men yet is independent and strong. Few things are more important to her than men. Not surprisingly, men like her. At work, she is especially good at creating an atmosphere that is conducive to work. She makes things happen. She comes across as reasonable and responsible. She does well in a leading position, treating others tactfully and inoffensively, but can be vulnerable to patronizing. She thrives on their acceptance of her, on their looking up to her. It is almost all she needs. Her best marital partner is a youngest brother of sister(s). She is strongly oriented to having children.

Youngest sister of brother(s): She powerfully attracts men. Her attractive traits include feminine, friendly, kind, sensitive, tactful, submissive without being subservient, a good companion of men, and a good sport. She is an ideal employee and self-starter. She lacks a strong desire to excel. Consistent with the complementarity that predicts the best marital partners for other sibling positions, her best choice would be the oldest brother of sister(s).

Intermediary sibling positions: They describe the characteristics of people who have both brothers and sisters. This configuration results in a mixture of profiles, such as a person having qualities of both an oldest brother of brothers and of sisters. The age of the siblings is also considered. For example, a third-born child, a son, has two older brothers fairly close in age and a younger sister maybe four or five years younger. In this case, he is likely to develop more of the characteristics of a youngest brother of brother(s) than an older brother of a sister. The sibling positions of the parents of these children can bias the situation as well.

Only child: A male only child is used to being the favorite of his parents. Consequently, he expects acclaim and to get support. He expects this from others as well as from his parents. He is not ready for a peer relationship but seeks out mother and father figures. The only way he can assume features of a sibling position is by learning them mostly from his father. A female only child tends to be more capricious, extravagant, and possibly selfish than other females. Growing up, she must appear quite precocious and sophisticated, but at the same time must remain the child. She understands the psychology of older people better than that of her peers. Like the male only child and his father, she can learn from her mother's sibling position about such things as how to relate to a man. Important to note, the sibling positions of the parents of an only child have more influence on the only child's eventual makeup than they do on children with siblings. One last point is that if siblings are six or more years apart, they tend to grow up like only children.

Twins: The profiles of the oldest and youngest brother will blend for each of the twin boys. The profiles for oldest and youngest sister will blend for twin girls. Identical twins have a more intensive problem than fraternal twins in that separation for outside friendships or marriage can be harder. Identical twins can empathize to a degree unknown to other siblings. If the twins have other siblings, if they are same-sex or identical twins with younger siblings, they will have features of oldest profiles. If the siblings are older, they will have features of youngest profiles. Twins tend to be glued more tightly together than nontwin siblings, which makes them more likely to remain attached for life.

Sibling profiles are always modified, sometimes to an extreme, because all other things are never equal, differences in basic level of differentiation are the most important modifying influence. A moderately differentiated oldest brother of brother(s) can be a leader but is vulnerable to being self-righteous when anxious. A poorly differentiated oldest brother may exhibit very few characteristics of an oldest profile. The aspects of the profile that remain in a poorly differentiated oldest may not be evident except under certain circumstances. For example, when I was a Navy psychiatrist and taking care of a ward filled with young men diagnosed with acute schizophrenic reactions, a small fire broke out near the back of the ward one afternoon. I was called to the ward immediately, and as I was moving rapidly down the corridor of the ward, I alerted patients as to what was happening and asked for help. By the time I got to the fire, a corpsman was already extinguishing it. I also saw that five or six patients had responded and were standing around me ready to help. I realized later that all of them were the oldest children in their families! A poorly differentiated youngest sibling, male or female, may be unusually helpless and childlike, always depending on someone else to make decisions.

Sibling position also has an interesting impact on people's political views. Not surprisingly, oldest children tend to support establishment views. Youngest siblings, in contrast, are more prone to antiestablishment views, even to being radically rebellious. Again, level of maturity in each case plays a key role in whether someone dogmatically adheres to one political view versus another. It is compelling to see how much the emotional system can affect which lever a person pulls in the voting box.

The influence of basic level of differentiation on sibling profiles notwithstanding, the most fundamental characteristics of a person's sibling position always seem to be there. Oldest siblings typically volunteer to assume responsibility and like being in charge. When I was director of the Bowen Center, I was sitting at a faculty meeting one day, looking at the twelve faculty members assembled around the table, and thinking about their sibling positions. Every faculty member knew the sibling positions of the other members from people doing multiple presentations about their own families over the years. As I looked out on the group, I reflected on the fact that there were eight oldest siblings and four youngest ones gathered there. I realized how much I could depend on this group of oldests to take responsibility and see a job through to its completion. I also realized that it would be a very different organization without the youngest siblings being part of it. They were not as quick to take the lead, but they always contributed to various projects getting done. The Bowen Center needed both groups. One tended to push a bit; the other tended to soften and loosen things up a bit.

Therapists' knowledge of sibling position can be extremely useful in their work. Some understanding of the importance of sibling position characteristics and the reciprocal interactions in the family that support them can help maintain emotional neutrality. Watching the interplay of oldests and youngests, seeing how mutually reinforcing the process is, helps a therapist not to slip into cause-and-effect thinking.

One case I treated early in my practice was a nuclear family with an oldest brother of a brother and two younger sisters married to an only child. It was tempting to feel sorry for the wife and blame the overly controlling husband for the marital issues. She was significantly depressed and indecisive, and her self-esteem was in shambles. Living in the midst of his extended family and away from her extended family aggravated the situation. Seeing the reciprocity between the husband liking to take the lead and make decisions and the wife stating that she felt relieved not to have to lead or make decisions helped me maintain my neutrality. The wife was an only child but fit the profile of a younger sister of a brother. She had sided with her mother, who was a dysfunctional younger sister of a brother, against her overly domineering, oldest sibling father and, consequently, developed less of a "self" related to her functioning position in the system. The husband of the family I was treating was a physician and a kind of superstar in his family, strongly supported emotionally by his parents. They gave him additional pseudo-self-based strength in dealing with his wife.

My ability to remain emotionally neutral—not pretend not to take sides but really to see both sides—helped both spouses want to stay in the family therapy. Understanding the family dynamics in each extended family and how it was playing out in the marriage—part of those dynamics were related to their sibling positions—helped me to stay objective and neutral. The wife began to be in better contact with her own family, saw the replicating emotional processes, and, as a consequence, began to be more decisive and less helpless in relationship to her husband and others. This turned an overfunctioning-underfunctioning marital reciprocity into a more conflicted pattern for a time, but the couple got through it, and the wife's functioning improved significantly. Initially, the husband reacted to the change in his wife by wanting to get a different family therapist. The wife said, "Go ahead! I'm going to stick with this one." The husband backed off and decided to continue with the same therapist as well. Taking that stand with him reflected her ability to function with more "self" in the marriage.

Another example of what I am trying to convey about sibling position and its relationship to differentiation of self comes from a presentation I made in 1971 at a conference in Washington, D.C., that Walter Toman attended. I presented a paper about my then two-year effort to differentiate more of a self in my family of origin. Part of Toman's response to my paper is that a youngest child is more likely to do a public presentation about his own family. My response to him was, "I am not as much of a youngest child as I used to be." What I was trying to convey is that my beginning efforts to be more of a "self" in my family of origin, function in a more mature way, had somewhat changed my particular youngest brother of brother(s) profile. I had become a slightly more mature youngest. My presentation was one of the earliest public presentations of efforts to function with more "self" in one's family of origin. Part of my effort toward more maturity was to take on some leadership responsibility in the network of people interested in Bowen theory. I was not trying to impress my elders with my presentation, a tendency of youngest brother(s)—at least that was not my primary purpose.

Toman also emphasizes how the sibling positions of a person's parents can modify the sibling profiles. As I will describe in my family of origin in the Epilogue, Dad was a youngest brother of two sisters (with a much older half-brother), and Mother was the oldest sister of a next younger brother and then two other sisters. Mother could slip into overwhelmed and helpless postures during highly stressful periods. Her less functional periods notwithstanding, she was still the emotional leader of my immediate nuclear family of origin. She set the emotional tone, and Dad went along. Dad's next older sister felt extremely protective of him, as did his mother. As I described the earlier in this chapter, Mother's sensitivity to her own mother's upsets and that she inherited a highly protective feeling for her younger brother. My parents coped with their immaturities in their relationship with emotional distance. Father distanced into alcohol and left the kid responsibilities mostly to Mother. Mother's functioning position in her family of older sister of a brother, Dad's functioning position of youngest son with two older sisters, the distance in my parents' marriage, and Mother's programmed high level of child focus and associated overprotectiveness all contributed to the intense symbiotic link between Mother and my oldest full brother that impaired his functioning. That dynamic also fostered some functional oldest traits in me, despite my position as last-born. Understanding that process helped me get beyond blame about my family situation.

To conclude, some people reject Toman's sibling profiles on the grounds that they are fatalistic. Rather than considering them fatalistic, the predictability that the profiles have can be regarded as testimony to the value of viewing the family as an emotional unit. Toman could have titled his book "Sibling Position" but chose the title *Family Constellation*. I do not know how he decided on that title, but I believe it implies that understanding the predictability of the profile of a given sibling depends on viewing the family as a whole. For example, the younger brother of an older brother and the sibling positions of his parents all affect the profile that the older brother develops. Bowen theory refers to people having functioning positions in their family systems. A particular functioning position affects the development of children and their adult characteristics. The relationship process creates and sustains these functioning positions. Using the lens of systems thinking to view the family as a unit explains the predictability of the profiles. The predictability is humbling in the blow it deals to how much free will human beings possess. An important factor in people rejecting Toman's sibling profiles is their wanting to see people as more autonomous in their emotional functioning than they really are.

I believe that the reactivity to ideas like Toman's is part of a larger process that stems from relatively recent knowledge of emotions and their evolutionary roots. The more that is being learned in this area, the more it appears that emotions are the most dominant force in human behavior. However, this idea has not yet penetrated public consciousness, and a very small minority of people truly grasps this idea.

The limited recognition that emotions can be so dominant is perhaps not surprising when one realizes that as recently as the 1930s emotions were considered unscientific. A link between the emotions, the stress response, and the brain had not been demonstrated (McEwen, 2002). James Papez (1937) proposed a mechanism of emotion in the brain, but the brain was not really considered an emotional organ until 1952, when Paul MacLean extended Papez's research (McEwen, 2002). Furthermore, only in the last few decades have numbers of neuroscience studies of emotion equaled or surpassed those of neuroscience studies of cognitive processes. This has given science a greater appreciation of the pervasive impact of emotion on all aspects of human functioning. Neuroscientists have now begun to see that the reciprocal interplay between subcortical emotional processes and cortical cognitive processes is critical to understanding feelings and subjectivity (LeDoux & Pine, 2016).

Aristotelianism gave birth to viewing humankind as the "rational animal." Human beings seem to have carried this idea to a far greater extreme than Aristotle ever intended. Economist Bernt Stigum (2003) makes the point that Aristotle did not imply that people necessarily make rational choices, only that they had the ability to make them. Ideas like Toman's challenge rationality and free will being dominant in human functioning. One thing that makes it difficult for people to recognize how powerfully emotions influence cognitive processes is that beliefs, attitudes, and decision making can be strongly influenced by emotions that are out of awareness. Haidt (2012) refers to such processes as intuitions, which are a kind of cognition. Emotions are filled with cognitions, but we may not experience the emotion as a feeling, making the influence of emotion hard to identify. Emotionally influenced intuitions are part of our automatic responses. One such automatic emotional response—though it seems rational to the person doing it—is confirmation bias, which is seeking evidence that confirms what you already think.

Bowen theory emphasizes this idea even further by recognizing that an emotional system in families and other societal groups powerfully regulates human emotional functioning. The togetherness force for oneness, sameness, and agreement renders all human beings—less differentiated people more so—highly vulnerable to adopt what others believe or automatically reject what others believe. Everyone can see that when someone is enraged they may act irrationally, but the impact of emotion on mental processes is usually subtler than that. The concepts of sibling profiles shaped by family configuration and the multigenerational transmission process have much in common at this very basic automatic level of response. *Homo sapiens* is perhaps best described as an emotional animal with some potential to apply reason to decision making.

Bowen speculated from time to time that humankind could potentially control its own evolution, "a little bit, maybe." I think he meant that if the application of natural systems thinking could eventually penetrate the public consciousness, culture would become a much stronger selective force in shaping human behavior.

CHAPTER THIRTEEN

Emotional Cutoff

Murray Bowen added the concept of emotional cutoff to Bowen theory in 1975, one of the last concepts he added (Bowen, 1976). It describes the way adult offspring handle their unresolved emotional attachment during and after leaving home. Both emotional distance and emotional cutoff function to manage the chronic anxiety generated by the fundamental dilemma in relationships described in Chapter 3: the need for emotional closeness and the aversion to too much of it. The distinction between emotional distance and emotional cutoff is that cutoff focuses specifically on how the distance plays out between the generations. Cutoff is a major contributor to what people commonly refer to as the "generation gap." The term *distance* is generally used to describe nuclear family emotional processes. The fundamental emotional processes at work are the same in distance and in cutoff.

One reason emotional cutoff is so important to understand and recognize is that it can make the difference between a successful an unsuccessful course of family therapy. If people are using a significant degree of emotional cutoff to deal with their families of origin, it can be very difficult to gain the needed perspective on current relationships with their spouse and children. *Bridging the cutoff*, as it is commonly termed, can tone down the intensity of current relationships enough to permit some objectivity and consequent progress. It is difficult for people to see their false assumptions about what constitutes a good marriage and good parenting—the way things "should be"—if they close off looking at their immediate families of origin and multigenerational families where the roots of those assumptions took hold. It is a little easier to see such processes if you are not living in the midst of them day to day. Seeing them in the family of origin can greatly facilitate being able to discern the components of similar emotional processes in one's immediate family.

Like so many aspects of applying systems theory, recognizing a process for what it is, what is factually playing out, is usually the first step in addressing that process. I describe in the Epilogue listening to Murray Bowen in 1969 lecturing about the concept of emotional cutoff and suddenly realizing, "My gosh, that is what I am doing: cutting off from my family of origin." I had not realized that I had been doing it and immediately decided that I wanted to do something about it. It was one of my first experiences of listening to an objective description of a relationship system process and recognizing it as an alternative to how I had been thinking about a situation. It was a gift. Of course, I knew little at that point about the details of the attitudes, sensitivities, and behaviors that created the cutoff, but I was at least convinced that it was happening, it was important, and I could do something about it. Fundamentally, I had been retreating for several years from the intensity of the relationship between our Mother and my schizophrenic brother. Another motivator was realizing that my cutting off might be making their situation more difficult. I described some of how that was the case in the Epilogue.

We all have some degree of unresolved attachment to our family of origin—it is part of human nature. Unresolved attachment refers to the emotional fusion that existed with one's family while growing up, which is not resolved simply by leaving your family and forming new intimate relationships. People carry the unresolved attachment with them and replicate it in some form in the new relationships. In response to a question by an attendee at a conference about what emotional intensity and cutoff looks like, I quoted the following statement from a letter written by the Unabomber, Ted Kaczynski, to his brother. The letter was sent from Ted's cabin in Montana in the summer of 1991, five years before his capture: "I have got to know, I have GOT TO, GOT TO, GOT TO know that every last tie joining me to this stinking family has been cut FOREVER and that I will never NEVER have to communicate with any of you again. . . . I've got to do it now. I can't tell you how desperate I am. . . . It is killing me" (quoted in Kovaleski, 1997).

Bowen theory does not assert people should not cut off from their families; it says that this is what people do and that it has its advantages and disadvantages. The principal advantage is that it can provide some peace from difficult and painful interactions with one's family; the principle disadvantage is that it intensifies future relationships and the problems associated with an even more anxiety-driven fusion. As discussed in more detail in Chapter 19, Ted Kaczynski had a very fused and problematic relationship with his family, which he blamed on the family.

The less "self" people have developed in the emotional attachment with their families by the time they leave home, the greater the vulnerability they have of their relationship with the family generating chronic anxiety from then on. The anxiety can be managed or coped with in two basic ways. One way is not to threaten the dependency on one's parents and theirs on you by leaving home. This is the "failure to lift off" syndrome. If people stay close to parents, besides avoiding the anxiety of being more independent, they can also manage the anxiety by isolating themselves, such as by retreating to some space in the house and minimizing interactions with parents and other family members. They can also retreat into some level of depression or psychosis, or even deceive themselves that a problem exists. Such situations can remain stable for years if the parents tolerate it and do not push for change. Some cases become malignantly unstable, such as the Sandy Hook shooter, Adam Lanza, and his mother (discussed in detail in Chapter 21).

A second basic way of dealing with the chronic anxiety is physically running away from the family and never going back. In the extreme cases of running away, people may become peripatetic nomads, vagabonds, or hermits. A superb dramatic film portrayal of this type of emotional cutoff is the 1970 movie *Five Easy Pieces*, starring Jack Nicholson. It powerfully portrays the intensity of the lead character Bobby Dupea's unresolved attachment to his family of origin, depicting what plays out when he returns home and how those same emotional sensitivities play out in his adult relationships, especially with women. Dupea was a relationship nomad, staying in a relationship until the problems become too intense and then moving on to a new place and a new relationship. The principal point is that all the family members contribute to the emotional cutoff, primarily the parents and the one that runs away. All of this is fueled by blame and self-blame. People who run away from their families sometimes stabilize their lives by joining some type of cult group or some type of substitute family. Substitute families are generally less reliable as support systems than one's own family.

Many gradations of cutoff exist between the extremes described above. Additionally, people commonly combine these two basic coping strategies, such as by having some physical contact with family but avoiding potentially emotionally charged situations and keeping interactions superficial. The case example presented in Chapter 2 of the man who dreaded visiting his family of origin because he felt they treated him like a child is an example of an unresolved emotional attachment in the moderate range of differentiation. He chose to live in a city physically distant from his parents and tried to use internal mechanisms to insulate himself from any emotional intensity when he was back home. He tried to keep visits home short and sweet. The parents' equal contribution to the cutoff is evident in that clinical example as well.

People who have developed a reasonable level of "self" and the associated good level of emotional resolution in the relationship between offspring and parents by the time they leave home grow away rather than break away from the family. This allows parents and adult offspring to remain in good communication, whether living in the same area or thousands of miles apart, and remain an ongoing resource for each other.

It is sometimes amazing how superficial interactions can make things look fairly normal. People who had highly conflicted relationships with parents in their teen years may have things smooth out considerably if they marry and have children of their own. The problem is that they then replicate those problematic interactions with one or more of their own children or in the marriage. This replication with the next generation indicates the lack of resolution of the attachment with the previous generation, even though things look mostly normal. A husband or wife can often see the spouse's unresolved attachment to parents better than the spouse can, for example, observing how sensitized the spouse is to upset in the in-laws and automatic behaviors that come into play to reduce it. The spouse has done it this way so long that it just seems normal. It is likely, however, that these automatic behaviors are playing out with the couple's own children as well, sometimes on an even more intense level. Another possible scenario is one spouse cutting off from his own family and joining the mate's family. Another fairly common scenario is cutoffs between siblings after one or both parents have died. These cutoffs can be addressed by understanding the triangles that existed with the siblings and the parents when they were alive.

A misunderstanding that many students of Bowen theory develop is viewing emotional cutoff as one end of a continuum and emotional fusion as the other end. This is a faulty conceptualization. People who remain emotionally dependent on their parents, with or without significant financial dependence on them, can have just as much unresolved attachment as the people who physically distance. As with all aspects of Bowen theory, many degrees of lack of resolution exist in both coping strategies for playing it out. The ideal is as much resolution of the emotional attachment as the current evolution of *Homo sapiens* allows. People can gain significant emotional well-being from a relationship with only a mild degree of emotional fusion existing between them.

Another important distinction is the difference between going toward a goal and running away from a problem. This may not always be easy to decipher, but it is an important distinction nonetheless. A given decision may contain elements of both. Moving toward a goal is part of differentiation of self; cutting off from an anxious family situation is part of an anxiety-driven togetherness process. In the normal process of things, people grow up and leave their families to form new emotionally significant relationships. This may carry them halfway around the globe. This can reflect mature goal-directed activity or an intense desire to get away from family. By the same token, people may decide to live in the area where they grew up and that can reflect mature goal-directed activity as well—perhaps they decide to enter the family business. Staying put may also represent anxiety about leaving the safety net. Geographic moves are important to examine, but it is also important not to jump to conclusions about them.

The initial approaches to family therapy based on Bowen theory focused on people working on differentiation of self in relationship to their spouse and children. This approach dominated during the 1960s. During that decade Bowen was working to apply what he was learning about families in his research to his own family of origin. He did a presentation about that effort at the Family Research Conference in 1967. It was later published as part of volume of the conference presentations edited by family therapist Jim Framo (Anonymous, 1972). This began a shift in focus by therapists and families in therapy toward work on differentiation of self directly in the family of origin. This turned out to be far more important than even Bowen realized at the beginning.

People were attempting to convert cutoffs to deal with the unresolved attachments to their families of origin into differentiation of self in the family of origin. Although it was not automatic, as people made progress in their family of origin they also started making progress in their current family systems. They began to see processes in their current families that had been operating outside of their awareness. The details of this process will be left to Part II of the book. This transformed the long-trusted idea of the therapeutic relationship in conventional theory-based psychotherapy, meaning that progress occurred based on something that transpired in the relationship between therapist and patient, into progress occurring based on what happened between the family member and the family of origin.

Psychoanalysis had heavily depended on the transference relationship in therapy. This was found to no longer be necessary. The therapist could stay outside the transference by not focusing on or responding to interactions that encouraged transference. Armed with motivation and a theory that makes more objectivity about family relationships an attainable goal, people could work on the original transference with parents, even if parents had died. In the case of deceased parents, much can be gained by working on relationships with people who were close to the parents, such as aunts and uncles.

The therapist or "coach" is sort of alongside the family member, helping apply Bowen theory to real-world relationships. In coaching sessions, there is no rule against a family member expressing feelings such as disappointment or anger with a coach and having those feelings discussed, but that is not the prime focus of the coaching. The coach learns how to maintain differentiation in consultations with a family member primarily by making progress on differentiation of self in family member's own nuclear and extended family. Clinical experience helps, but that alone is not enough. Effective coaches must have gone down the road they are trying to help others go down.

I hope that all I have described here about emotional cutoff helps explain why Bowen elevated emotional cutoff from family of origin into a distinct concept. Perhaps the point worth reiterating to close this chapter is that emotional cutoff is not a pathological process, but it is important to understand the consequences it can have for oneself and for others.

CHAPTER FOURTEEN

Societal Emotional Process

Emotional regression has been addressed at the family relationship level, but the concept of societal emotional process extends that application to groups as large as entire societies. Bowen included societal regression as a concept in Bowen theory in a 1976 paper. (The name changed from *societal regression* to *societal emotional process* to clarify that societies go through periods of progression as well regression.) A stimulus to develop the concept occurred in 1972 when the U.S. Environmental Protection Agency invited Bowen to do a paper on the human reaction to environmental problems. The idea is that the family emotional system, which is subject to progressions and regressions in functioning as chronic anxiety fluctuates in the system over time, can be extended to explain phenomena in the larger social arena.

Societal regressions are more than an emotional process. Psychological processes are key factors that drive them as well. Virulent propaganda is used to stir emotional reactivity in tribe members, cementing unity (emotional fusion) and inciting its members to reject or even cleanse the society of "other" tribes. Emotional process lurks not only underneath family processes but also underneath political and economic processes.

Many people sense the emotional underpinnings of the false beliefs that can drive regressions but still remain vulnerable to succumbing to emotion-triggering rhetoric. In face of heightened chronic anxiety, emotionality fuels the descent of political and economic systems into dysfunction. It would be valuable for this perspective to be more solidly anchored in the public consciousness than it is currently. Given how vulnerable the human species is to irrational thinking, I propose changing our species name from *Homo sapiens* (wise man) to *Homo dysrationalis*. Psychologist Keith Stanovich, whose work was cited in Chapter 5, introduced the term "dysrationalia," which means capable of wisdom, but commonly falling short of it (1993). Glorifying ourselves as *the* rational species contributes to perpetuation of the insane but pervasive notion that our species merits dominion over Earth and all its inhabitants, flora and fauna.

Many people, including some Bowen theorists, reacted negatively when Bowen introduced the idea of societal regression in the early 1970s to describe the state of society. Critics responded by noting that mean and nasty things have occurred throughout human history and that contemporary society is progressing, not regressing. The concept accepts that there can be elements of progression present even in a period of overall regression and also that there have been other periods of regression throughout history.

From Dawn to Decadence (2000), a book by historian Jacques Barzun, supports the idea that contemporary society is indeed in a period of "decadence" or what Bowen theory terms emotional regression. Barzun emphasizes how cultures change in a period of decadence but does not explicitly address emotional process. The quote below summarizes Barzun's assessment of the pervasive societal changes that reflect decadence:

> The general relaxation of conduct so widely complained of since the mid-century. The attack on authority, the ridicule of anything established, the distortions of language and objects, the indifference to clear meaning, the violence to the human form, the return to primitive elements of sensation, the growing list of genres called Anti-. . . . And all this was going on long before the moral, sexual, and political rebellions that shook the western world in the 1960s. (p. 727)

He summarizes the current state of things by stating that, despite great advances in technological capabilities, we live in a time of cultural sunset, depleted energies, and more confusion. It is a culture of entitlement. The book examines history in the Western world from 1500 until the present and describes previous periods of decadence from which societies eventually emerged. He predicts that we will eventually emerge from the current period as well.

Barzun arrived at his perspective through the meticulous examination of history. Bowen arrived at his perspective in a very different way: observing that over approximately a fifteen-year period the court system in the United States was addressing the problem of juvenile delinquency in ways increasingly similar to the characteristic regressed patterns of emotional functioning that played out in families with a juvenile delinquent member (Bowen, 1978). He also noted an increased incidence of delinquency cases between the early 1950s and the early 1970s. Society appeared to have shifted from family patterns that tended to foster internalized problems to patterns that fostered externalized or acted out problems, as is the case with juvenile delinquency. A more permissive society is conducive to generating character disorders (borrowing for the moment from conventional psychiatric terminology) over neuroses. This is not to suggest that acting out behaviors are more regressive than neurotic behaviors, only that changes had occurred both in the level of anxiety in society and in the way it manifested.

The overly permissive family pattern conducive to delinquency begins with overly devoted parents, a pattern that became more exaggerated and present in more families during the 1950s. In recent years, other terms have been used, such as *helicopter parenting* and *snowplow parenting*.

The pattern begins as illustrated in Figure 14.1. The diagram depicts two overly devoted parents, as symbolized by the fairly heavy arrows going from the parents to their teenage son. Typically, the mother is more focused on the son than the father is, but as described in Chapter 3 on triangles, the father is just as fused into the triangle as the mother: her functioning affects his and vice versa, and the child's functioning affects both parents and vice versa. Both parents and child foster an exaggerated fusion process. The shaded oval in the symbol of the son indicates that he has become unhappy or distressed in some way.

Figure 14.2 symbolizes the next phase of the family emotional process. The mother's anxiety-driven feeling reaction in response to her perception of the child's distress is to do more of what she has been doing since early in the child's life, which is to try to relieve the upset by anxiously giving him even more love, attention, and support. The teenager's distress triggers in her a fear that she has not done enough.

Figure 14.3 illustrates the next phase of this process of more intense fusion and the particular form of emotional programming to which it contributes. The son's distress and frustration increase (shaded oval has expanded to symbolize his increasing distress) because he has been programmed in the relationship by the mother's ongoing efforts to smooth his path in life and has learned to expect a solution for his distress from outside himself.

In the next phase (Figure 14.4), the son responds to his mother's increased anxious focus on him by feeling justified in demanding even more from her to relieve his distress. He has learned to blame the problem on her, a consequence the mother has unwittingly fostered. The mother responds out of her own unsureness and fears about what could go wrong and tries to meet her son's unrealistic expectations by meeting his demands (Figure 14.5). This reinforces the son's sense of entitlement and automatic blaming of others for his unhappiness. Although the mother may become angry and rejecting of the son later on, her overall message is, "I'll love you no matter what you do." Figure 14.6 symbolizes the next aspect of the process. The son begins to feel that this is breach of promise: "Mother has promised me she can solve my

Overly-devoted
A.
More love
B.
More love
Expects solution from outside himself.
C.
More love
Unrealistic demands
D.
Tries to meet demands
Unrealistic demands
E.
More love
Tries to meet demands
Unrealistic demand
More demands
F.
Firm stand attempt to control son through punitive measures
More love
Tries to meet demands
Unrealistic demands
More demands
G.

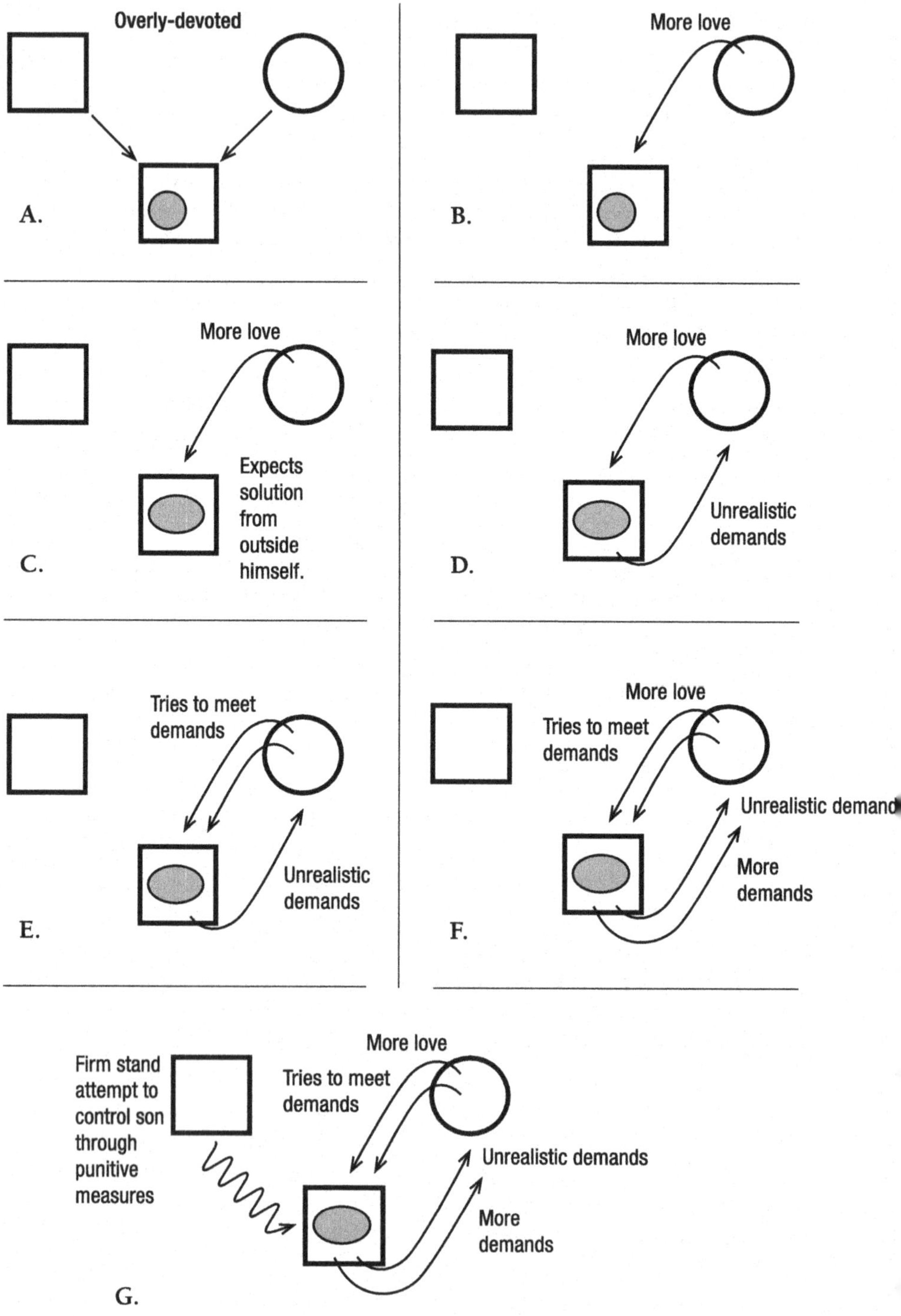

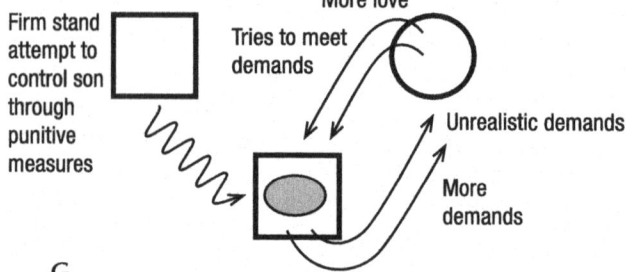

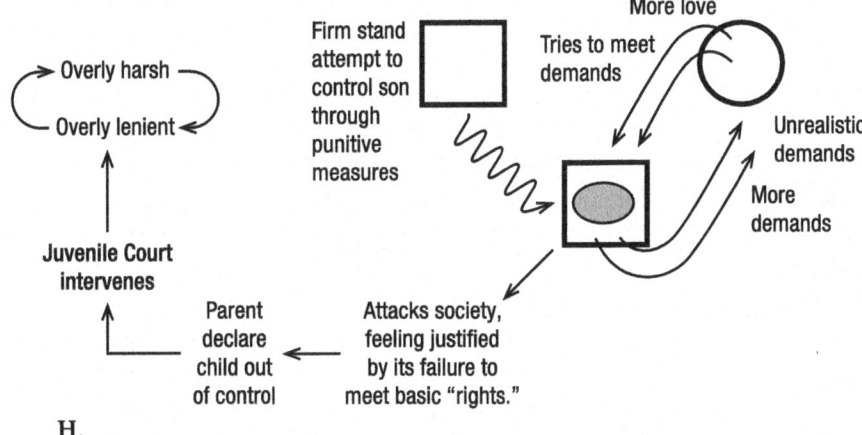

H.

Figure 14.1 (A.) *The arrows from the two parents to a son symbolize an anxious focus on him by overly-devoted, permissive parents. The shaded circle inside the symbol for the son indicates his heightened vulnerability to chronic anxiety related to the child focus process.*
Figure 14.2 (B.) *The son's verbal and nonverbal expressions of any discontent triggers a feeling in the mother that he needs more love, which she then showers him with.*
Figure 14.3 (C.) *This type of mother-son interaction emotionally programs him to expect solutions for his distress to come from outside himself.*
Figure 14.4 (D.) *The enlarged circle in the symbol for the son indicates higher anxiety in response to his mother's anxiety-driven efforts to fix his distress with accompanying increased unrealistic demands on his mother to solve his distress.*
Figure 14.5 (E.) *The arrows back and forth in the mother-son relationship indicate an escalating cycle of the mother giving in and going along with her son's expectations.*
Figure 14.6 (F.) *Increasing permissiveness intensifies the unrealistic demands.*
Figure 14.7 (G.) *The father responds to the anxious interaction between his wife and son by anxiously and harshly attempting a firm stand with the teenager that includes threats of punitive measures.*
Figure 14.8 (H.) *As the son grows into his mid and later teens, he expands his demands into self-righteously expecting the larger society to meet "basic rights." The parents eventually declare their son out of control, at which point the Juvenile Court intervenes to punish the son's disruptive transgressions in society. However, decision-making by the courts has become more like that of the parents of such "juvenile delinquents," fluctuating between overly lenient approaches that do not work and anger driven overly harsh punishments, which make the son feel more justified in his anger with his parents and society.*

problem, but she hasn't!" Parents can usually describe this interactive process in detail but feel that the son's problems are at fault. The only option they see for solving this problem is to get the boy to change.

In the next escalation (Figure 14.7), the father eventually has had enough of what he sees as the son's efforts to manipulate the mother and her going along, and he becomes harsh and punitive in trying to control the son. The climate of permissiveness then shifts to overly harsh tactics by the parents, such as threats of punishments like grounding, no car privileges, strict curfews, or being sent off to military school. The son is feeling harassed, treated unfairly, and misunderstood. The son has usually become adept at getting around the parents' efforts to exert more control. It is common to have long periods of permissiveness punctuated by briefer periods of harshness characterized by threats that are erratically enforced. A variation of the pattern that programs for acting out behavior is the father siding with the teenager and undercutting the mother's efforts to hold the line. She does not have enough "self" to take an effective stand with her husband.

The son's delinquent behavior gets more and more extreme. A supportive like-minded peer group accentuates the son's problem but does not cause it—the core of the problem is in the parental triangle. The son develops little solid self, and the parents are functioning with little solid self in relationship to him. The son moves out into the world with a strong sense of entitlement. He then expands his upsets to attacking society, and his delinquent acts become more extreme. The feeling-overwhelmed parents declare the child out of control and the juvenile court intervenes.

Bowen's clue to societal regression stemmed from his reviewing juvenile court decisions in the fifteen or so years preceding the early 1970s. The decisions showed a growing pattern of fluctuating between overly lenient and overly harsh legal decisions. He noted that the process is very similar to what plays out in the families of the delinquents. Figure 14.8 summarizes the flow of the overall process from the family to society. The regression unfolding in the larger society reinforces the unsureness of families struggling with juvenile delinquent symptoms. Families affect society, and society affects the families.

Not all the teenagers that act out are dominated by the attitude of entitlement. Some feel distressed about who they are and what they do, but much of that attitude results from buying into the parents' view of the problem. This does not mean that they won't be devious, lie, exploit, and manipulate the parents' unsureness like an entitled child is so adept at doing.

"Tough love" approaches have appealed to many families in these situations, and some young people respond to that approach, but the downside is that tough love supports the parents' view that the problem resides in their child. The effort is to teach the parents to be firmer, but the approach addresses only superficial aspects of the family problem.

The courts are not the only social institutions affected by and participating in the regression. Barzun (2000), recalling the campus unrest of the 1960s, describes this process going on at the level of higher education as well:

When the rebellious were still in their colleges and universities, their way of protest was to occupy a building, especially the president's office, and vandalize ad lib, not excluding the destruction of research notes and equipment. On their side, administrative officers behaved with the final degree of caution which is cowardice. They complied with summons to discuss non-negotiable issues, swallowed all insults. (p. 765)

Barzun is not blaming the administrators or the protesters. He describes unrealistic demands by the students met by unsure responses by the administrators. This is the same dynamic that plays out in families that spawn acting-out offspring. At the same time, schools are being called on to be overly devoted and overly protective of their students. In loco parentis had been a useful guiding principle for teachers and administrators in the past, but Barzun was observing unsure administrators caving in to unrealistic student demands. It is important to distinguish between the content of the demands, which may have merit, and the process by which the protesters went about it, such as by interfering with the legitimate rights of others.

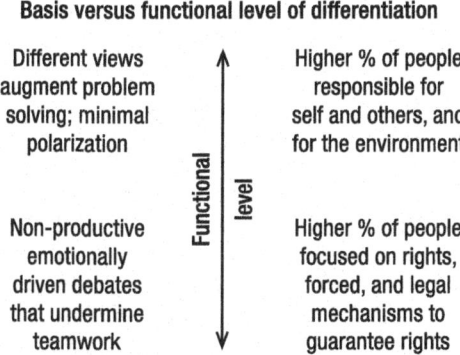

Figure 14.9 *This diagram summarizes what happens when an anxiety-driven increased togetherness process in society results in a decrease in society's functional level of differentiation. Prominent changes are an increased emphasis on rights over responsibilities and a level of polarization in society that interferes with problem solving.*

Figure 14.9 summarizes the most fundamental aspects of the difference, according to Bowen theory, between regressed societies and ones functioning on a higher level. Emotional regression in the family and in society reflects an anxiety-driven decrease in *functional* level of differentiation, not a change in basic level of differentiation. As a society drifts down into a deeper level of regression, the characteristics of a higher percentage of people are described in the lower right part of the diagram and the difficulty people have working together is described in the lower left part of the diagram. One of the obvious places these regressed features manifest currently is in the halls of Congress. Constituencies support more legislators that represent extreme positions. Neither side is necessarily right, but polarization prevents thoughtful compromise and problem solving. When a society emerges from a regression, functional level goes up and the changes that occur in people and in their communications are described in the upper left and right of the diagram.

The fundamental process at work in emotional regressions is that principle-determined decisions and actions give way to a more feeling orientation. This happens in the family, and it happens in the larger society. Other manifestations of this shift from principle to feeling include a rising incidence of violence, with much of it being domestic violence, as well as more we-they factions characterized by extreme self-righteousness, rapid changes in mores (these changes are considered regressive because a more pressured feeling orientation replaces a more rational and contemplative process), less stable intimate relationships with overall higher divorce rates (this can fluctuate over time), more focus on rights than responsibilities, more crime, more litigation, more substance abuse, a rise in teen pregnancies, permissiveness, radical dogmatic fundamentalism, a more pervasive attitude of entitlement, less responsibility for the environment, quick-fix legislation to relieve the anxiety of the moment, omnipresence of conspiracy theories, and a rise in terrorism. People blame their troubles on others rather than accepting their own responsibility for what unfolds. As a culture becomes unstable, it has a strong impact on families, particularly less differentiated families. A stable culture supports pseudo-self and associated calmness that is a significant part of all of us. People are more vulnerable to their social context than they usually recognize. A minority of better-differentiated people in a society can float above the regression that surrounds them. They offer fact-based thoughts and ideas about what is transpiring in the larger society, but their contributions are commonly ignored or overruled by the regressed majority.

The end of regressions reflects an increase of functional level of differentiation. This occurs in families in several ways. One way is that things have gotten so bad for a family and resources have so dwindled that one family member says "I cannot do this anymore, we cannot keep going along with the way we have been." It amounts to an I-position taken out of desperation. In my description of the James Madison family in Chapter 6, that family never emerged from the regression. Decisions about their ne'er-do-well adult son never departed from giving into him. Had the family fully exhausted their financial resources, James or Dolley would have been forced to draw lines on the degree to which Payne was draining the resources, simply because there were no more resources.

Another way of a family emerging from a regression is the preferred one: a structured effort by a family leader toward functioning with more "self" in the system, which can reverse a regression. This occurs when a family member gains a systems understanding of the regression and has the courage and motivation to function with more "self." This is generally what family therapy is all about. Unfortunately, not everyone is motivated to do this.

Probably the most frequent way regressions end is that the level of chronic anxiety drops. It is often not clear why this happens. It is common in family therapy for anxiety to decrease because the family has taken the step to get some help and they can talk about things in a more neutral setting. This does not represent an increase in basic level of differentiation, but it is a reduction of anxiety and a functional increase in differentiation. This is where a therapist's theoretical understanding of the family emotional process and associated emotional neutrality makes a difference. Families commonly function better when they interact with someone who can do that.

It is obviously a far more difficult task for one motivated person guided by a good understanding of theory to influence society. One person can make some difference in smaller social systems, such as a business or community organization. In a democracy, when a regression becomes severe enough and the majority of the population moves away from principle and more to feeling-based quick-fix solutions, the people elevated to leadership positions typically mirror that orientation. It becomes the blind leading the blind. In nondemocratic societies, ruthless authoritarian leaders often emerge to restore some semblance of order, and the populace goes along. There are obvious downsides to such a development.

Bowen's prediction for the current emotional regression in the United States was that the regression would reverse when the pain of taking the easy way out exceeds the pain of taking a more principled long-term-view direction. If this occurs, it will likely take several more decades for it to happen. Bowen speculated that the type of human being that emerged from the regression would have more capacity for systems thinking about human behavior and for living in harmony with nature.

Barzun (2000) observed that a regression had been unfolding in Europe leading up to the time Columbus discovered the New World. The regression quickly subsided after that discovery. He implied that the discovery sort of lifted people's spirits, expanded their horizons literally and figuratively. Some people think that human ingenuity and technology can bail us out of our current problems.

Comprehending what might end the current regression in society can be aided by understanding what set it in motion. Bowen was certain that a regression was under way and had been since shortly after World War II ended, but was less certain about what was driving the chronic anxiety that fuels regressions. He did suspect, however, that what is driving our current regression is unique compared to previous regressions in human history. He believed that the fundamental process at work was a disturbance between humankind and nature. He suggested that at least three conditions contribute to that disturbance: (1) the rapid depletion of natural resources, (2) the population explosion, and (3) the absence of new frontiers. As a regression deepens and associated symptoms emerge, that further increases chronic anxiety. The irony of these processes is that they require that people be thoughtful and work together to solve problems, which is very difficult to achieve when the functional level of differentiation is down.

One last aspect of Bowen theory to apply to societal emotional process is the individuality-togetherness life force balance. This idea can be extended from the family to the societal level. Bowen theory holds that optimal functioning for a society is a 50-50 balance, with neither force overriding the other. This even balance implies a flexibility to adapt to change. Each of the forces can be more or less influential for a time period appropriate to the circumstances at hand. In an anxiety field that drives a regression, the instinctive default mode for the group is toward more togetherness to relieve the anxiety. If the anxiety is sustained, a new balance can occur, such as 55 or 60 on the togetherness side and a reciprocal 45 or 40 on the individuality side. This represents the decrease in functional level of differentiation, which renders a society somewhat less adaptive to the challenges at hand. This manifests in a bias for society to support togetherness solutions for the challenges it faces more than individuality-guided solutions. Below are the characteristics of each side of the equation:

Individuality
Plead for principle
Autonomy of self
Maintaining a predetermined course despite anxiety
Rights of individuals to determine their own life course

Togetherness
Harmony
Caring for others
More rights (permeated with an air of entitlement)
Humanitarianism
Responsiveness
Sensitivity

Looking at the list, the tendencies on the two sides of the balance obviously each has its merits. These descriptions are unrelated to political parties. The important thing is the flexibility to move back and forth in a way that is most adaptive to the circumstances at hand. In a regression, this flexibility is reduced to one degree or another. The positions are increasingly vulnerable to polarization and conflict as anxiety increases and the regression deepens. The more thoughtful segment of the population retains adaptive flexibility, but the more feeling-oriented side is less inclined to listen. The process is similar to the feeling system flooding and impairing the functioning of the intellectual system when chronic anxiety is high. People can be just as dogmatic about autonomy for self as about togetherness.

Another aspect of the regression is that those in power impose an increasing number of rules and regulations that many people react to as onerous and rebel against. The idea is that a degree of this is necessary to maintain a safe and orderly society, but in a regression togetherness forces an associated polarized push for more of it. One example is the worldwide obesity epidemic. People are warned on an almost daily basis of the health risks of obesity. The warnings make sense, but it is similar to parents continually warning their children about the risks of substance abuse. People justify their warnings by citing the true dangers that exist, but this is, in part, an anxiety-driven emotional process unfolding. It easily degrades into parents or the government overfunctioning, typically thinking this is good parenting or good governing. I am not dismissing the addictive qualities of opioid drug use, but it is fundamentally an emotional process. As societies drift into deeper and deeper levels of regression, an increasing number of people predictably will numb themselves to the frenzy of life in some way. Telling them not to do it probably does not help much. People often respond to such a statement with a comment like, "Well, we have to do *something!*" Such a comment is part of the anxiety-driven symptom process in society, paralleling what goes on in families.

Before closing this chapter, I again emphasize the deep biological roots of emotional regression, by presenting a brief description of an emotional regression in the ground finches of the Galapagos Islands in 1982–1983 and its eerie similarity to the financial crisis of 2007–2008 in our own species. Peter Grant and Rosemary Grant (1985), evolutionary biologists at Princeton University, began studying the ground finches that lived on one of the Galápagos Islands in 1973. They returned year after year and accomplished some very important research that has enhanced understanding of Darwin's theory of evolution by the mechanism of natural selection. The small part of their work that I describe here began when an especially powerful El Niño occurred during 1983. The impact on the islands was an extraordinary amount of rainfall. This resulted in incredibly abundant food resources for the finches. The staples of their diet, seeds and caterpillars, increased exponentially. The abundance had a very interesting impact on the birds.

Earlier research had investigated the normal social structure of the ground finches. The males joust for territory, and then, once the male that will control that territory is sorted out, male-female courtships begin. Once a relationship is formed, the pair cooperates extensively in the process of raising the young. The female offspring that are born do not normally breed until their second year of life. In years in which El Niño does not occur, the conditions can become quite dry, resulting in fewer food resources and consequent lack of breeding for most of the birds—the birds concentrate on survival rather than reproduction. In wet periods, the breeding process resumes in the orderly manner described above.

However, in the extraordinarily wet year of 1983, something unusual happened. In the midst of the superabundant resources, the birds began a copulating frenzy. Some birds produced up to twenty-nine eggs in seven clutches and fledged twenty young! This level of reproduction had not occurred in the first ten years of research observation. The mothers, normally monogamous, became bigamous, even polygamous. Females commonly abandoned their begging young offspring. Furthermore, the young females in their first year of life were copulating with males. As for the males, they staked out poor territories but still managed to mate. Not surprisingly, with all this frenzied breeding going on, the population exploded. Everyone had enough to eat. However, eventually the rain stopped, and resources dropped precipitously. Huge numbers of the expanded population died.

Bowen theory's way of conceptualizing what happened to these birds is that, in face of unusually abundant resources, the orderly social structure of the frenzied birds regressed. Stable families disappeared. Population increases in periods of good resources are not unusual in nature, but that being paired with a decline in social structure is fascinating. It is not a stretch to refer to this as an anxiety-driven emotional process. It is difficult to be certain if birds experience feelings, but they possess an emotional system, regressions of which manifest in the relationship system of the birds.

Now consider the financial crisis of 2007–2008 and what appears to be an emotional process very similar to the one involving the ground finches of Galápagos. First, my conclusion is that the financial crisis reflected societal regression and that, like the finches, human beings do not seem to cope well with excess. The core biology at play in human beings and likely the ground finches involves the pleasure and reward systems of the brain. Cognitive processes enter into the process as well in human beings, but it is hard to discern if they play a role in the birds. In both species, optimal stimulation of the pleasure and reward systems in the brain is an essential motivating system. However, high levels of stimulation interfere with impulse control.

It is perhaps no surprise that the ability of ground finches to regulate their behavior so as not to disturb normal social interactions would be heavily dependent on the environmental context where they reside. Many examples exist of significant changes in environmental conditions powerfully affecting the flora and fauna that inhabit that area. A way to think about what happened to the birds is that the usual range of resources in their environment had covered up their inability to gratify themselves destructively if the resource constraint disappeared. Evolution had not endowed them with that level of adaptive behavior. Perhaps the immediate gratification behavior of many members of our species in face of excess resources provides a clue to the potential power of the emotional forces that drive human behavior as well. *Homo dysrationalis* may be far more dependent on environmental context to aid self-regulation and consequent stable social organization than people fathom. An antidote to facing the limited control over one's own emotional system is blaming one's irrationality on others. Indeed, much finger pointing occurs in a regression.

Some of the basic elements of the financial crisis were the breaking of the housing bubble, subsequent high default rate in the subprime home mortgage sector, and consequent threatened collapse of large financial institutions. It seems like many who worked on Wall Street never once questioned the ethics of their activities and were too focused on the enormous rewards that allowed their firms to pay out huge bonuses. Meanwhile, the mortgage and banking industries found ways to place almost anyone with—or even without—a credit score in a home. Investment banks, the mortgage industry, rating agencies, and investors were all complicit in the trillions of dollars of losses that occurred. Washington, Congress, presidential administrations, the Federal Reserve, Security Exchange Commission, and others all played their roles in not providing adequate oversight. Federal spending energized the economy. One gets the impression that the Federal Reserve refused to inflict pain! City, county, and state governments participated as well. They too wanted to preserve proliferating operations but not raise taxes—they borrowed to fill the gaps.

The groups just mentioned certainly played their roles, but since 1980 Americans have been consuming more than they have produced and have made up for it through considerable borrowing (Federal Reserve, 2015). Household debt began increasing in the early 1970s along with personal disposable income, but the debt increase surpassed income increase in the early 2000s. Several decades of easy money and innovative financial products resulted in virtually anyone being able to borrow any amount for any purpose. That trend continued until the financial crisis hit.

The immediate gratification impulses of the people who defaulted on their loans were the other half of the problem. People might say that the trusted institutions should be held most responsible for what happened, but *Homo dysrationalis* works on Wall Street too. It is not about intelligence but about frenzied emotionality that drove feelings and subjectivity to override reason, reflection, and a long-term view. These are hallmarks of an emotional regression. The vulnerability to the financial crisis would have been less if the functional level of differentiation of society had been higher during the buildup to the storm. The feeling system overwhelmed principled decision making.

To summarize societal regression in a nutshell, the major processes at work are the following: (1) more decisions to allay the anxiety of the moment, (2) more cause-and-effect thinking, (3) a greater focus on rights to the exclusion of responsibility, and (4) a decrease in the overall level of responsibility. We can forgive the finches for not recognizing that there's no such thing as a "free lunch." Can *Homo dysrationalis* do better? Time will tell.

PART II

The Process of Differentiation

CHAPTER FIFTEEN

Key Ingredients in the Process of Differentiation

> *I believe and teach that the family therapist usually has the very same problems in his own family that are in the families he sees professionally, and that he has a responsibility to define himself in his own family if he is to function adequately in his professional work.*
> —Murray Bowen, Family Therapy in Clinical Practice

The word that leapt out at me in reading Bowen's above quote is *responsibility*. It makes complete sense that family therapists must address their own problems to be effective in helping the families in their clinical practice. The theory and method that Bowen recommends for addressing one's own problems are radically different from Freud's theory and method, but the two pioneers both thought it essential for therapists to address their own problems. Therapists that yearn for techniques to treat families are bypassing the importance of addressing their own functioning. Addressing one's own emotional functioning is the Holy Grail for being an effective therapist.

I suggest broadening Bowen's idea to the following: not only do family therapists have the responsibility to define themselves in their families, but so does every person who comprehends that a human family functions as an emotionally interdependent system and, consequently, that each family member's emotional functioning powerfully affects the health and well-being of other family members. Differentiation of self promotes one's own health, well-being, and productivity, and it promotes the health, well-being, and productivity of others. Lack of differentiation can promote the opposite, particularly in an anxious system.

I make this point about responsibility to emphasize the importance of trying to improve one's basic level of differentiation. I do this in the spirit of Charles Darwin's thinking on the moral sense (Keynes, 2001). Darwin believed that as human beings gradually advance in intellectual power and are able to address the more remote consequences of their actions, they will increasingly regard the welfare and happiness of their fellow human beings and extend that regard to the lower animals. Forester Peter Wohlleben in *The*

Hidden Life of Trees extends Darwin's idea to flora as well as fauna: "When the capabilities of vegetative beings become known, their emotional lives and needs are recognized, then the way we treat plants will gradually change, as well" (2015, p. 244). Darwin and Wohlleben both predict that humankind would raise the standard of morality higher and higher as we better appreciate the remote or hidden consequences of our actions. Their prediction is already manifesting in society to a degree, but we are still falling far short of what is necessary for helping human beings to live in more harmony with one another and with the natural world.

In reference to Darwin's and Wohlleben's predictions, focusing a Bowen theory lens on human behavior enhances people's capacity to see the consequences of their actions. As a clinician, I am impressed that, as people come face to face with the deleterious consequences of some of their actions due to lack of "self," no one needs to tell them to function with more "self." People want to do it—it is a kind of instinctive morality.

Bowen theory is not a *prescription* for what people "should" do; it is a *description* of what people do. The theory is an attempt to move toward a science of human behavior, a theory based on verifiable functional facts about human behavior that can make predictions. Being descriptive rather than prescriptive, it may be confusing to conflate the responsibility to improve one's ability to function as a "self" with morality. What I am suggesting is that Bowen theory contributes to what E. O. Wilson described in his book *Consilience: The Unity of Knowledge* (1998). Differentiation of self is one bridge for a consilience between science and the humanities that Wilson is advocating. A science of human behavior can inform the development of a culture's values, morals, and ethics, matching their content with what is known factually to enhance the emotional functioning both of individuals and of the group.

In preparing to write this chapter on the process of differentiation of self, I reread the chapter in *Family Therapy in Clinical Practice* (1978, pp. 467–528) that describes Bowen's efforts to differentiate a self in his family of origin. The denouement he describes occurring during a trip to his hometown where his parents and most of the family still lived came after a twelve-year increasingly enlightened effort to be in close contact with the family without emotionally fusing into the system. He wrote that chapter several years after he presented a shorter description of his visit at the Family Research Conference in Philadelphia in 1967, which I referenced in the introduction to this volume. The chapter is a must-read for any student of Bowen theory. The possibility of differentiating more of a "self" in one's family of origin as an adult is one of Bowen theory's most important contributions.

After reading the chapter—and having read it many times over the years—I am in awe of Bowen's preparation for being in contact with his then fairly anxious family system and yet remain outside the emotionality or family emotional field, and then to successfully implement his plan. He did something no one had ever done before. Theory led the way, particularly the concepts of what it looks like to be in contact with but outside an emotional system, triangles, and chronic anxiety. No one had done it before because no one had ever had a theoretical framework to guide the endeavor. Bowen generated that framework from family research and then had the courage and conviction to apply it to his own family. A palpable improvement in his family's functioning after his time at home helped validate the accuracy of the theory.

In August 2015 I made a presentation about Bowen theory at a summer weekly forum held on the island in Maine, where I have lived since 2011. I had worked for several months to present the core ideas in a way that would be heard by a non-mental health professional audience of people largely unfamiliar with Bowen theory. I wanted the ideas to resonate with the audience. I was not trying to convince anyone about the accuracy and usefulness of Bowen theory, but if people disagreed with the ideas, I wanted them to be clear what they were rejecting. A year later at a social function on the island, I sat at dinner with a woman who had attended that talk. She told me she liked the talk very much and that she had had various kinds of therapy in the past. She added, "The ideas are very interesting and compelling, but I don't think I could apply them to my family." I responded by saying, "With some help, I think you could." I said that because when people respond positively—not all do—to presentations about Bowen theory, it usually means that the ideas resonate with them. They glimpse how the ideas match their own experience, which typically motivates people to learn theory and try to apply it successfully in their own lives.

Resonance with the ideas notwithstanding, the task of differentiating a self in one's family system can seem overwhelming at first blush. Many people have read about the ideas and tried to apply them in their families but usually get stuck at some point early in their effort. People being fairly reactive to the emotionality in their own family is the rule rather than the exception. The reactivity can manifest in idealizing or denigrating the family and many gradations between. Therapists or coaches who have been down the differentiation road in their own family, is almost always necessary for a successful effort. I often referred to Murray Bowen as the only "uncoached coach" that I ever met. (I amplify a bit how the therapist or "coach" helps further below.)

I thought again about the woman's comment at dinner when I revisited Bowen's presentation about his own family. Many people read Bowen's paper and think they could never do what he did in their families. People commonly miss that the theory applies to all families, but not everyone has to proceed like Bowen did. No one family is exactly like any other. The principal reason people run into problems in applying theory to their families is failing to approach their family with a sufficient understanding of a natural systems framework to help make sense out of what they are encountering. If people can think systems about family interactions, see the family as an emotional unit, new options for approaching the family come into view. One person's options may be very different from another's.

Viewing the family as an emotional unit is a radically different mind-set than one guided by individual theory. Individual theory tends to promote diagnosing family members rather than seeing the flow of emotional forces in the system that regulates everyone's functioning. It is critically important to keep in mind that the goal is not to fix one's family but to interact with more ability not to fuse emotionally into the system than has been the case in the past, to do a better job of maintaining "self" when in close emotional contact with the family. Achieving this goal is of more use to the family than anything else a person can do. Staying outside the system feels distinctly counterintuitive to people who have worked long and hard to fit into their families by being supportive and understanding and to quell selfish desires. Differentiation of self is attractive to a family—notwithstanding the frequency of immediate and automatic efforts by other family members to undercut it—because of the emotional neutrality associated with it. Well-differentiated functioning is a firm direction for oneself that is accompanied by an absence of judgments, blaming, and trying to change others. It contributes to others being thoughtful as well.

I now move on to describe six ingredients crucial to the success of functioning as more of "self" in one's family.

OBSERVE AND THINK ABOUT EMOTIONAL PROCESS

This involves observing oneself and one's relationship system to gain knowledge about the part self plays, the parts others play, the reciprocity, the triangles, and the other patterns of emotional functioning in a relationship system. Bowen theory is a lens that helps focus on important observations. It is sometimes hard for people to fathom that it is possible to be interacting in a relationship system and to observe your impact on the emotional functioning of others and their impact on you. In fact, you can surmise how you change the system and how the system changes you. An example of doing this occurred in a phone conversation with my mother in the aftermath of my brother's suicide. The conversation occurred a few weeks after her worried sister and husband pressured her to leave her apartment outside of Philadelphia and live in their house in western Pennsylvania. This was several months after my brother's death.

Up until that time, the relationship between Mother and me had, for better or for worse, generally been conflict-free. In this phone call, however, she was uncharacteristically negative and critical of me. I felt quite defensive at first, but it soon dawned on me that the tension in our relationship at that moment was a part of Mother and me being one side of a triangle involving her next oldest sister.

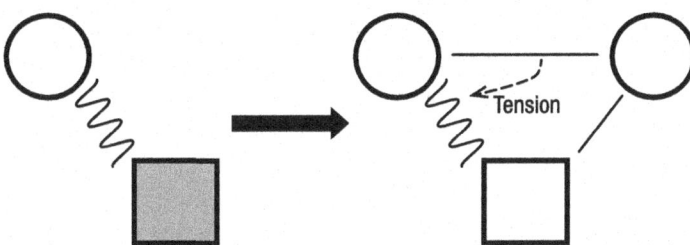

Figure 15.1 *This diagram depicts an unexpected and tense interaction with my Mother and the value of the concept of a triangle for reducing my reactivity to mother's accusations about me. The jagged black line on the left side of the diagram symbolizes Mother's harsh criticism of me. The diagram on the right my conceptualization of the triangle at work. Tension between Mother and her sister was playing out in Mother's relationship with me.*

This process is diagrammed in Figure 15.1. I cannot say this is exactly how I experienced it in my mind, but I recall picturing it in some fashion. My intellectual system was able to access the mindware of the triangle that I had learned about from studying Bowen theory. The left diagram symbolizes when I was thinking of the conflict as something pertaining to just Mother and me and experiencing my initial anxious defensive response (shading) to her criticism. In the right diagram, the third person to the far right being my aunt; this symbolizes my hypothesis that the interaction between Mother and me was embedded in a triangle. I also symbolize (no shading) the calming effect on me once I started thinking triangle. It was not personal; it was about the laws of triangles. An anxious triangle commonly has one negative side. The tension unexpressed and unaddressed between Mother and her sister was manifesting as conflict between Mother and me. I was able to see the flow of emotions in the triangle (process thinking) and escape focusing on her criticism of me (content thinking).

Part of the reason I could hypothesize a triangle being at work is that I knew from decades of experience with Mother and this sister that their relationship placed a premium on harmony, no matter how high the worry level in my aunt and how intense Mother's reaction to it was. Each would automatically say and do things to avoid conflict between them, and the issues in their relationship were never addressed. Her sister was the overfunctioning one, a mother figure for her generation, and Mother was drifting more and more into an underfunctioning position with associated symptoms (depression and childlike neediness) as I described in the epilogue.

When I realized that Mother and I were on the negative side of a triangle, the threat level I was experiencing plummeted. I refer to this dramatic reduction in my anxiety in response to a more objective view of what was playing out as a "systems miracle." The shift from cause-and-effect to systems thinking interrupts taking things personally. It is like a new information-processing highway has miraculously opened in the brain.

Armed with perspective on the triangle, I asked Mother in an off-handed way if she was enjoying the time with her sister. My tone, which was calm and friendly, as much as the content of what I said, is what communicated that I was not caught in the triangle. Continuing to be reactive to Mother's criticism would have kept me caught in the triangle. She did not answer the question, but her critical tone disappeared. I surmised from that change in her that I had successfully detriangled. This means I was able to communicate being outside the emotional process of the triangle at that point in time. It is not necessary to explain Bowen theory to one's family to detriangle. A dividend is that my detriangling allowed us to move on to a more personal conversation about how she was doing and how I was doing. It was a calming exchange for Mother because I think she benefited from contact with someone outside the triangle. It did not change the interaction between Mother and her sister, as there were plenty of other family members in western Pennsylvania to side with my aunt that her worry about Mother was justified.

DISCRIMINATE BETWEEN THINKING AND FEELING

My initial response to Mother's tone of voice and content was a subjective feeling reaction, which I recognized as such. Having the mindware of the triangle concept available provided an objectivity about the process that was unfolding. It allowed me to think as well as feel in response to what was happening. Using only dyadic thinking, one might say that Mother was trying to pick a fight and I did not take the bait. Failing to think in terms of triangles would have left out seeing that both Mother and my aunt played a part in the tension between us and that any reactivity on my part would be reinforcing the triangle. The recognition of the triangle provided a level of neutrality that was not feigned and would not have been possible by thinking that Mother wanted to pick a fight with me. Constrained by dyadic thinking, I could easily have gotten stuck (miffed, for example) in why she was trying to pick a fight, which is content focused and not process thinking.

Bowen theory is a lens that describes variability—between people and in the same person over time—in the capacity to distinguish thoughts from feelings, objective thinking from subjective thinking. It is unknown at this point exactly how the brain accomplishes this, but Bowen theory considers it a function of its concept of an intellectual system. (Again, this capacity seems to use brain operations that are different than those involved with intelligence.) The expansion of the number variables that systems thinking includes, by observing the relationship system in which one is embedded and seeing its reciprocal relationship to one's internal experiences, seems to be the important element in freeing people from cause-and-effect thinking and intense feeling states (which can obscure fact-based thinking) that often accompany cause-and-effect thinking applied to human behavior.

RECOGNIZE THE IMPACT OF ANXIETY ON FUNCTIONING

Anxiety can powerfully affect thoughts, feelings, and actions. Acute anxiety occurs in response to an immediate or imminent real threat. People are keenly aware of acute anxiety. Neuroscientist Joseph LeDoux equates Bowen theory's concept of acute anxiety with fear (LeDoux & Pine, 2016). Fear is a feeling state accompanied by fight, flight, or freeze behaviors and the physiological changes that support those behaviors. Chronic anxiety occurs in response to threats that are uncertain or distant in space and time. Such threats are commonly more imagined than real and associated with relationships. LeDoux terms Bowen theory's concept of chronic anxiety as simply *anxiety*.

Clinical and personal observations have led me to the conclusion that human beings are commonly less consciously aware of chronic anxiety than of acute anxiety. One piece of evidence for this is that if people develop some type of heightened chronic-anxiety-related clinical symptom, they frequently reflect on the period leading up to the development of the symptom and only then realize that they were stressed during the days, weeks, or months before the symptom manifested.

If my clinical judgment is correct that people have less subjective awareness of chronic than acute anxiety, Joseph LeDoux and Daniel Pine's (2016) research may shed light on why this is the case. Their research supports previous findings that the subcortical circuits that support acute anxiety are different from the ones that support chronic anxiety (Walker, Toufexis, & Davis,

2003). They also conclude that the subcortical circuits for anxiety trigger behavioral and physiological adjustments but do not mediate the subjective experience of anxiety.

LeDoux and some other neuroscientists now think that the subcortical circuits trigger cortical circuits that mediate the subjective experience of anxiety. LeDoux and Pine (2016) also think that both nonemotional and emotional states of consciousness emerge from the cortical networks that mediate consciousness. These conscious networks are not yet well defined, but it is possible that the subcortical circuits involved in acute anxiety are stronger than those involved in chronic anxiety. It is also possible that different cortical circuits mediate the subjective manifestations of acute versus chronic anxiety.

Being aware of chronic anxiety in oneself and in the relationship system is important. For example, recent research by Nicole Powell and colleagues (Powell et al., 2013) has demonstrated the importance of social stress in promoting the chronic inflammation that plays a key role in a wide range of clinical conditions. Epinephrine and norepinephrine, hormones that are increased as part of the body's stress response, affect bone marrow precursor cells in such a way as to result in proinflammatory white cells becoming numerous in the blood stream. Like hypertension, chronic anxiety could one day be known as the "silent killer."

People can get into a position in their important relationship systems that compromises them but not be consciously aware of the toll it is taking on them. From a Bowen theory perspective, an anxious relationship system and a person's anxious reaction to it is likely key to stimulating a chronic stress response that promotes chronic inflammation somewhere in the body. The specific place in the body the inflammation plays out would be governed by other biological and psychological variables. Presumably a chronic stress response and other mechanisms of brain-body connection also affect physiological systems besides the immune system that can contribute to organ and tissue dysfunction. Bowen theory is unique in describing how specific relationship interactions affect family and other important social relationship systems to generate chronic anxiety. Knowing about these specifics helps in becoming more aware of chronic anxiety (such as with the triangle example with Mother and my aunt) and for doing something about it. It is an odd paradox that our most intimate human relationships can heal (comfortable interactions) or promote clinical dysfunction (anxiety infected interactions).

My experience with studying psoriasis helps illustrate the difficulty being adequately aware of one's level of chronic anxiety. I got interested in the clinical manifestations of psoriasis in the 1970s and also the biological processes creating those manifestations, which led to a published paper (Kerr, 1992). Learning that many of the biological processes involved in psoriasis are similar to those operating in other clinical conditions contributed to my suggesting a new concept in Bowen theory called *unidisease* (described in Chapter 23). The unidisease concept holds that a wide range of diseases have a number physiological processes in common, such as inflammation, and the activity of those processes may better predict clinical course than the disturbances (pathology) present in the organ and tissue. Elevating the idea to a concept in Bowen theory is appropriate because it provides a bridge between chronic anxiety generated by family emotional process, a chronic anxiety-driven chronic stress response, and the stress response impact on physiological processes involved in most clinical conditions. It reinforces the idea that how family members interact can affect health as well as well-being.

Mother's psoriasis surfaced initially as an inflamed knee joint (psoriatic arthritis). She later developed what is referred to as plaque psoriasis on her skin. She was the first person to alert me to the idea that being stressed could bring on flare-ups of psoriasis. She had come to that conclusion over time. There were periods when she had no plaques at all, which she equated with calmer than usual periods in her life. Her comments about the role of stress were helpful to me when I realized in my late twenties that I had psoriasis too.

Psoriasis became a biologically based biofeedback system for me. Routinely, plaques developed on my elbows without my being subjectively aware that I had been in a more chronically anxious state. I call it biofeedback because I came to trust the appearance of the plaques as a more reliable indicator of my level of chronic anxiety than my subjective experience of the anxiety. When the plaques appeared, it helped me realize that I had been more tightly wound, more overly pressured—more vigilant, as I sometimes describe it—for an extended period of time than I had recognized.

Years ago when I was a medical intern, my chief of medicine said, "The secret to good health is to get a chronic illness and learn to live with it." He meant that a not immediately life-threatening illness can motivate a person to manage better the many factors that can affect exacerbations and remissions of a chronic illness; chronic stress is one of the important factors. The first step in addressing chronic anxiety is recognizing its presence.

The internet is full of advice for how to recognize when you are chronically stressed. Many of the phenomena people are advised to track have to do with physiological manifestations, such as tight muscles, twitching, upset stomach, sniffles, teeth grinding, recurring dreams, menstrual cycle changes, and losing hair. These signs of a disturbed physiology are commonly not associated with strong feeling states. At least, the feeling state does not rise to the highly gripping level that fear can.

One potentially useful marker for heightened chronic anxiety is feeling-driven attitudes and fantasies. It helps people to learn to observe better how what occupies their mind changes when they are more chronically anxious, for example, a person obsessing about the unfairness of life, or a husband being flooded with fantasies about another woman—these are indicators of heightened chronic anxiety. Given the difficulties of close human relationships, some degree of chronic anxiety is inevitable in all of us. Its impact on mind, body, and behavior, however, is frequently underestimated.

A quick aside here to clarify that Bowen theory holds that a history of exposure to abuse, trauma, and neglect as a child, which people commonly cite as causes of later-life problems, may correlate with but do not cause those problems. Bowen theory holds that if anxiety-driven symptoms exist in the present, an important relationship system disturbance exists in the present. This clarification is important because even people with exposure to Bowen theory often do not make this distinction. I am not insisting that the Bowen theory view is correct, but it is a valuable alternative to the conventionally held view. It is valuable because one cannot change the past, but one can make progress on what is playing out in the present and, consequently, reduce symptom-fueling chronic anxiety.

According to Bowen theory, exposure to events such as trauma and other adverse experiences as a child suggests that the person grew up in a poorly differentiated family. Trauma, abuse, and neglect are indicators or symptoms of a chronically anxious family system. The anxiety-driven intense emotional programming during childhood and limited development of "self" that are so prevalent in poorly differentiated families often render one or more children in such a family more vulnerable than others to relationship instability and associated chronic anxiety during adulthood.

Sibling variation in emotional functioning occurs in poorly differentiated families as well as in well-differentiated ones, and this may help explain why two siblings exposed to an environment filled with trauma, neglect, and abuse can have significantly different adult outcomes in terms of living fairly stable and productive lives. It is also the case that two siblings who have grown up in families with no evidence of abuse, trauma, and neglect can have significantly different adult life adjustments. Abuse, trauma, and neglect are not necessarily a part of every poorly differentiated family.

What probably helps most in reducing chronic anxiety is emotional objectivity and associated emotional neutrality. I would rate applying systems thinking in one's own life along with acting on the basis of the objectivity and neutrality that accrues from that effort as more effective than the myriad techniques available for stress reduction. It is even more effective than having a calming, non-fact-based belief system. I am not opposed to stress reduction techniques or calming beliefs, but such techniques alone seem not to solve the chronic anxiety associated with life's most difficult challenges, such as successful intimate relationships. It is one thing to improve one's ability to calm oneself based on a stress reduction technique, but it is quite another thing to grasp the specific triggers for anxiety in one's emotional environment and the ways self can trigger anxiety in others. Gaining more emotional objectivity and neutrality are key steps toward being able to function with more "self" in relationship systems.

ENGAGE EMOTIONALLY DIFFICULT SITUATIONS

When I was doing a child psychiatry fellowship, I had a supervisor based in the community who thought I was doing great work. At least he thought that until he attended a midyear faculty meeting at the department of psychiatry for the purpose of reviewing the performance of the fellows. This meeting occurred in January 1970, about two months after my brother's suicide.

The consensus of the faculty was that I was a potentially good trainee but that I did not seem enthusiastic about or take full advantage of my training experience. Some faculty members speculated that Murray Bowen, who was also supervising me at the time, was unduly influencing me away from psychoanalytic thinking. However, the majority thought I was depressed in reaction to my brother's suicide and could benefit from individual psychotherapy. When I had my regular meeting with that supervisor after the faculty meeting, he said he was taken completely by surprise by what he heard. Furthermore, he was persuaded that I would benefit from individual therapy to deal with my reaction to my brother's death. What happened next took me by surprise.

I told my supervisor that Murray Bowen was coaching me in dealing with my family in the aftermath of my brother's death and that it had been helpful. My supervisor abruptly got up from his chair, stood behind his desk and passionately exclaimed, "Mike, you can't solve your difficulties by dealing directly with your family. It's too difficult. You have to do it in the safe haven of a therapist's office!" At that moment, I especially realized what a gutsy pioneer Murray Bowen was in dealing with his own family and helping others do the same. He had bucked a powerful tide in the psychiatric profession. I soon realized that my supervisor's opinion was more prevalent in the psychiatric department than I had appreciated. The gist of the attitude was that your family caused your emotional problems, so it is the last place you want to go to try to work out those problems. That attitude encouraged cutting off from the family.

My supervisor's words "too difficult" particularly caught my attention. I thought later that of course it is difficult if you lack a theory to guide you. Armed with a theory, Bowen had the courage to engage the emotionally difficult and did it because that is where you learn the most about yourself. This approach means that you do not have to develop a transference relationship with a therapist to work on your intrapsychic problems. Changing in relationship to the people who shaped the original transference (Bowen theory uses the term *fusion* rather than *transference* to emphasize the reciprocity involved) that surfaces in one's adult relationships changes intrapsychic as well as relationship processes. In the early years of the family movement, many people did not accept this idea that relationship changes in the direction of functioning with more "self" would result in internal changes, biologically and psychologically. This method of working out one's problems in the real-world relationships rather than in a therapeutic relationship also greatly decreases the frequency of sessions necessary to make progress.

MAINTAIN MORE OF A "SELF" WITH OTHERS

This means being present and accounted for in a relationship system but outside the emotional process when that is important to do. The classes of behavior that reflect an inability to maintain "self" include intruding into the emotional space of others, pressuring others to function more to your liking, caving into the intrusiveness of others into your emotional space, and avoiding good emotional contact with others. Many invitations come our way each day to lose "self" by becoming part of a triangle. The invitations include a wide array of verbal and nonverbal cues. People talking about other people, conveying information about them to a third party, is wired into the social fabric.

Yuval Harari provides an important perspective on triangles to retard slipping into the notion that triangles are bad or pathological. He writes the following in his book *Sapiens*: "All apes show a keen interest in . . . social information, but they have trouble gossiping effectively. Neanderthals and archaic *Homo sapiens* probably also had a hard time talking behind each other's backs—a much maligned ability which is in fact essential for cooperation in large numbers" (2015, p. 23). A gossip system can be one manifestation of triangles. Harari suggests that, along with gossip, new linguistic skills that modern *Homo sapiens* began acquiring about seventy millennia ago (sentences and myths) allowed for imagined realities as well as objective reality enabling them to gossip for hours on end. Harari refers to this period as the Cognitive Revolution, which lasted almost 60,000 years. The gossip system provided reliable information about who could be trusted, which allowed small bands to expand into larger bands, which facilitated more sophisticated cooperation. He adds that the vast majority of the now many forms of human communication is gossip. Much gossip involves rumors about other people and their personal lives, particularly their wrongdoings. The World Wide Web has greatly expanded and intensified gossip networks. Hearing rumors about others can powerfully affect our opinion of and way of behaving toward them.

Bowen theory assumes that triangles have emotional roots that may be more ancient in evolution than the linguistics skills unique to Homo sapiens. Many animal researchers, such as Frans de Waal (2007), have observed coalition formation in the species they study. De Waal used the term *triadic awareness* to describe the ability of a chimpanzee to recognize that how two other chimps are interacting could affect him or her. Chimps selectively spend time with certain other chimps to form alliances that can enable the chimp, for example, to rise to a higher status in the group. Such behaviors are enhanced by chimp intelligence. This does not preclude, however, subcortical processes, which are older evolutionarily, playing an important role in coalition formations to help individuals get what they want.

It is unknown at this point how far back in evolution the roots of triangles extend as they operate in the human species. As described earlier in Chapter 3, Bowen theory conceptualizes triangles as the "molecule of an emotional system," the smallest relatively stable relationship system. Such a view seems more encompassing than what is captured by descriptions of coalitions and alliances in other primate and mammalian species. Triangles in Bowen theory are a pattern that binds system-generated anxiety in one part of the system and that helps to stabilize the system as a whole. Triangles do more than just building coalitions, but much is not understood about their evolutionary roots at present.

One could argue that three people could interact without it being a triangle. Exchange of information about others not present is not necessarily a bad thing, which is a point that Harari makes. The emotions and intelligence that support group formation and tribalism can operate in the service of coordination and cooperation. It is anxiety-generated emotional reactivity that turns useful gossip into having a potentially toxic impact on others. Awareness that in an anxious emotional field anxiety is flowing through interlocking triangles is essential for improving one's capacity to be a "self." Being aware of interlocking triangles and the impact of anxiety on them is key to maintaining "self," which in turn enables one not to fuse into an emotional system.

THEORETICAL THINKING AND SCIENTIFIC INQUIRY

People's efforts to improve their ability to be a "self" in their own families help them make the theory their own, not just something they read in a book. Success in functioning with more "self" in one relationship enhances the chances of being successful in other relationships. Another effort that promotes one's ability to increase "self" is pursuits that enhance theoretical thinking. I borrow the term *scientific inquiry* from biologist George C. Williams (1966) to characterize such pursuits.

Williams defines *scientific inquiry* as any combination of theoretical thinking, empiricism, and intuition that suits the investigator. I prefer Williams's term to *research*, because at this point in the development of Bowen theory, it is difficult to conduct research projects that meet the standards of science. One reason for this is that it is possible to observe functional facts of emotional process and to describe large networks of seemingly linked occurrences, but it is hard to put numbers on it or to find ways to prove one's observations. As I've mentioned before, people prove Bowen theory to themselves by applying it successfully and getting a predicted result.

A common and useful approach to the above lack of numbers relates to Williams's description of scientific inquiry, namely to search for inconsistencies between what is regarded as good scientific research and Bowen theory. I, for example, have conducted a considerable number of interviews of cancer patients and their families and have delved into the biology of cancer. I have concluded from my studies that emotional process could play a role in the onset and clinical course of cancer. However, I cannot prove my findings about cancer to others, nor can I do that with the many other clinical entities that I have systematically "inquired" about, such as autism, sociopathy, schizophrenia, depression, and the addictions. However, not discovering inconsistencies between scientifically accepted cancer research and a Bowen theory perspective on cancer helps support my conviction about the accuracy and usefulness of a Bowen theory perspective on cancer and other clinical entities. What this amounts to is knowing where you stand and knowing reasonably well where others stand who are doing different types of research on the same subjects and have other points of view on how to explain their findings. Understanding other points of view and seeing that they do not contradict Bowen theory helps to maintain "self" in one's professional life.

CHAPTER SIXTEEN

Personal Vignettes of the Process of Differentiation

RESEARCHING ONE'S FAMILY OF ORIGIN

In this chapter I will describe my effort to use most of the ingredients described in Chapter 15 in my effort to increase basic level of differentiation of self. Actually, it is more accurate to refer to the process as increasing solid self, which is one component of basic self. Progress in the family of origin does not transfer automatically to nuclear family relationships, but it helps considerably in nuclear family efforts. One reason the transfer is not automatic is that many important aspects of the relationships with one's parents and siblings replicate in the relationships with one's spouse and children, but one's spouse is not one's parent. Spouses bring aspects of their own unresolved attachment to their family of origin that must be observed and addressed. Another reason progress in family of origin does not transfer automatically to the nuclear family is that a person lives day in and day out with them, which makes the emotional process more intense and more difficult to observe objectively.

I have left out the nuclear family in the vignettes that follow to protect the privacy of those individuals, all of whom are living. All the members mentioned in my family of origin are now deceased, with the exception of my next oldest brother. I do not discuss vignettes that involved this next oldest brother for privacy reasons as well. The exception is a vignette involving my wife Kathy, which she fully endorsed my including.

Research on one's family makes a unique contribution to people's efforts to increase their basic level of differentiation of self. I described the multigenerational transmission process in Chapter 11 and the unique perspective it can provide. However, people must do research on their own families to acquire this perspective. Such a project enables a macroscopic view of family emotional process. People can often make some progress on differentiation without doing much multigenerational research, but it makes a unique contribution to the effort to develop more "self." Studying the multigenerational emotional system of one's family, coupled with gaining enough knowledge about evolution to convince oneself that the human emotional system has been shaped by billions of years of evolution, greatly facilitates making the transition from cause-and-effect to systems thinking.

I began multigenerational research on my family coincident with embarking on the process of learning Bowen theory. Such an effort involves gathering as much objective knowledge as one can about the family from a wide range of sources, such as genealogical records, birth certificates, death certificates, obituaries, census records, newspaper articles, real estate records, old letters, family bibles, and other sources. A particularly important aspect of the process is gathering remembrances of deceased relatives from a wide range of living relatives (parents, siblings, aunts, uncles, great-aunts, great-uncles, grandparents, close and distant cousins, and family friends). For many people, such an effort involves being in more contact with more family members than had been the case previously. Knowing something about how the lives of cousins, great-aunts, and great-uncles, for example, have unfolded gives one a unique sense of the mold from which one has been sprung. The purpose of this research is to have enough reasonably factual information to be able to view one's immediate family of origin in the context of at least four generations of multigenerational emotional process that shaped it. The most pertinent facts derived from the research on the maternal and paternal sides of the family are recorded on a family diagram as was described in Chapter 11.

I had interacted with many relatives in Mother's and Dad's families while growing up, but large gaps existed in my knowledge about the family, particularly three and four generations back. I had limited knowledge of my four grandparents (all but one of whom were deceased when I was growing up), their siblings, my eight great-grandparents, and the descendants of more distant branches of family. Murray Bowen often said that if people could develop "person to person" relationships with every member of their extended family, they would grow up in the process. The effort is an antidote to egocentrism by helping people to reflect on perspectives other than their own.

Being able to compare your family unit with units from other branches, some of which will reflect more stable and productive functioning than your immediate family and others less so, provides clues as to how multigenerational emotional process shaped your own immediate family of origin. The comparisons reveal the inevitable increases and decreases in emotional interdependence (fusion) of the various lines in any family. Family branches that are less stable and productive reflect a multigenerational increase in degree of emotional interdependence and associated higher than average level of chronic anxiety; those that are more stable and productive reflect a decrease in emotional interdependence and lower than average level of chronic anxiety. Being able to think about changes in levels of emotional interdependence as a key element for understanding variation in the emotional functioning of families is a step toward a more tolerant view of the human condition. No one has had control over how this process has played out, even though everyone participated in it.

People often lament or are angry about what may have been a particularly difficult family situation that they grew up in but with little clue about how it got to be that way. This narrow perspective renders people vulnerable to blaming their families for whatever tribulations they experienced in them. They may also descend into self-blame to explain their experiences. Some understanding of how things got to be the way they were over a few generations does not fully resolve feelings that are the legacy of a difficult environment while growing up, but it provides some equanimity. A quantum jump in equanimity occurs when people see that they do many of the same things their parents did but without slipping into guilt and anger with that revelation. Like it or not, people do not leave their families but take their families with them. It helps to remember that significantly dysfunctional branches of a family are not inferior families, just poorly adaptive families. Chronic-anxiety-driven emotional reactivity and subjectivity sap much of individual autonomy in such families, which makes for the unstable ship.

As I began my research and began to ask questions of various relatives about the family, I was impressed with how many versions of family history I got from different family members, particularly in reference to what people were like. This is probably not a surprise to most readers, but I had not really reflected on the phenomenon until I began the systematic research. So how do you gain more objective knowledge about the family when you are getting different stories from different people?

Many useful facts for deciphering emotional process are easily gathered through records of one sort or another, but the information about the emotional history of a family is greatly enhanced by the memories of living members. A tried and true principle of rational thinking is to seek multiple points of view before coming to a conclusion. I discovered that, by talking with enough people over time and reflecting on their many recollections, I could develop my own view of the family history by keeping the distinction between fact and opinion at the forefront of my mind. I developed my viewpoint without assuming it was the final word. This was an important early step toward becoming more of a "self" in the family. A manifestation of that change was that what one family member said to me about another less easily swayed my view of the person being described than in the past. In the past, I had been barely aware of how much one person's comments about another could affect my viewpoint about that third person. Now I could better discern opinion from fact. Another dividend of this effort to know more about the family was that, by being interested in a wide range of relatives and spending more time with them, it contributed to the family beginning to think of me as an individual in my own right, not just my parents' youngest son.

I visit the point many times in this book that rigidly holding onto a belief stems from challenges to that belief triggering a strong emotional response that closes down any chance of a more open mind. Interestingly, recent neuroscience research has shown that challenges to strongly held beliefs increase the activity of the default-mode network in the brain and also trigger a bold signal in the insula and amygdala (Kaplan, J., Gimbel, S. & Harris, S. 2016). The researchers conclude that their results highlight the role of emotion in resistance to changing to one's beliefs. The study of one's multigenerational family and the broad perspective it provides on the variation in emotional functioning in every family, as well as the recognition of how much all families are alike—the same processes at work, but with differences in degree—make one's family and the human condition in general more interesting. Being interesting is an antidote to feeling threatened. Threat triggers negative (critical) or overly idealized (defensive) emotions about one's family. The change in emotional state that comes from making it interesting helps to open one's mind.

The importance of talking to many close and distant relatives was brought out by what occurred when I began increasing my contact with my maternal extended family. As I sought information about my maternal grandmother, who died when I was a toddler, no one, including Mother, mentioned her significant drinking and depression in the later years of her life. It was not until I talked with an aunt by marriage in my mother's generation that I learned about my maternal grandmother's problems. When I told Mother what I had learned, she finally fessed up that indeed that was the case. Quoting Mother, "She was a saint but did drink a lot!" I guessed that Mother's earlier reluctance to mention her mother's drinking was related to protectiveness of her mother, wanting me to think well of her.

My grandmother's decline in functioning may have been related to feeling overwhelmed by the birth of a fourth child. In teaching, I sometimes draw an analogy between family process and a pinball machine tilting in response to a player applying too much motion to it. A family may adapt to having a certain number of kids but have its functioning drop dramatically when one more child is added—it is one more than the family organism can manage without a significant increase in symptoms. Mother was beginning to enter adolescence at that point, which helped me better understand how Mother's sensitivity to the unhappiness and distress of others might have been intensified by responding to her mother's distress. That dynamic was most strongly replicated in her relationship with my oldest full brother. Importantly, this understanding helped me be less judgmental and more tolerant of certain traits in Mother that also affected my development. What choice did Mother have about the nature of her emotional programming? A key to the shift in my thinking was being able to think about Mother as a child of her mother, not just as my Mother. I had similar experiences on my Dad's side, which I describe in Chapter 16 and the epilogue.

Researching one's own family results in more than a "roots" experience, although that is part of it. The phenomenon of the roots experience came more into the public consciousness with the publication of Alex Haley's 1976 novel *Roots* about his ancestry. Gaining a picture of the lives of one's ancestors over many generations is clearly valuable for bolstering one's sense of identity. People commonly have a strong emotional response to connecting with the past. Another emotional impact of researching one's own family is that making emotional contact with close and more distantly related members of one's family can have a unique calming effect. I term it *unique* because it is not something that usually occurs to that degree with nonfamily groups. People are usually treated as members of the family club in making these contacts. Because you are related to a somewhat distant branch of family but were not caught up in their emotional system as you grew up, they typically welcome your interest and readily discuss issues in their family with you. It is easier to be objective about more distant branches than about your more immediate family of origin.

As described in Chapter 13 about emotional cutoff, many people find their relationships with their family of origin so problematic that they want considerable distance from them. Some recoil at a suggestion that they could gain something by getting into closer contact with family. One man I saw in my family therapy practice announced, "The only reason I would go to see my family is to rehabilitate them!" People without much "self" can be quite vulnerable to being in closer contact with their families. This can manifest in strong negative opinions about their family. One person Murray Bowen encouraged to have better contact with his family exclaimed, "I went to see my family and was diagnosed with diabetes soon thereafter!" Bowen's rejoinder was, "Good, good! Keep going home until you don't get diabetes no more!" (M. Bowen, personal communication, July 1979). (Bowen had a penchant for colloquialisms.) His comment reflected his repeated clinical observation that people can learn to get less reactive to their families once they quit trying to change their families and, with the aid of theory and coaching, focus on changing self rather than others. People can get so focused on what is wrong with others that they are barely aware of how much they want to change them.

One's immediate family of origin is part of a larger multigenerational family. If people are highly reactive to their immediate families, such as their parents and siblings, they often find that by establishing contact with more distant branches of their family, such as with the siblings of their grandparents or their descendants, a more relaxed climate exists in those branches that can foster good connections and more objectivity. Beginning to view one's immediate family of origin in this larger context can take the edge off anticipating contact with one's parents and siblings.

One particularly memorable perspective generating experience in researching my own family occurred in April 1972 in a cemetery in Minneapolis, where many members of my father's family are buried. The moon was full that day and visible in daylight when I was at the cemetery. Snow was still on the ground, and men were walking on the moon. By the time of that cemetery visit, I had gained a great deal of information about Dad's grandparents, his parents, and their siblings. Part of this information came from records, such as birth and death certificates and old newspapers, and part of it came from listening to multiple stories from Dad's sister (Dad had died in 1962), sister-in-law, her daughter, and some distant cousins who were either old enough to remember my grandparents' family or had heard things from their parents and other family members that I never knew. While at the cemetery, I reflected on the many tribulations that I had learned my Dad's family had experienced. I asked myself whether I was all that different from them and decided we were far more alike than different. It was a leveling and comforting feeling.

A related experience was driving with my mother around her hometown in about 1975. Unlike Mother, many of her closest relatives had stayed in the home area to raise their families. Her third-born sister had stayed, and many of her children and grandchildren lived in the area. We had seen many of them during this particular visit to western Pennsylvania. Reflecting on the experiences of that visit as we drove, Mother said, "I can see now that I was in too big a hurry to get away from this town and to push my children to take advantage of opportunities I did not think were possible here. As I look at my sister's children and grandchildren and see how well they are doing, I can see the advantage of being more patient." I do not know if Mother was thinking about my schizophrenic brother at that moment, but I suspect she was. I found it very satisfying to hear about her reflections and pleased that I had played some part in it by taking more interest in the family than would have been the case without Bowen theory. It was amazing to realize how much of my knowledge about Mother had been colored by bias and reactivity until I began to learn more about her and her family. This was an important element in resolving my unresolved attachment to her.

Expectations about how one's family should be and harboring disappointment about expectations unmet are common. Family research revealing the universality of family difficulties gives credence to the adage "it is what it is."

That recognition can reduce counterproductive anxiety-driven urges to push to make things how they "should be." That alone can reduce family anxiety and help each family member be a little more thoughtful. This is not about giving up but about growing up. It is useful to remind oneself that being more of a "self" usually brings out more of the best in others.

I believe that the amount of chronic-anxiety-driven unrealistic expectations that people have of themselves and others usually exceeds realistic expectations, particularly in intimate relationships. It is hard to see this when you are living it, but theory can help bring it into focus. Through family research, I came to understand that what happened in my parent's families of origin had powerfully shaped my life. I had known that intellectually, but there was something about connecting the intellectual knowledge with the emotional experience of being, for example, at the cemetery that was important. Many people say that they realize that their parents did the best they could. The comment is often conveyed with an attitude of forgiveness. Awareness of multigenerational emotional process provides solid evidence for going beyond forgiveness as a feeling to knowing objectively that one's parents did the best they could. I think this is not a Pollyanna attitude but a conclusion based on recognition of the limits multigenerational emotional process imposes on human emotional autonomy. Nor, of course, does this attitude absolve people of responsibility for their actions.

On Mother's side, by spending time with a few of my elderly great-aunts who still lived in western Pennsylvania near where they were born, I learned that four of their male siblings (there were five males in that ten-children family) did not marry until in their forties and after their mother died. Male adult children who remained quite involved with their mothers well into adult life were fairly common in Mother's family of origin. It was primarily an emotional dependence on their parents, not a financial one, but it struck me that males slowly leaving the nest was in the emotional fabric of Mother's family. The situation with my great-uncles was not as extreme as my oldest full brother's was but more common than I had realized. This realization provided a useful perspective for not blaming Mother or my brother for the unresolved interdependence between them. As I write in the epilogue, I had the attitude initially that the situation between Mother and my schizophrenic brother "shouldn't be" that way, but as I learned more about the multigenerational family it cleansed me of that attitude. Many people would say my brother did not lift off because of his schizophrenia. From a Bowen theory perspective, something more basic and multigenerational had unfolded that eroded his developing "self" and rendered him vulnerable to such an outcome.

THE VALUE OF A COACH IN THE PROCESS OF DIFFERENTIATION

An important experience related to coaching occurred in 1969, soon after I began coaching sessions with Murray Bowen. I was living in the Washington, D.C., area with my wife and firstborn daughter. Mother and my oldest full brother were living together in an apartment in a Philadelphia suburb. I was planning a weekend visit there. My oldest brother from Mother's first marriage and his family would be involved in the visit as well. I had a coaching session with Bowen on the Monday before my weekend visit. Bowen helped me think about entering what could be an anxious emotional field and its potential impact. I recall expressing confidence that I could deal with the situation.

I made the visit, and it turned out that I had no clue how much I had fused into the emotional system that weekend at home. My wake-up call for what had happened did not occur until I had a scheduled meeting with Bowen the Monday morning after my weekend visit. I opened the session with what turned out to be a long monologue describing my visit home. It lasted the better part of a half-hour. It ended when I finally looked at Bowen and noticed a slight smile on his face. My reaction to seeing his facial expression was, "What the hell is he smiling at—this isn't funny!" Well, bingo, my head cleared. I did not realize until that moment how anxious I was in describing my visit and how anxious my family and I were when I was there. I also realized that I had been more chronically anxious in anticipating the visit than I had realized. I had been more emotionally fused into the system anticipating the visit as well as during the visit than I had realized.

The experiences of becoming aware of how anxious I had been over the weekend and how anxious I was in the first part of the consultation with Bowen helped me gain an inkling of what it would be like to be in contact with the family emotional field but outside of it. It was an excitingly, novel experience because before I had no sense of what that would be like. I had greatly underestimated my level of chronic anxiety and, in retrospect, had done so for years.

Something I have never forgotten is that Bowen did not need to tell me that I had been caught in the system; he simply did not get caught in my anxiety, and that was enough to get me out of it. He was emotionally neutral and present to me during the session. A series of experiences like this over time gradually helped me know more about what I am like when I am more chronically anxious and what it looks like in the family. Being able to recognize more behaviors that are associated with chronic anxiety in others and in me was a valuable step.

SEEING MY UNRESOLVED ATTACHMENT TO MOTHER REPLICATED IN MY MARRIAGE

I described an example in Chapter 8 on emotional objectivity of seeing a reciprocal process play out between my mother and me, the incident involving the stairway. A dividend of what unfolded after gaining more emotional objectivity about that interaction with my mother resulted a few weeks later with my wife. I was sitting with her on the couch in the living room, and she was distressed about something—I do not recall what it was, and the content is not that important anyway. I listened and responded to what she was saying, but then I suddenly realized that what had unfolded between Mother and me was now unfolding between my wife and me. She was distressed and conveying an expectation that I should do something to remedy the situation. I was feeling anxious and guilty, and I was paralyzed about what to do other than to sit and listen. Realizing the reciprocal interaction that was unfolding, after listening for fifteen or twenty minutes I turned to my wife and said, "I realize that you are upset, and I would like to be able to say or do something to relieve it—in the past such an interaction could go on for an hour or two, and the emotional climate even linger over a few days—but I have something I need to do upstairs and am going to do that now." I got up from the couch and climbed the stairs. My legs felt like they weighed a hundred pounds each, but I made it to the top of the stairs and managed to attend to what I said I needed to do.

This may seem like a minor incident, but it captured one of the more fundamental patterns in our relationship: she got upset about whatever, and I would get passive and fumble around saying things in the hope it would relieve the situation, all the while wanting to distance emotionally. Seeing that pattern between Mother and me enabled me to see the identical reciprocal interaction between my wife and me. When I chose to walk up those stairs, I was not blaming my wife and not distancing emotionally. The slight resolution of the unresolved attachment with Mother had enabled me to see it in the marital relationship. My wife later said, "As I watched you walk up those stairs, I did not like it, but thought you were finally being your own person." These were only very early steps of progress in the relationship with Mother and in the marriage.

AFTERMATH OF MY BROTHER'S SUICIDE

An extremely important period for me in working on differentiation of self was in the aftermath of my schizophrenic brother's suicide, which occurred in November 1969. I describe the emotional process in my family of origin in the epilogue of this book, but that piece ends with the suicide and the ensuing three months. Here I describe the later winter to late spring of 1970. It is possible that my efforts to maintain "self" during that period saved my mother's life.

During the first three months after the suicide, despite efforts by one of her sisters, Kitty, and Kitty's husband, Dick, to persuade Mother to go back to their home in western Pennsylvania, Mother insisted on staying in Swarthmore in her apartment. It was very difficult emotionally for all of us, but especially for Mother, of course. She talked openly on the phone about what it was like. It was difficult to listen, but I listened. I was again struck by how she seemed to know that the apartment was the place she needed to be to get through this. Kitty called often, as she was very worried about Mother, but had to accept Mother's decision.

Things turned for the worse in the middle of February 1970. Kitty and Dick drove to Swarthmore to spend some time with Mother, their first trip since the funeral. This time, under considerable pressure from them, Mother agreed to go back to western Pennsylvania, to the town of Sidman, where she grew up and Kitty and Dick still lived. They were hoping she would stay there permanently. However, when Mother got to Sidman, her functioning declined markedly. She became childlike, not unlike a steep decline in her functioning that had happened years earlier when my parents lived for a few years on Maryland's Eastern Shore, a period I describe in the epilogue in which Mother's functioning nose-dived. Kitty, Dick, and the three of their five children that lived near them were all anxiously focused on Mother. When I would visit Sidman, which I did several times during the next four months, Kitty and her family would corner me in the kitchen, out of Mother's earshot, and lament, "Your mother is not good, Michael, not good." The anxiety was palpable.

A family physician was very involved with Mother's case. He saw her frequently and prescribed tranquilizers, antidepressants, and sleep medications for her. Mother was pretty drugged up and lethargic. The doctor and all of Kitty's family were operating on the assumption that Mother's emotional state was a depression caused by Billy's death.

Systems theory helped me see things differently. It was a shaky time for Mother, and she was extremely vulnerable. I saw the decline in her functioning as related to living in the midst of such an anxious emotional field in Sidman. These were people who meant well but, in Bowen theory terms, were overfunctioning and Mother was underfunctioning. She was acting helpless and lost, and they were treating her as if only medications and time could fix that.

During the period in Maryland, we would take Mother up to Sidman to spend weeks with Kitty, and she would recover there. Removing her from the anxious environment in Maryland to what was then a calmer healing environment in Sidman worked consistently. The problem was that when she came back to Maryland, she would inevitably go into a nosedive again within a matter of months. Three months after Billy's suicide, mother was taken out of an environment in Swarthmore in which she could manage and placed into a highly anxious environment in Sidman, in which she could not thrive. As I reflect on both of those periods, mother's vulnerability to dysfunction in an anxious environment in which she was the focus indicates her own tenuous level of "self."

One of the complications of this situation was that, even though Mother was unable to make a decision to move back home, she would call Bob, my oldest brother, from Mother's first marriage, and his wife, Marjorie, back in the Philadelphia area and tell them that she wanted to move back to her apartment. This triggered panic in Bob's family because, hearing the descriptions coming out of the family in Sidman and hearing Mother's distress on the phone, Bob did not feel capable of dealing with Mother if she was nearby in that emotional state. Marjorie was anxious about Bob in that regard as well. Bob watched a mole on his arm begin to grow larger and darker starting in early March. It was May before he had his doctor look at it. He was immediately referred for a biopsy: stage II malignant melanoma. An operation was scheduled for early June. When I heard the news in May, I was not surprised. These were not the best of times; these were the worst of times.

I made a trip to Sidman by myself over Memorial Day weekend. I had thought the situation through using Bowen theory as a guide and had plans for how to handle myself when I was there. I thought Mother could die in this situation, and Bob's cancer diagnosis was weighing on me as well. I thought his cancer was related to the emotional upheaval of the family. It was a very regressed situation.

I arrived in Sidman on Friday night and found mother so spaced out on medications that useful communication was impossible. I finally said to her, "You are on so much medication, I can't talk with you. Please do something about that." She took no more medications and by the next day was much more available. We took a walk around town and talked. Vintage Mother, she expressed her worry about the impact of her problems on Kitty and said she wanted to go home but did not feel as if she had the strength to do it. I listened but did not take a side on what decision she should make. I did say, "It sounds like you want to go home." I had also made a decision prior to the trip to visit by myself all three of Kitty's children living in the area. I had gained a reputation in Kitty's family for not taking Mother's problems seriously enough. The kids were hearing that from their parents. I wanted to communicate by my presence that I was there and was appropriately concerned about Mother's situation and Kitty and Dick's dilemmas dealing with it. My cousins were glad to see me and, I think, felt reassured by my visit.

Later in the day I invited Kitty to take a car ride with me. I drove and vowed to myself to keep driving until the climate of uneasiness between Kitty and me broke. It took a while. She said, "Michael, dear, I am so worried about your mother. I know that she wants to go back home, but I fear that she can't do it." She had much more to say, of course—we were driving for over an hour—but my response was, "You know, Kitty, when this is over, maybe you could write a book about it!" Well, she laughed and things loosened up between us. She appreciated my being there.

At the end of that day, Kitty, as her custom on a holiday weekend, served dinner at her place. All the cousins living in the area and their kids were there, about twenty people in all. About ten of us were at the table at any one time. I sat down at the early shift, and Mother sat across from me. Kitty and Dick were there, too, along with a several cousins. Not long into the meal, I spoke and described my ride with Kitty that afternoon. I could see Kitty react to my bringing it up, but she did not say anything. I said, "Kitty was telling me how worried she was about Mother and that she is at her wit's end about how to help her." Mother immediately got up and left the table. She circled through the living room and eventually returned to the table when she heard others talking. Two of my cousins had a lot to say about the situation, agreeing that it was taking a toll on Kitty and Dick, not just my Mother. The conversation was not tense, which was striking because these sorts of things tended to get murmured about behind closed doors, out of earshot of the parties most directly involved. The conversation went on for more than a half hour and then shifted to humorous things, which the family is very good at. Mother did not say anything, but she was listening carefully.

My plan ahead of time was to bring up the subject of Mother in the group in a calm and matter-of-fact way. I had hoped people would respond—they did, and I was very pleased. I was unsure what impact it might have but thought my being present, not critical of anyone, and not pushing for a particular solution might help. I saw the anxious interplay between Mother and Kitty as a reciprocal interaction that imprisoned both people.

The next day—Sunday—was a fun kind of day with softball outside, a trip with Mother to a favorite place of hers in Sidman, and a pass by where she once taught school before marrying her first husband. I returned to D.C. on Monday.

I talked with Mother by phone on Tuesday or Wednesday night, and she announced that she had flushed all of her pills down the toilet and that she was going back home. Her voice was clear and firm. Dick and Kitty had agreed to drive her back later that week. She had called Bob and, without conveying a helplessness or neediness, told him of her decision and plans. Bob was to have his surgery on the melanoma later in the week. Mother expressed her love and concerns for him but said, "I'm sure everything will be all right." It was.

I went up to the hospital near Swarthmore the night before his surgery to be with Bob and his family. The melanoma was easily removed, the edges proved to be clean of tumor, and a skin transplant went smoothly. When I saw Murray Bowen early the following week, he was on his way out the door of the psychiatry department. I told him that the doctors were expecting a cure for Bob. Murray smiled and said, "Predictable!" He meant that the lancing of the boil of family tensions boded a good prognosis for Bob. Bob died thirty-eight years later of unrelated causes.

Mother made an excellent adjustment after returning home to her apartment, where she lived until her death sixteen years later. Billy had been buried in the same cemetery where my Dad was buried and where Mother was to be buried when she died. My parents' infant daughter who died soon after birth was buried there as well.

I visited the cemetery many times with Mother until she died and occasionally after Dad, Mother, and Billy had all died. Each visit was a time to reflect on the extraordinary emotional power of the interactions among the three of them and to remind myself how much my life had benefited from the amount of family anxiety that was tied up with Billy. (You may notice that one of the people I have dedicated this book to is Oscar William "Billy" Kerr III.) Murray Bowen occasionally commented, "We all grow up on the backs of schizophrenia!" He meant that Billy had inherited the weaknesses of the family, and siblings like me were thus somewhat freer to inherit the strengths. It is a phenomenon that plays out in every family to varying degrees.

SEEING AN IMPORTANT TRIANGLE

Another triangle I observed and addressed was related to my oldest brother, his wife, and Mother, with Dad and the rest of us siblings caught up in it. The triangle formed in the late 1940s when my oldest brother got engaged to the woman whom he married in 1950. I will not detail the content of the issues involved other than it was a religious bias. Mother did not want my brother to marry this young woman. She threatened to boycott the wedding and to cut my brother out of my parents' will. Dad was not opposed to his son's marriage but sided with Mother. My brother was not dissuaded and married this young woman. Mother backed down on all of her threats. This negative attitude about my brother's new wife continued after they were married. It was not overtly conflicted between our sister-in-law and Mother but more about negative comments behind her back. Dad continued to outwardly side with

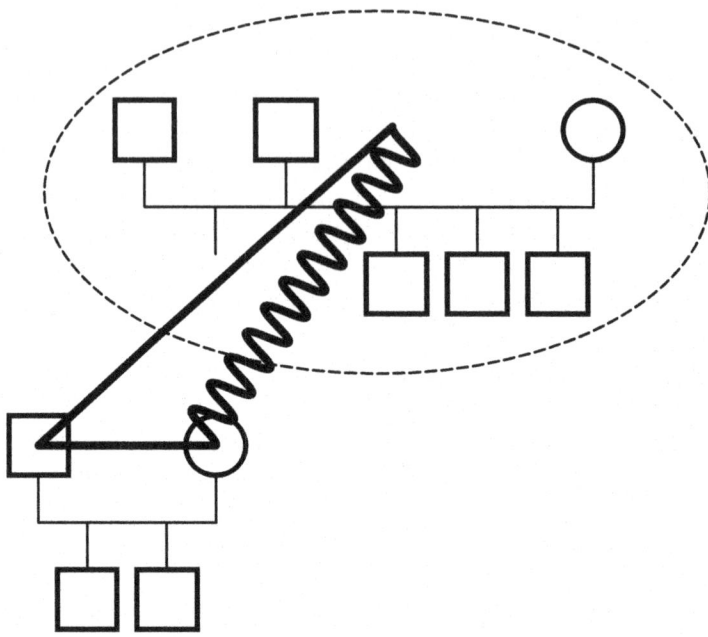

Figure 16.1 *This diagram depicts how the concept of the triangle applied to my family of origin's relationship with my half-brother and his wife. The triangle depicts the negative side as between my family grouped at one corner of the triangle, my sister-and-law in the outside position, my family being negative about her, mostly by talking about her behind her back, and a positive relationship between my brother and our family. My brother gained some support from the family taking sides in his marriage.*

Mother, and the three of us younger boys were drawn into to seeing it from Mother's point of view.

Figure 16.1 symbolizes the triangle that I came to understand after being exposed to Bowen theory. The symbols in the top half of the diagram are for Mother's first husband, my parents, and the three sons from this second marriage. The symbols for my oldest brother (half-brother), his wife, and their two young sons are in the lower half of the diagram. The diagram's squiggly line between my sister-in-law and my family of origin symbolizes the negative relationship between her and my family of origin. No conflict is symbolized between our family and my oldest brother because the family remained positive about my oldest brother and blamed the situation on the woman he married. The dashed circle around my family of origin symbolizes that we were generally of one mind that my brother's wife was the problem.

I included the simple diagram in describing this family process to emphasize how important learning about the triangle concept was to seeing the situation in what was for me a radically new way. I do not remember if Bowen pointed this out to me as being a triangle or if I figured it out for myself, but I think it was the latter—no matter, he figured out the concept and I applied it.

The first dividend from this new way of thinking was observing on a trip home the many subtle negative comments my oldest brother made about his wife. I had never noticed that before. Much of it had been conveyed nonverbally. I also observed that no one in the family challenged his comments. He did this not in front of his wife but during times when she was not with him. I had not seen until then how my oldest brother helped create and sustain this triangle. The reader might ask whether I could explain this triangle to the family as a way of addressing it. Experience has shown that trying to explain emotional process to one's own family on a rational level does not work—people tend to get defensive. Trying to explain it to the family usually reflects one's own anxiety.

I made the observations about the triangle while still living in Washington, D.C., on one of my fairly frequent trips home. Realizing that the triangle involving my oldest brother and sister-in-law had interfered with my relationship with her, I made a point of trying to make better personal contact with my sister-in-law on my trips. The other thing I made a point of doing was visiting my sister-in-law's mother, who lived in the same area where Mother and my brother and family lived. Naturally, my sister-in-law appreciated that. My sister-in-law's mother died when I was later serving in the Navy and living in the Midwest. My wife and I and our then two daughters came east to attend the funeral. This was a clear statement to my family that I was not buying into all the negativity about my sister-in-law. Being present at such times in one's family goes a very long way to opening up the relationship system. It was clear to my oldest brother and to Mother that I was no longer on board with the negativity. My effort changed my relationships not just with my oldest brother and his wife but between mother and his wife as well. Things softened on both sides, and my sister-in-law eventually became Mother's right arm in her later declining years.

This is a case where I did not make detriangling statements but took detriangling actions, such as making it to the funeral. One fun little detriangling statement I did make was when I was home for a visit and Mother and I went over to my brother's house for an evening visit. During the conversation, Mother criticized my brother for not buying his wife a dishwasher. I had not appreciated how much Mother could needle him about such matters before and found it interesting. I watched my brother visibly tense up and not respond verbally to our mother's comment. With a smile on my face, I said to my brother, "Didn't you hear what Mother said?" I felt totally neutral about my brother-Mother interaction and wanted to communicate I was aware of it but not reactive to it. My brother relaxed when he saw me smiling.

OBSERVING INTERLOCKING TRIANGLES
INVOLVING DAD YEARS AFTER HIS DEATH

Earlier in this chapter I described hearing about my maternal grandmother's later life decline in functioning and how that provided insight into some of Mother's emotional programming in relationship with her mother. A very different circumstance came along that helped me learn more about Dad's emotional programming. Dad's next-oldest sister was the last surviving member of her generation, outliving Dad by almost thirty years. She lived in Washington, D.C., and my wife and I frequently had dinner with her at our house or at her apartment. One night after we had had dinner, she and I were talking. She touched on a subject that I had not known about until a few months earlier, when Mother had talked about it with me for the first time. In a kind of confession mode, Mother told me that she had had an abortion in early 1939. This was about a year after my next-older brother had been born. Mother felt very guilty about the abortion and for some reason finally decided to tell me about it. She apologized to me passionately for having done it. She went onto to say that after the abortion she insisted that she and my Dad try to have another baby. She did, and I was that baby. Needless to say, I told her no apologies were necessary because I would not be here if she had not had that abortion. That was all she told me about the abortion.

I do not remember why my aunt chose to focus on that subject that evening after dinner, but what she told me turned out to be incredibly useful. Since Dad had died seven years before I began learning about Bowen theory, I did not have the same opportunities that I had with mother in gaining a better understanding of him, but what my aunt told me that night helped. She said that when she heard Mother was pregnant a year after having had my next-older brother, she was very upset about the news. My aunt said, "I told your mother in no uncertain terms that my baby brother already had too much responsibility on his shoulders with three children and that she should abort that baby!"

I had not realized until then how fiercely protective my aunt was of Dad. Pieces fell into place. My aunt pressured Mother, along with my Dad, to abort the pregnancy. What struck me even more powerfully was that Mother had given in to that pressure. I have described how protective a person Mother could be, and I realized she and Dad were a perfect fit. Dad's functioning position in his family of origin was a bit of a doted-on prince surrounded by three women who were fiercely protective of him, not just my aunt. Dad married a woman with fierce instincts to protect the male from being overloaded with responsibility.

As I reflected later on that conversation with my aunt, I realized that until that time I had not been as emotionally neutral about the interaction between my parents as I had thought. I realized that to some degree I blamed Dad for being an underfunctioner in relationship to my mother. I was freed up from that feeling as a result of these two conversations related to Mother's abortion. I finally understood that Mother and Dad were a perfect emotional fit: each played an equal part in perpetuating their pattern, and each had been programmed as kids to do just that. If I ever doubted that important feelings could be recognized and resolved by working on family relationships in the here and now, this experience cured me of that doubt.

INTERLOCKING TRIANGLES INVOLVING MOTHER AND MY NUCLEAR FAMILY

I made reference briefly in the introduction to a process of working to resolve the emotional attachment with Mother. The process reached a major turning point when I recognized that my perception of her as "fragile," and an associated fear that Mother would fall apart if I disagreed with her on something important, was a major obstacle in my relationship with her. I now describe a three-year process that led up to that awareness and associated change in my behavior with her. The process I describe in Chapter 8 about my reaction to Mother standing at the top of the stairway when she visited with us in D.C. occurred in early 1970. The process I describe now unfolded between 1975 and 1978.

In early 1975, my wife and I decided to have a third child, this time through the process of adoption. I informed Mother soon after we had made this decision, and much to my surprise, she was very upset about it. Reminiscent of what my Dad's sister had said in no uncertain terms to Mother when she was pregnant with the baby she agreed to abort, Mother said to me: "You have way too much responsibility already and should not have another child!" She added, "You are letting your wife dictate to you!"

Between Mother's initial reaction to my decision and the end of 1978 when we adopted our son, I went through what I would characterize as three phases. During the first phase, which lasted about a year, I was very reactive to Mother's criticism of the decision and would counter her arguments with my arguments. It accomplished nothing other than my realizing that getting so reactive to her was pointless. In the second phase I was less defensive and did not try to change her mind. A time I particularly remember was Mother and me having a weekend visit with my cousin, Mother's sister's daughter, and her family. Mother and I did not talk about the adoption issue in traveling to see my cousin and family, but when I went to bed early one of the nights of our visit, I overheard Mother bad-mouthing my wife and me to my cousin and her family.

As I lay in bed listening, it helped me to think of Mother as triangling her anxiety into the family system rather than just feeling angry with Mother. I also thought that I would have to rely on my cousin and her family not to be negative toward me based on what Mother was telling them. This experience was one of a number of examples of my using theory to decrease my reactivity to Mother during that second phase.

The third phase began with the incident I referenced in the introduction, which occurred a few months before the actual adoption. Mother was having a visit with my Dad's sister on one of her trips to D.C. to spend time with my family and me. I went down to pick her up at my aunt's home and bring her back to our house. No sooner was she in the car to begin our ten- to fifteen-minute trip to my house than she launched into a diatribe, accusing me of making a stupid decision about the adoption and blaming it on my wife's influence on me. I was fairly calm in face of her intensity and said, "I understand your point of view." Mother responded, "Well, if you understood me, you wouldn't do what you are doing!" I remember thinking that she wants me to do what *she* wants, not what my wife wants.

I am not sure if the awareness that I perceived her as fragile floated into my head while I was listening to her on the trip home or if I recognized that in retrospect, but I saw that trying not to react was an insufficient response to her. I did not feel angry with her, but after five or ten minutes I pulled the car over and in a very firm voice said, "Mother, I am not willing to listen to your attacks on my decision making and blaming my wife for my decision any longer. This will stop now!" If I came across as angry, it was a controlled anger that I was using to make my point. She shut up, and we drove the rest of the way home in silence.

When we got back to my house, I decided that I was going to bed. I remember being concerned that Mother would dive into the scotch and be a mess the next day, but I walked up the stairs to the bedroom and fell asleep fairly quickly. I recall thinking at the time, "This woman can bloody well take care of her own emotions."

I was up before Mother the next day and greeted her as she came down the stairs the next morning. She spoke first and said, "Michael, are you still mad at me?" I responded, "Do I have reason to be?" That is when she said, "Finally, you told me what you think." When our son was born and we brought him to our home two days later, I called Mother and told her the news. Within a few days, we received a package in the mail, an infant sweater with the words on it, "Grandma Loves You."

A common critique of Bowen theory is that there often seems to be too much focus on the relationship with the mother. What about the father? I have already emphasized that the father is an equal contributor to what plays out in the parental triangle with each child. The intensity of the relationship between Mother and me is inadequately explained without including the nature of the relationship between my parents and the characteristics of the relationship with my Dad. Dad died before I knew anything about Bowen theory, but as I explained earlier in this chapter, I got clues about aspects of my unresolved attachment to him through his sister's story about the abortion. In my last personal vignette, I illustrate how the core of the interactions with my wife replicated the unresolved fusion with Mother.

GAINING MORE EMOTIONAL SEPARATENESS IN THE MARITAL RELATIONSHIP

The example earlier in this chapter of seeing reciprocal interaction in the marital relationship occurred in the early fall of 1969. The current example occurred years later in the middle to late 1990s. A number of other efforts at differentiation of self in the marriage on both of our parts occurred between those two dates, but they all involved triangles with our children and, as I mentioned at the beginning of this chapter, I do not describe them to preserve our children's privacy.

My wife had been away for nearly six weeks not long before the following incident occurred. She was in Africa observing chimpanzees at Gombe Stream National Park in Tanzania. We exchanged letters during this period, and that was a useful experience during this longest period of physical separation in our marriage. I am not sure how to assess the impact that period may have had on the possibility of making new observations about our marital interaction after she returned, but it could have played some role.

My wife and I were alone in the house—I do not remember the content of what we were discussing, but the process I observed remains vivid in my mind. We were having a tense interaction. At some point during our exchange, I saw very clearly that I was shutting down and starting to distance in the face of what I perceived as her intensity. This part was all very familiar from myriad interactions over the years. This time it was different—I suddenly thought of her intensity as her reaction to my distancing and associated disdain. Up to that time, I realized, I had justified my distancing by viewing her intensity as causing it. I had not realized until then that I was a 50 percent contributor to her intensity and she was a 50 percent contributor to my withdrawal. At that point I had been teaching this cocreation idea to students of Bowen theory for over twenty-five years, but I had not observed it fully in my own marriage until that day.

Perhaps equally important, I saw during this interaction with my wife that my unresolved relationship with Mother was replicating in the marriage—it was crystal clear. One legacy of my fairly intense fusion with Mother was a more than moderate need for attention and acceptance from the emotionally significant female in my life; another legacy was a powerful desire to escape from being overwhelmed by a significant other's expectations of me. When I put those two ideas together, I thought to myself, "God put this woman on Earth to help me resolve my unresolved attachment to Mother!" I knew, of course, that God had not done that, but the thought captured the awareness that this was not something my wife was doing to me but a reflection of a more complex process. I would term what I have just described as gaining more emotional objectivity.

An outcome of these observations was a significant increase in emotional neutrality about my wife and our interactions. The action part was simply calming down, not withdrawing, and watching the emotional intensity in my wife diminish in an amazingly short time. I think that what I had accomplished with Mother played an important role in being able to see the same process in my marriage. One effort facilitated the other, but it was not automatic. I still had to observe it unfold in the marriage and then develop a new way of being with my wife based on this new way of thinking.

I took the lead in this instance, but many other occasions occurred over the years in which she took the lead. She had developed her own interest in Bowen theory not long after I did and had many coaching sessions of her own with Murray Bowen. She worked hard to apply it in her family of origin and in our nuclear family. It was humbling when she saw some emotional process playing out in our nuclear family, between us or in triangles with our kids, which I had been blind to. This is typical of differentiation of self in one's own family: different people can take the lead at different times, and then others will follow. One person can accomplish a lot on his or her own, but a spouse making an effort as well is a cherished dividend.

Many people have asked what is an unresolved emotional attachment and what does it mean to resolve it. Probably the most important point to make in responding to such a question is that no one fully resolves an unresolved attachment. The lack of resolution is rooted in the fact that emotional fusion, fueled by the togetherness force, is at the core of human nature. Our species is not social simply because of cultural forces; our sociality is firmly anchored in biology. It is no surprise to anyone that fusion reaches its peak in the family emotional system, but it plays out to some degree in all social relationships.

The important point from a Bowen theory perspective is that the members of a sibling group predictably vary in the degree of resolution of their emotional attachment to the family organism at the point they leave home. This appears to result primarily from variation in each sibling's developmental experience: one sibling, as my oldest full brother did, can grow up in a more intense parental triangle than the other siblings. Each sibling is part of interlocking triangles with the other siblings' parental triangles: the projection process is a family affair.

How much resolution can occur based on a structured, long-term effort to increase one's basic level of differentiation of self? The only answer I can give with certainty is enough to make a difference, enough to make the effort worthwhile. Our family emotional system programmed my oldest full brother and me to have more need for attention and approval than the average sibling who grew up in a more differentiated family than ours. My oldest full brother's need for attention and approval was simply greater than mine. My efforts on differentiation with my family of origin and nuclear family have not resulted in any quantum leaps along the continuum of differentiation on my part. They represent relatively small changes, but ones that have resulted in more stability in important relationships and more productivity in a range of areas.

I wrote Murray Bowen a letter when I was living in the Midwest during my tour in the Navy between 1971 and 1973 in which I thanked him for developing a theory that had already contributed much to my emotional functioning. He responded with, "How do you know that you couldn't have accomplished more with psychoanalysis?" It was a vintage Bowen response, and it was useful. As I reflect on that period now, I realize that I had no idea how much I still had to learn about better managing my emotional functioning. All manner of life challenges lay ahead of me over the next four-plus decades that would alert me to how much I still had to learn about differentiation of self, even when many had come to consider me an expert on the subject. In many ways, the effort to be a more differentiated person results in seeing how undifferentiated one is, and that is not necessarily a bad thing.

CHAPTER SEVENTEEN

Clinical Example of the Process of Differentiation

Figure 17.1 is a hypothetical family diagram of a composite clinical case describing how progress in the process of differentiation unfolds over several years in a clinical family. I present the case for three primary reasons: (1) to illustrate how one spouse can take the lead in differentiating more of a "self,"

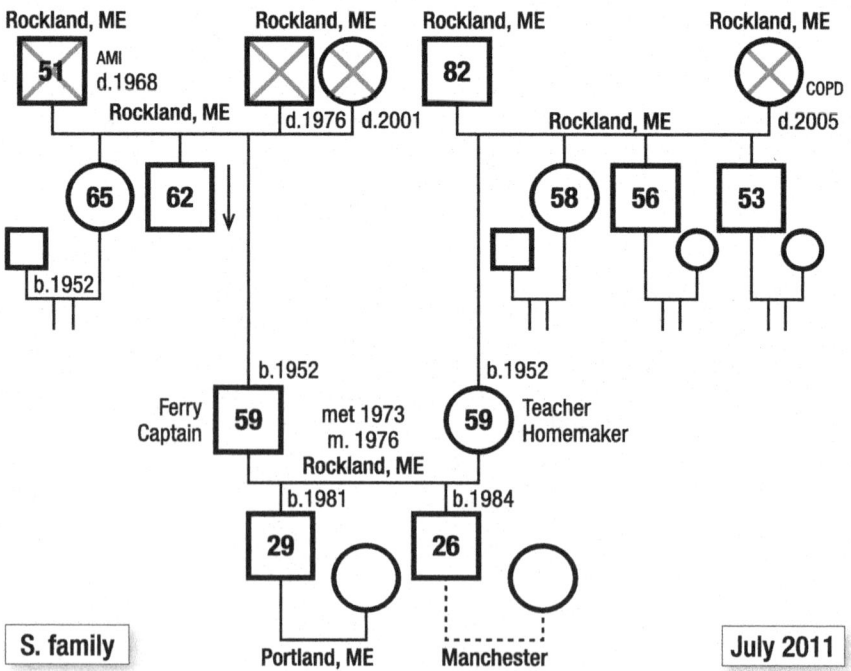

Figure 17.1   *The family diagram for the composite clinical case, the 'S' family. The downward arrow next the husband's older brother symbolizes fairly extreme underfunctioning throughout his life. That brother was diagnosed as having schizophrenia.*

(2) to illustrate that the process of differentiation is not a predictable or step by step process, and (3) to illustrate how one family leader's efforts benefit the family as a whole.

Generally speaking, the process of differentiation begins with people getting exposed to the ideas through the person representing them (the coach) and deciding to stay with the approach over time, but typically with some reservations early on. It is most important for the coach to be aware during this period of the extent to which family members are thinking in terms of cause-and-effect versus systems. People begin coaching embedded in cause-and-effect thinking and, with the help of the coach, can gradually move toward systems thinking. The coach helps by conveying emotional neutrality and interest but, most important, with helping a family member distinguish between individual and systems thinking. This is accomplished through the coach's questions and explanations. It is fundamentally an educational process but always with awareness of what may be transpiring emotionally in the relationship between coach and family member. It is always important for the coach to represent a way of thinking but not to try to sell it.

Family members can be in coaching for long time and believe they are gaining something from the process but still not be gaining anything more than they could from a conventional individual therapy approach. For example, a family member may be focusing on managing himself better in relationships but not have a handle on a relationship system perspective. The gains from Bowen theory based coaching do not occur until the family member observes relationship process and his or her part in that process. It is fundamentally an exercise in overcoming observational blindness to see what has been right in front of a person's eyes all along.

As a person becomes acquainted with systems thinking and takes a serious interest in it, this prepares the person to make observations about system process somewhere down the line. The observations could occur in a routine interaction with a spouse or parent or may occur during some sort of family upheaval in which what is unfolding is much more obvious. For example, in another clinical case a mother had been trying to apply systems thinking in her nuclear family for many years but did not begin to see the process clearly until one of her children went off to college and was placed on probation after a drinking episode. It is hard to predict when such observations will occur, and this takes patience on the part of a coach, who cannot get anyone to differentiate more of a "self"—it happens when the coach is doing a good job, the family member is motivated, and the right context occurs.

The husband in this clinical case, Mr. S., initiated the therapy. He was the fifty-nine-year-old ferryboat captain on the family diagram. A fellow member of his meditation group suggested the referral. Meditation had long been a part of this husband's efforts to improve his emotional functioning. His principal concern was the unsatisfactory state of his marriage. This had been the case for several years, and he did not want a divorce. He wished his wife would be more active, especially in activities in which both of them were involved, and nicer to him. Meditation had been useful to him in a variety of ways, but it had not helped him make progress in the marriage.

They couple lived and grew up in Rockland, Maine, a place both their families have lived for several generations (see Figure 17.1). Mrs. S. is the oldest of four siblings; her father is still alive, but her mother died in 2005 from complications of pulmonary emphysema. All of her siblings live in the Rockland area. Her family gets together often, and there is a lot of focus on helping her aging father. Mrs. S. is the mother figure of her generation. Mr. S. is the youngest of three siblings in his family of origin. Notably, the middle sibling, a brother, has been quite dysfunctional since his late teenage years, has been diagnosed to have schizophrenia, and lives in a group home in Rockland. He never married. Not much contact has occurred between the brothers in recent years. The older sister also lives in Rockland, is married, and has two grown children, one of whom is married. Mr. S. stays in close contact with his sister. Mr. S's father died of a heart attack when Mr. S. was only sixteen years old. His mother remarried a few years later, but the second husband died after just a few years of marriage. Mr. S's mother died in 2001.

After hearing Mr. S's reasons for seeking therapy and gathering much of the data on the family diagram, I suggested to Mr. S. that both he and his wife come to the next session. I suggested this because the marital relationship was his primary concern. He agreed and thought she would be willing. At the first conjoint session, she was very clear that she came because her husband was unhappy and that, if coming to therapy together would help, she would do that. She had no particular agenda for herself other than that. Dealing with her husband's expectations of her and the desire not to disappoint him troubled her the most. She said she liked to do a lot of things on her own, but he wanted to do a lot of things together. She said her husband would be retiring in a few years, and she was nervous about how that might escalate the tensions in their relationship. The husband reiterated that he wanted more tenderness and openness in their relationship. He added, "I feel I have lost her approval" and that there had not been a sexual relationship for a year or more.

There were several more conjoint sessions during the next several weeks. Mrs. S. said that the degree of involvement she had with her father and siblings was a problem for her husband. She described her position in the parental triangle as "being recruited by Dad to help with Mom." Mrs. S. said also that her sister had been having many marital problems and that she felt a lot of obligation to help her sister. She had several pithy descriptions of the marriage, including, "I want him to do what he wants to do, but he wants to make me into someone else. Furthermore, we both think we are right!" She added, "He gets angry if I don't do what he wants, and I clam up."

The husband thought that historically he and his wife had been very close but now it was different. He said, "I want change, but I doubt it will happen." He said he could act independently, but that is not what he really wanted. In essence, he wanted more togetherness and she was easily overwhelmed by it.

Five or six conjoint sessions over the next few months helped reduce the marital tensions some. Important points in those sessions included his view that his wife chooses her family over him, and that angers him. Mrs. S. acknowledged that she had little interest in sex at this point, but that he is more needy in that regard.

Over the next few months, occasional conjoint sessions occurred, but he also came alone many times. It was very clear to him (and me) that he wanted the therapy more than she did. At one of the individual sessions, he explained that he had been a premature baby and had spent several months in the infant intensive care unit. He added, "I believe that I'm so needy with my wife because of that experience. I didn't get the love and attention I needed." I challenged him on the view that that was at the core of his neediness, but he was not persuaded.

The wife soon dropped out of coming to the sessions entirely. Interestingly, he had some outpatient surgery. He commented, "My wife loved to take care of me and I loved the attention." I commented that what he described indicated that he had married a woman who seemed ideal to meet his needs, but it was getting lost in their tense interactions. He listened but, again, was not all that persuaded. My impression was that Mr. S. tried to take a hard look at himself, but it was not helping when it came to the marital relationship.

During a session not too long after the outpatient surgery, we visited his trauma theory related to the infant nursery experience. I suggested an alternative Bowen-theory-based view that he was replicating with his wife a version of what transpired between his mother and him when he was growing up. In this and later sessions, he described how angry he was at his mother for being so intensely involved with his brother. He felt there was not enough left over for him. He could readily see his mother's overinvolvement with his brother, but had a harder time seeing how involved she had been with him as well. My statement to him was, "You were the outsider in the triangle with your brother, and lucky you, but your mother was heavily involved with you too, just less so." I speculated that his mother likely felt some guilt about his unhappiness, just as his wife does. At that point, I encouraged him to get back into contact with his brother, which he eventually did. He did not think his brother was all that enthusiastic about their weekly lunches, but being with his brother and listening to him brought back some vivid memories of their childhood that were useful. He began to think a little bit in the direction of him being better off not being the target of so much overmothering.

By the end of that year, after about six months of twice-a-month sessions, he developed a recurrence of irritable bowel symptoms. He was very receptive to the idea that anxiety likely played an important role in the symptoms. He questioned whether he was being selfish in pressuring his wife to meet his needs. He recalled that they were closer when they were raising their sons, both of whom were doing reasonably well in their lives. Factoring in the impact of the kids was useful to him in trying to understand their marriage. He said that he was pressuring his wife to come back for conjoint sessions, but saw fear in her. His younger son told his dad, "Mom is a warm and loving person, but shut off."

During the spring of 2012, turmoil increased in his wife's family related to her sister's deteriorating marriage. Mrs. S. was also developing some physical symptoms at that point. One medical opinion was that she was using too many anti-inflammatory drugs. Mr. S. noted that both his wife's mother and maternal grandmother had ended up living out their lives in bed. He feared that would be his wife's fate as well.

Things got much worse for Mrs. S. medically, and her doctor hospitalized her in the late spring of 2012. She was very sick at that point. She was diagnosed to have acute tubular necrosis resulting in kidney failure. She had to be treated in the intensive care unit. It was not clear that she would live. Tensions rose between Mr. S. and his wife's family. They were quite critical of him. After a number of touch-and-go weeks, Mrs. S. began to improve some. However, Mr. S. was appalled to hear her ask, "Why did you keep me alive; I'm tired, it's too difficult."

She was discharged to a rehabilitation facility after a three-month hospital stay but had developed an additional problem, what her doctors diagnosed as stress-induced cardiomyopathy. Mrs. S was able to come home in early summer but was not fully recovered. Mr. S. had been able not to work during much of the hospital period but was now back at work and back to regular attendance at his meditation class. Mr. S. admitted hoping that this whole hospital experience would change something in their marriage and with her family. He was discouraged that same old patterns had quickly returned. During this period I constructed a diagram using PowerPoint that I e-mailed to him (Figure 17.2).

I sent this to Mr. S. in an effort to help him think about the laws of triangles and not use cause-and-effect thinking. He did not derive much benefit from it, but I enjoyed trying to conceptualize the process. I had earlier suggested a book he might read: Jonathan Haidt's The Righteous Mind (2012). I don't push people to read, but I often describe the content of something that I have been reading if it is relevant to Bowen theory. If they take an interest, I give them the reference. Mr. S. particularly appreciated Haidt's metaphor about the rider (rational mind) and the elephant (automatic emotional processes; see Chapter 5). The recent events of his wife's very serious illness and the tensions surrounding it in the family had given him a new

Clinical Example of the Process of Differentiation 205

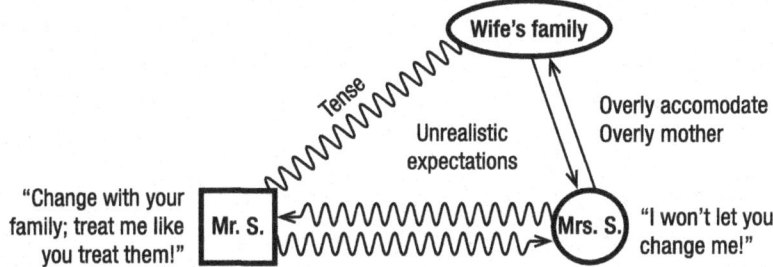

Figure 17.2 *I drew this diagram in a family coaching session with Mr. S. of a triangle involving Mr. S., his wife, and her family of origin to help him think about emotional process rather than get reactive to the content of the issues. The jagged lines between Mr. S and his wife indicate a high level of tension and conflict about her relationship with her family. The jagged line between Mr. S. and his in-laws was a fairly constant level of tension between him and most members of her family.*

perspective on the power of emotions, which was in line with the rider being rather weak in comparison to the elephant.

Mr. S. described what had happened to his wife as humbling. He also recognized that he had traditionally tended to think of himself as "right," but now he saw himself as opinionated. I considered these useful insights on his part but nothing that could not be gained from therapy based on individual theory. He had yet to get to a systems framework.

By early 2013, Mr. S. had come to the conclusion that if his wife had not gotten sick, he would likely have separated from her. He did recognize that the marriage was smoother if he decreased his expectations of his wife but felt that attitude left the relationship kind of dead and him feeling isolated. He was still stuck in cause-and-effect thinking, not really seeing reciprocity in their relationship. This was so even though he had become more keenly aware of what he reacted to in his wife's demeanor and behavior. He made a "rule" for himself not to judge his wife, but the idea was not based on the emotional neutrality that systems thinking generates. He had a glimmer of reciprocity in describing himself as having a "hidden agenda" in his approaches to his wife and her reacting to his expectations, but the yearning that she act more like he wanted her to act was primarily in play.

Another thought during this period included trying to make sense out of his wife becoming so ill. He remained distressed that she did not seem to be doing as much as she could do to recover her health. His stomach symptoms continued, which he still regarded as a reflection of his anxiety.

By the fall of 2013, he reported a very clear statement by his wife: "I don't want anyone telling me how to live my life!" They were now sleeping in separate bedrooms. For whatever reasons, Mrs. S. started taking a little better care of herself in terms of following her doctors' advice. Mr. S said he was better able to contemplate his tendencies to try to change others and that thinking about that seemed to help control it a little bit. He also got a better handle on his anger: "I am angry at my mother for making my brother her favorite." These are all valuable insights, but he tended to regard them as "bad" traits rather than placing them firmly in a systems framework.

Toward the end of 2013, he reported that he was becoming slightly less reactive to his wife's family and that he and his wife were trying to be more affectionate with each other. He was now describing himself as a "polite prick." He also noted that he was happier when his wife was recuperating. He did not know how to interpret that, but he thought it was important. I did not speculate about the reason for that but thought it was interesting.

By the spring of 2014, he said that things in the family were calmer, but he still felt a void. His brother was now sick. He commented that he and his brother were alike in being stubborn, sarcastic, and wanting "what we want when we want it." Mr. S. was certainly facing up to his undesirable traits, but the marital relationship was still bothersome. In terms of some relationship insights during that period, he posed the question to himself of whether he transferred his negative feelings about his mother to his wife when his mother died. He also wondered how much the death of his wife's mother affected their marriage. "We lost two triangles that may have stabilized our marriage," he suggested. It seemed a plausible and useful perspective that was informed by systems thinking.

Mr. S. was definitely beginning to broaden his perspective in a useful way. He was thinking systems about the big picture, but, as will be evident shortly, still was not able to bring it into the day-to-day interactions of the marriage. His older son said, "Dad, you are less oppositional, you think differently." Mr. S added, "The unexamined life caught up to me." He was referring to the turmoil of the last few years.

Mr. S's brother died in April 2014. He had lung cancer and emphysema. In June 2014, he described his wife as nearly back to normal health, like she was before all the events of the late winter and spring of 2012. He had become even more convinced that the death of his and his wife's mothers had increased tension in their marriage. He made a very interesting comment in one of our sessions in the early summer of 2014: "I acknowledge Bowen theory, but I don't feel it." He added that I have shifted thinking from, "Why can't my wife be on my side?" to "Why does she react like this?" All this seemed to be very definite progress toward systems thinking, but without being quite there yet. I interpreted his comment about acknowledging Bowen theory as accepting it intellectually but recognized that he had not changed emotionally.

Mr. S's bowel symptoms increased during the summer of 2014, and a dividend for him was seeing his wife's deep concern. He was beginning to feel she really did care, did have his back. He and his wife also had an interesting conversation about her family. It was triggered by Mr. S's effort to stay in contact with his wife's sister's husband after they separated. Mrs. S's family was quite upset about his doing that. His wife commented in a matter-of-fact way, "In our family, you have to be on our side—or else." It was one of the most objective exchanges they had had about her family. Mrs. S. was not defensive, and Mr. S was not attacking.

Another interesting observation Mr. S. made that indicated his effort to think systems was that his younger son was now mad at his mother's family. Mr. S. viewed the son's reaction as an interesting triangle: he was taking sides with his mother. More evidence of Mr. S. using systems thinking was a series of phone calls from his sister about how furious she was at her daughter's husband, citing his behaviors as a cause of their recent marital separation. At first Mr. S. tried to enlighten his sister about Bowen theory by telling her she was caught in a triangle with her daughter and husband, siding with her daughter and blaming the marital problems on her husband. His sister did not take kindly to this idea, which helped Mr. S. back off and see the futility of trying to explain Bowen theory to his emotionally wrought sister. He saw that he was trying to get out of a triangle with his sister and her daughter by explaining to her that she was in a triangle with her daughter and her husband. The incident helped Mr. S. better realize that you communicate Bowen theory by living it, not by trying to teach it to close family members, particularly when they are upset. In October 2014, Mr. S's discouragement was again triggered by a comment by his wife that conveyed that she did not care how long she lived.

During that same time period, Mr. S. recalled something his mother had told him when he was teenager, something he had not thought about since. He recalled his mother trying to reassure him by saying, "I love you, but your brother needs me more." Based on his knowledge of Bowen theory, this statement now made sense to him. He was on the outside of a triangle with his mother and brother—it was not about his mother rejecting him but about how intensely fused she was with his brother. This new perspective helped resolve much of the anger toward his mother. Mr. S.'s experience highlights an important difference between systems/relationship thinking and cause-and-effect/individual thinking. His feeling of anger toward his mother was linked to the bias that her lack of giving him as much attention as his brother was an important cause of his emotional problems. It felt that way. He lived his life in the grip of that feeling, and it affected how he interpreted his wife's behavior toward him. Comprehending that his mother was more fused to his brother than to him and that this was to his advantage, coupled with his newly acquired understanding of the laws of triangles, allowed him to link his anger to being in the outside position of the triangle. The trauma of it all was driven by his interpretation of the basis for the feeling, which he now perceived as simplistic. He had a new way of thinking that helped him toward a new way of being.

A major event occurred in early January of 2015. He was diagnosed with prostate cancer. It was clear that the news affected his wife as much as him. He made the decision for radiation, then radiation implants, and anti-testosterone therapy. He was amazed at how calmly he had taken the news. He believed that the stresses in his life played a role in developing the cancer and quipped, "Anxiety makes the world go round." When a friend said he was shocked by the news of his cancer, Mr. S. replied, "It is just who I am."

In a February 2015 session, Mr. S. told me something very interesting, which I thought had contributed to his ability to have remarkable equanimity in dealing the cancer. During the recent Christmas holidays, his sons were home, along with the older son's wife and younger son's girlfriend. Anticipating the whole family being together, he had planned an outing that would involve his wife as well as sons and their female partners. He told his wife and she had agreed. Then a few days before the planned outing, his wife got a call from her sister. The sister said that the family had planned an important event that would include their father. It turned out that the date of this event conflicted with what Mr. S had planned. She told her husband she felt she had to be there for the event with her father and siblings. Mr. S. was incredibly furious at her. In fact, he reacted so strongly that it frightened him. He had not realized the depth of his anger up to that point. Yes, his wife had agreed to the outing that he had planned, and he could be legitimately upset about her backing out in favor of her dad and siblings, but his reaction went far beyond what he would have expected.

As Mr. S. thought about this over the next few weeks, which was also in the midst of getting the cancer diagnosis, he concluded that it was the depth of his fusion with his wife that explained the rage he had felt. "I was so very angry and bitter with my wife. What gave me the right?" By the fusion he meant that he had acted as if she should do what he wanted her to do, that she was some kind of extension of him. That attitude appalled him. He saw it as truly absurd, beyond the pale. Having the insight about the triangle with his mother and brother had helped him get to this point in thinking, but he thought the cancer diagnosis was important too. It was a wake-up call: he knew he had to change the way he had been living his life all these years. His wife had paid a price, and he was paying a price. He saw the fusion for what it was. "I see the core of my anger as related to fusion," he explained.

I was fascinated and impressed with what he had to say. My thought was that he had finally made it all the way to systems thinking after close to four years of effort. This experience heralded a series of systems observations that following over the next few months. Most involved marital interactions—I have given examples of this earlier. One such observation occurred as he was standing in the kitchen of their home talking with his wife. They were having a bit of a tense discussion about some subject. Suddenly he realized that what he perceived as a tense expression on her face reflected his own facial expression and tone of voice, which in turn were intensified by what he saw in her. At that point, his thinking shifted radically from "you don't understand me" to "we just have differences in viewpoint." He relaxed, and they had a productive exchange. He soon came to think of the relationship problem as, "It's not you, it's us!" This change in thinking reflected an emotional change in Mr. S. Thanks to a systems perspective, a clear view of the reciprocal interaction, the emotion became decoupled from his attitude about his wife. He went on to explain that he realized that, through all these years, something hidden was going on in the relationship, governing it. That would be the emotional system and its coupled subjective attitudes.

His medical woes were not over. In June 2015 he was diagnosed with a carcinoid tumor in his bowel. The doctors thought it had likely been there for a long time and that it may have contributed to his bowel symptoms. He noticed how his wife was there for him, which was very comforting. He posed the question to me (and to himself), "Is my need for fusion greater than others?" I replied, "Not much. Fusion is a part of who we all are." In reflecting on his illnesses, bowel disturbances, the cancer, and the new tumor, he had concluded that his illnesses began or were exacerbated when he wife had been hospitalized three years earlier. He added, "There is more than randomness to my getting cancer." He was pleased by how well he seemed to be adapting to the challenges of it all.

He helped me recognize another important dynamic in this whole process, one that I think I had been vaguely aware of from the beginning but had failed to articulate adequately to myself. He had concluded that he had played an important role in his wife getting so sick in the spring of 2012. "The strong pressure I was putting on her to be who I needed her to be and her very high sensitivity to my expectations and disappointment broke her down," he said. I saw that I had been complicit in this process. I was alongside as he strove to change her, was aware of its strong impact on her, but I failed to define a "self" to him about that process, meaning I should have communicated as clearly as possible that trying to change the other person is not differentiation of self. I can't say that it would have prevented her illness if I had addressed that process with him vigorously, but it might have. He added that he was now giving his wife space to make her own decisions about medical therapy. He observed that she had been taking better care of herself since he quit overfunctioning in that way.

By September 2015 his medical illnesses appeared to be under control. He said, "I see our marriage as wonderful." I often say to people who have been pressing their partner for more togetherness, and who commonly perceive trying to be more of a "self" in the relationship as tantamount to giving up and distancing, that being more of a "self" will lead to more emotional closeness but will be different than what you might expect. I think this is what Mr. S. meant by "wonderful." If he distances in the marriage now, she pursues. That was a big change. It is evident that she wants to be with him as much as he wants to be with her.

Affirming a comment I made to him maybe two years earlier, "You have had *the privilege of having two women in your life, your wife and your mother, that have been devoted to your welfare,"* he acknowledged that this was absolutely the case. He sagely observed that romantic love is filled with high anxiety. From a Bowen theory perspective, the intensity of the emotional fusion generates the chronic anxiety that makes a relationship unsatisfactory. His comment seems right on. There was now slightly less fusion in their marriage.

In June 2016, the tumors were all reported as indolent. He noted that he was able to stay engaged with his wife even in face of disagreement. He felt far less judgmental about his wife's family, saying, "So what if they want to defer to their aging father!" He had a lot more personal insights that I do not detail here. Some of the changes in his wife were captured in her comments about missing him when he was away for any period of time and apologizing for how anxious she would get at times. His son said, "Dad, you have changed completely." A friend of the family commented, "Your wife is back—she has that twinkle back in her eye." His wife also said to him, "You don't even walk the way you used to."

What stands out in the group of people, parts of whose stories I tell in this hypothetical case presentation, is their strong motivation and willingness to engage the possibility that the person seeking therapy may be part of the family problem. This includes people who self-blame as well as people who blame others. Systems thinking is a paradigm shift comparable to what glider pilots thrive on: atmospheric uplifts. People can lift up out of an emotional field and view it from a refreshing new vantage point. It is refreshing because people can rest from trying to change others without giving up on a situation improving. Being in emotional contact with a system but outside of it allows for a substantive change in mindset. It is new mindware for viewing the complex social world of *Homo sapiens*.

CHAPTER EIGHTEEN

The Process of Differentiation

Theory, Method, and Technique

In this last chapter of Part II, I briefly review how the approach to family therapy based on Bowen theory has changed over the many years since it began in the Family Study Project at the National Institute of Mental Health (NIMH) in the 1950s. The overall approach to treating families involves theory, method, and technique. Quoting biologist John Tyler Bonner: "Science is about things. It is about rocks, stars, atoms, and living beings . . . it is about the relation of things; science is concerned with order. . . . One way to deal with these things is to make generalizations in the form of theories, laws, or principles" (1969, Introduction). Bowen theory is derived from functional facts discovered from observing how people interact in families. Those facts led to the conceptualization of emotional forces, such as togetherness, and patterns of emotional functioning, such as the triangle. The theory is the basis for the method used in treating families: facilitating the process of differentiation. A number of techniques for implementing the method have been developed over time. Those techniques are the subject of this brief review.

The first technique was developed at NIMH: family group therapy. This approach involved meeting with the whole family, parents and offspring together. Observations about the constructive impact of one family member functioning with more of a "self" were often made during family group sessions, but it was not the best approach for facilitating differentiation of self. Family group therapy can help reduce chronic anxiety in a family, thus increasing its functional level of differentiation, but increasing basic level is another matter. The problem is that having the whole family in a therapy session distracts from the central goal of parents recognizing that progress in the family depends on one or both of them exerting leadership, developing the ability to function with more of a "self." The focus on the parents is based on viewing the family as a system and on seeing that, if one member of the family can function with more "self," other family members will predictably pull up their functioning. The offspring often have useful observations to make during family group therapy sessions, but they are too dependent on the family, emotionally and financially, to exert leadership. It is unrealistic to expect that of them.

A second technique that has been used is therapy sessions that include the parents and just the symptomatic offspring. This approach reduces distractions, which helps bring the parental triangle involving that child into sharp focus. However, doing this with a psychotic-level family process is usually too intense to be useful. Not infrequently, psychotic symptoms are exacerbated in such sessions. Many Bowen therapists have tried this technique with less intense problems, such as behavioral acting out by an adolescent. However, having the three family members together in the sessions resulted in the parents sitting back and waiting for the adolescent to change as a result of the family therapy. The technique tends not to result in the parents making a project out of themselves. The therapist treating parents and adolescent separately is a variation of this second technique, but the same problem tends to occur: parents hoping the therapist will fix the child. The need to promote progress by holding parents' fingers to the fire is an apt expression here. This variation in technique can be helpful in reducing anxiety in both the parents and the child, again improving functional level of differentiation. Sessions with parents and child separately can be a useful short-term approach in crisis situations for reducing anxiety.

The most prevalent technique in use by Bowen theorists during the 1960s regardless whether the presenting problem was in the marriage or with a child was working with parents, usually in conjoint sessions. The therapists' questions were aimed at helping the parents see the reciprocal interactions in their relationship, to use systems rather than cause-and-effect thinking. There was also an effort to bring out factors beyond their relationship that were influencing it, such as a triangle involving the wife, her mother, and the husband. Variations existed in this technique, but the basic goal was to facilitate increased differentiation of self in the parents by each parent working on himself or herself in relationship to the other parent.

Many family therapists who are not guided by Bowen theory do conjoint marital therapy, but these therapists are using different theories and methods as a basis for their techniques. Spouses are commonly encouraged to talk directly to each other. A goal is for each spouse to talk to the other spouse about innermost thoughts and feelings. This often has a calming effect on a relationship. An exception is a highly conflicted relationship, where efforts to talk directly to each other typically exacerbate conflict. A guiding principle for many therapists doing marital therapy by having spouses talk directly to each other is a legacy of psychoanalytic thinking: the importance of people learning to recognize their feelings and express them.

Bowen theorists are different in using a technique that is guided by a goal of facilitating differentiation of self. Many therapists who did not understand differentiation of self were baffled by the Bowen theory approach, thinking it was encouraging people to suppress their feelings, that it was too intellectual. The Bowen theory guided technique in dealing with a couple is anchored in the understanding that intense feelings can override fact-guided thinking, thus interfering with gaining some emotional objectivity about relationship process and seeing patterns such as reciprocity.

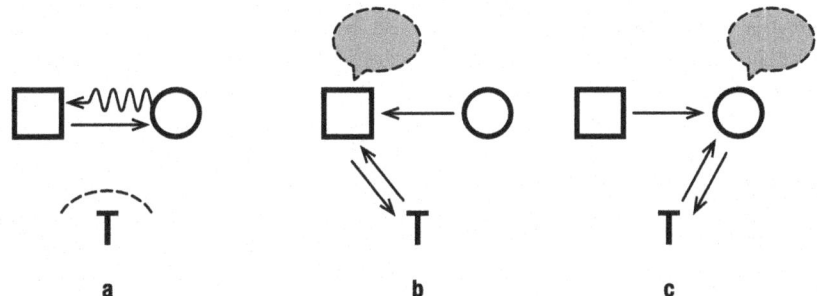

Figure 18.1 In panel a, the arrow from husband to wife symbolizes a comment made directly to her by him. The arrow with a jagged line from wife to husband symbolizes a reactive comment by her in response to what her husband said. In panel b, the reciprocally interacting arrows symbolize the family therapist conversing with the husband. The thought cloud above the husband symbolizes his thinking about a question the therapist has asked. The arrow from the wife to her husband symbolizes her listening to him without reacting. After a few minutes of thoughtful exchange between the therapist and husband, therapist shifts to a similar type of exchange with the wife. The goal of this technique is to help people think about emotional process as opposed the reacting to a discussion about it.

Figure 18.1 symbolizes the Bowen theory approach. Diagram a symbolizes the therapist encouraging the couple to talk directly to each other. The husband makes a comment to his wife (symbolized by the straight arrow toward the wife) and the wife is prone to react defensively to the comment (symbolized by the jagged line). People play out in front of the therapist the problem that brought them into therapy: being too reactive to each other to talk in a useful way. The therapist usually tends to point out what they are doing to each other. From the perspective of Bowen theory, this action-reaction process is part of emotional fusion, which it makes it more difficult for people to think about what being a "self" would be like in their interactions. One common element in this approach based on other models is encouraging each spouse to better understand the partner's needs and sensitivities, and then the therapist encourages each spouse to try to meet those needs and respect the sensitivities.

This idea as used in couples therapy has some merit, but it leaves out the important process of increasing levels of chronic anxiety that result from how the two people are interacting. The anxiety intensifies each person's needs, such as for attention and approval, and each person's sensitivities, such as to criticism. The needs and sensitivities of each spouse have commonly been part of what attracted them to each other in first place but have been accentuated by the heightened chronic anxiety to the point of becoming problems. The whole has become greater than the sum of its parts.

This non-Bowen-theory-based technique that I have been describing is typically based on thinking about one or both spouses as having particular neurotic traits or disorders (such as an attachment disorder) and seeing this as the explanation for the problems in their relationship. It is fundamentally trying to use individual thinking to treat a relationship system problem. It is not that therapists using the model are unaware of anxiety but that the anxiety is viewed as stemming from unmet needs rather than from interactions triggered by needs and sensitivities that have been blown way out of proportion. Neither spouse's particular traits cause the marital problem; the spouses cocreate the problem related to their equal difficulties maintaining a "self."

The Bowen theory technique is symbolized in Figure 18.1 in diagrams b and c. In diagram b, the therapist engages in an exchange with the husband (two arrows going back and forth between them), and the husband responds to the therapist. The therapist might ask a question like, "Mr. G., when you wife has that certain look on her face that you described earlier, what goes through your mind, thinking about it?" The circle above the husband's head symbolizes what is going on in his mind as he thinks about the therapist's question and how he then responds. As Mr. G. responds to the therapist's question to the therapist rather than his wife, the straight arrow from the wife to the husband symbolizes that she is listening and reacting less defensively. The fact that the husband does not direct his comments to the wife helps her to listen better and react less. The husband has less reactivity as well in discussing an emotionally charged subject with the therapist, a neutral party. The therapist then switches over to the wife and does the same thing, symbolized in diagram c. A whole session can be conducted by going back and forth between the spouses in this way.

The ability of the two spouses to listen to each other in a less reactive mode makes it more likely that they will be able to gain some objectivity and see a pattern like reciprocity in their exchanges. For example, the husband might say that when his wife gets that certain look on her face, he interprets it as criticism and shuts down. As his wife listens to him describe that to a neutral third person, she is more likely to see that her intensity ratchets up when she senses that he is withdrawing, and that the two forms of reactivity feed on each other in reciprocal fashion. This supports the idea of managing one's own reactivity rather than focusing on the other. Taking responsibility for one's own emotional reactivity and managing it better is an ingredient of being a "self."

Bowen developed one of the more fascinating applications of this theory-guided technique used in family therapy with a couple by conducting a clinical teaching conference at the Medical College of Virginia from 1967 to 1976 using the same technique. The teaching conference attendees, who were primarily mental health professionals, would gather in a large conference room each month and watch Bowen interview a couple on closed circuit television. The session was part of a series of sessions with that couple. In the first few years of the conference, the couple would leave after the interview, and Bowen would go to the conference room to discuss the interview and respond to questions.

After a few years of this format, Bowen invited the couple to attend the conference discussion after the televised and videotaped session so that they could listen to the group's discussion of their interview and participate in that discussion if either spouse saw fit. A powerful impact of this new format was that it broke down the doctor-patient barrier, or the idea that therapists are normal and patients are not.

However, a significant problem quickly emerged with this new format. Many audience members had strong emotional reactions to what had transpired in the interview, which often took the form of siding with one member of the couple. When some of these audience members who had fused into the family emotional process made comments during the conference, they would look at the family and try to engage them directly. This was in stark contrast to Bowen's interview, where he worked to stay detriangled from the spouses by making comments and asking questions in a neutral way that reflected seeing both sides of the marital problem. The members of the couple, as with most couples, were not immune from being affected by the bias and passion of an audience questioner. If you are in a tense relationship with someone and a third person takes your side, it is seductive to be emboldened by that. This, of course, is counterproductive for the couple's progress in therapy.

Figure 18.2 diagrams how Bowen decided to manage that process in the conference. The diagrams represent the auditorium where the conference was held. The Xs represent the attendees, which could include as many as fifty or

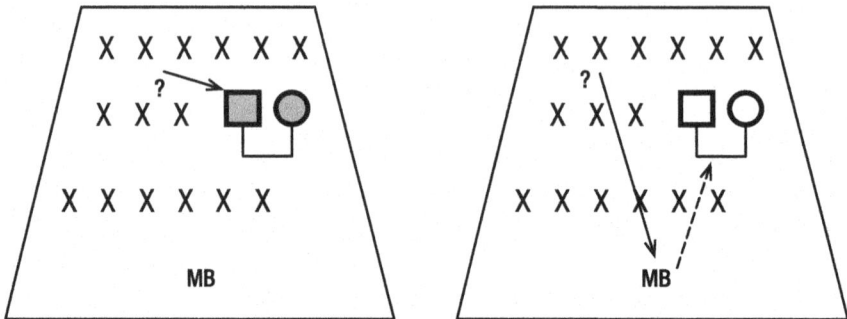

Figure 18.2 *This diagram illustrates how a technique first used to do family therapy with a couple is extended to manage the emotional process in a conference.* MB symbolizes the therapist in front leading a conference. The couple the therapist has just interviewed in a nearby television studio is sitting in the conference midway back in an amphitheater on the right side. The audience had watched the interview over closed circuit television from this conference room. The arrow from an audience member and question mark symbolize that an audience member has asked a question directly to the couple, making eye contact with them as they turn toward the questioner. The shaded symbols of the couple indicate their emotional reactivity to an emotionally charged question. The diagram on the right indicates how a conference leader tones down reactivity of this sort. The arrow from an audience member with a question in the right-hand diagram, at the conference leader's direction, is addressed to the leader, not the family. The leader then decides whether to ask the family to respond to the question.

sixty people. The couple that Bowen interviewed is sitting with the audience (square and circle). Bowen (MB) is at the front of the room.

The diagram on the left side represents the problem that Bowen quickly recognized. The arrow from an audience member to the couple represents that person asking a question to the couple directly, which prompted the couple to look at the questioner. This meant there was both auditory and visual communication between questioner and family, which can ratchet up reactivity. The shading within the symbol for each member of the couple represents their reactive response, not necessarily expressed, to a question from a person who was reactive to their interview in some way.

The diagram on the right symbolizes Bowen's approach to dealing with the problem. Audience members were instructed to ask their questions or make their comments directly to Bowen. He would then decide whether to ask the couple if they wanted to respond. Bowen would screen out the obvious emotionally charged, side-taking questions and respond himself to the questioner. He would pass more thoughtful questions onto the family, leaving them the option of whether to respond. The couple also related directly to Bowen, not to the questioner.

Some audience members were very reactive to the family and typically violated emotional boundaries with the couple at intermissions and lunch by commenting directly to them about their interview. Bowen repeatedly emphasized how toxic this could be to a family, particularly if the attendee had taken a side in the marital problem. Attendees were reminded about the importance of keeping their own emotionality contained and not inflicting it on the family. This did not mean they should not speak with the family at all. Some audience members understood, tended to ask more thoughtful questions during the conference discussion, and respected emotional boundaries. I attended many of those conferences and came to appreciate how important it was to recognize that a conference had its own emotional process and that it needed to be managed if the format was to work.

Before leaving the discussion of the Medical College of Virginia video project, there was another aspect of it that highlights Bowen theory's recognition of how difficult it can be to recognize the impact of emotional reactivity on one's thinking and attitudes in the moment. After the project had been running for three or four years, Bowen suggested that the family begin to review videotapes of sessions that were at least six months old. This would be their first viewing of the old sessions. They would do this review in the time between the regular ongoing monthly newly taped sessions. Bowen and a few therapists that worked with him reviewed the tapes along with the families. This was unlike a number of family therapists at that time who videotaped sessions in their office and then did "instant replay" with the family, pointing out problematic interactions. Bowen thought that it would be useful for them to view the tapes, but only several months after they had been taped. The thinking behind this approach was that the family would be in a different place emotionally after time had passed and could perhaps then view a replayed tape more objectively. The couples that took advantage of viewing older taped sessions learned much from appreciating how reactive they had been when the tape was made. This, not surprisingly, was true for some sessions reviewed more than for others. "Delayed replay" proved more useful to the families for recognizing their reactivity than instant replay.

Years ago, Murray Bowen showed a videotape of an interview he had done with a family. During the discussion after the tape, an audience member proclaimed, "That was not therapy, but a contemplative discourse between two well-intentioned people!" This comment highlights the distinctions I have been making about the difference between a technique based on Bowen theory and a technique based on other theories. With Bowen theory as a guide, the therapist is not trying to say and do things to fix the family but trying to relate to the family in the ways I have been describing such that the family figures out how to fix itself. If a therapist is emotionally neutral, is in good contact with the family but outside the family emotional process, and asks questions and makes comments that reflect this, a family will tell its story in a way that resonates and is useful. People do not need to be instructed on how to change; they need to learn what the obstacles are to change and to reflect on them. That is part of the process of increasing one's ability to be a "self."

I had a personal experience with the value of delaying watching a taped interview that helped me see for myself one of the key obstacles to my making progress. My wife asked Bowen to interview us as a couple and to tape the interview at MCV. We had been involved with Bowen theory for a few years at that point. I think she was thinking that we could capture on tape some of the progress we had made. The MCV conference crowd viewed the session and a discussion followed in the usual way. On the way to lunch after the discussion, a colleague from the Family Center in Washington. D.C., touched me softly on the arm in a way that convinced me that she had taken sides and was blaming my wife for the tensions in our marriage that we had discussed. The woman's touch and facial expression I interpreted as her feeling sorry for me. I realized how insidious emotional process could be. Fortunately, I was far enough along with Bowen theory experience at that point to be clear that someone taking sides on our marital issue is not doing us any favors. It is too easy to be emboldened to think you are right when someone else reinforces that view.

More important, I did not look at the tape of the interview again until a year later. When I finally watched it, I listened to myself on the tape and thought, "Whom does that guy think he is kidding?" It was humbling and useful to recognize how the emotional side of me influenced how I acted and talked on the tape. I was trying to look good. I do not think I would have seen my charade if I had watched a playback of the tape closer to the time we did the interview. As I said earlier, part of the process of differentiation is fathoming how undifferentiated you are!

In the mid-1960s, Bowen began to use the techniques of family therapy with a single family in treating several families meeting in a group (Bowen, 1971). He called it multiple family therapy. The techniques that have been discussed already were carried over into doing multiples, as he and others came to call them. The Bowen theory technique put three or four couples together in a group but minimized the families interacting with each other. It is a given that the members of each couple will be reactive to the problems that exist in the other families. This was not a group therapy model in which members of one family would exchange with members of the other families. The technique was to apply the technique of working with one couple with each couple individually for, say, thirty minutes and then moving onto the next couple for their thirty minutes. The rationale of doing this was that each couple would have the opportunity to listen to the other couples and to observe the therapist's interaction with each couple. The thought was that this might speed up their learning about the emotional process in their own family. Interaction between the couples was discouraged to reduce the degree of emotionality in one couple infecting or being a problem for other couples in the multiple. This is the same idea that was applied to audience-family interchanges in the MCV project.

Multiple family therapy seemed to add something to the process of facilitating differentiation of self in the nuclear family, but the logistics of coordinating multiple schedules for the sessions was one factor in Bowen theorists using it less over time. The technique itself remains a solid approach.

Family therapy with one person is another technique that appeared fairly early in doing Bowen-theory-based family therapy but underwent significant changes over time. The clinical case I present in Chapter 17 is one illustration of that process, where the vast majority of the sessions were with just the husband. Therapists who have done a decent job on differentiation of self in their own families are most able to overcome the primary challenge in doing family therapy with one person, which is being able to think in terms of the relationship system as a whole while listening to just one family member.

The difficulty staying objective about the overall family process when listening to just one spouse is highlighted by an experience I have had routinely. In situations where I had been seeing one spouse for a time and then the other spouse joined the therapy or came on his or her own, I have usually gained a somewhat different perspective on the emotional process in the family. This indicates that I was not getting an adequate picture of the family process from listening to just one member. The change in perspective was rarely dramatic, however, and I have gotten better over time at gleaning the larger system process when seeing just one person. The more people can develop their ability to think theory through by applying it in their own lives, the more adept they become at keeping a systems perspective when dealing with just one family member. This, of course, is critical to coaching a person on differentiation of self in family of origin, the most recently developed technique for increasing differentiation of self.

Another major vulnerability in doing family therapy with one person is that a person may come to see you as on his or her side and gain false strength or pseudo-self from that perception. Many spouses of people in psychoanalysis or other variations of individual psychotherapy come to feel like the outsider with their spouse and the therapist. Therapists thinking they should be an advocate for the patient in individual therapy contributes to this problem. In Bowen theory, even though therapists may be working with just one family member, if they are doing a good job of thinking systems, they are an advocate for the family. Certainly, on a feeling level, people commonly want their therapist to take their side, but most know at some level that what they will benefit from most is a therapist's ability to be objective about them and their families.

I have already discussed in much detail differentiation of self in one's family of origin and the role of the coach in such an effort. It is probably the most important innovation in technique thus far. The key is that coaches must have gone down that road in their own family to do an adequate job assisting others in doing the same. The combined clinical experience of skilled Bowen theorists over the last several decades has contributed in important ways to a better understanding of the process of differentiation. The most important thing I have come to realize about the process of differentiation is that the people who make the most progress are those who stop mixing theories. They have acquired a hard-earned conviction that minimizes them flip-flopping in highly anxious situations. *Flip-flopping* means mixing individual, cause-and-effect explanations and approaches with systems explanations and approaches.

It is a legitimate question to ask, What is the difference between conviction and close-minded dogma? A person can have conviction but still be open-minded, always alert to new information that could challenge the accuracy of Bowen theory. Bowen theory is unfinished. Bowen's frequent reminder to Bowen theorists is that theory can be changed by facts alone, not by personal opinion. That is the key to continuing to move toward a science of human behavior.

Differentiation of self is probably the most important concept in Bowen theory for humankind. Many colleagues have described differentiation of self as counterintuitive, and I agree with them. It seems paradoxical that the feeling system can aid cognitive processing in the brain but still be the primary impediment to sorting out what being more of a "self" looks like and having the courage to act on it.

Differentiation of self is important in all human relationship systems, from the family to the societal level. Clinical observations, however, support the idea that people must make gains in their own families before they are able to apply it effectively in nonfamily relationship systems, such as the workplace or a social group. In my opinion, this is because differentiation of self is hard and requires considerable motivation to stick with it over time. People are motivated the most to improve relationships in their families, more than in nonfamily relationships.

Family therapy is a way of thinking, not something defined by how many family members are in the room. If therapists are using systems thinking, they are doing family therapy. All of the techniques that I have described in this chapter that are guided by Bowen theory and differentiation of self have merit. Family therapy with one family member has been used much more since the innovation of differentiation of self in one's family of origin. This does not mean that this should be the technique choice for everyone. One prominent misconception about therapy guided by Bowen theory is that it takes a long time. If a therapist comprehends what it means to be in contact with a family system, but outside the emotional process, this is extraordinarily useful in short-term crisis intervention. If a therapist is dealing with someone who wants to commit to a long-term effort on differentiation of self in the nuclear and extended families, then that, of course, will take a long time. The primary innovation here is a new theory of human behavior that can be applied in many ways in many different settings. *The Atlantic Monthly* (September 1988, pp. 35–58) excerpted the book that Murray Bowen and I coauthored, *Family Evaluation*. When the editor told me what intrigued him about the book enough to excerpt it, he said, "Differentiation of self, something new since Freud."

A brief caveat before closing out this part of the book devoted to the process of differentiation. Articles and lectures can give people an intellectual awareness of systems thinking and the concepts in Bowen theory, but that alone is insufficient for operationalizing the concepts in one's own life. Seeing the hidden life of families requires the kinds of experiences that I described in Part II about the process of differentiation. Consultation with a coach who has been down this road in his or her own family greatly facilitates this effort. The task is to use systems thinking to distinguish process, such as relationship reciprocity and triangles, from content, such as "I can't believe that person treated you that way." I do not want to minimize the value of reading and listening to lectures about the theory, because many people have learned about Bowen theory and usefully applied it in settings that are less emotionally intense than one's personal life, such as in the workplace or a nonfamily social group. Reading and lectures can also motivate people to learn more about the ideas; it can help long-term students of Bowen theory clarify some of their thinking about the theory and, at a minimum, keep people in touch with systems thinking while living in a cause-and-effect world.

PART III

Applying Bowen Theory to Families in the Public Eye

The terrible and exasperating thing about humans is how goodness and gentleness, and utter depravity and disregard for human life, can be contained within the same person, and in terrifyingly close proximity. . . .

Good God, it would be easier if this were not the case. If murderers were of a wholly different species, if they were beasts who we couldn't talk to, relate to, understand in any way, if they were incapable of love or light—it would be far easier. But this is not the case. They are almost always people precisely like ourselves, flawed and good and weak, capable of acts of courage and horrible mistakes.
—Dave Eggers, foreword to Norman Mailer's
The Executioner's Song

I introduce Part III with a quote on the difficulty reconciling the sometimes two strikingly contradictory sides of a human being's nature, and about how much the best and the worst of us have in common, because the quote is relevant to the case studies presented in this part. Three of the four cases are about murderers: the Unabomber, Ted Kaczynski; Adam Lanza, the Sandy Hook shooter; and Gary Gilmore, executed in 1977 for the wanton murders of two men in Utah. The fourth case study is of John Nash, subject of the book *A Beautiful Mind* (Nasar, 1998) that inspired the movie of the same title in 2001. Nash was a genius mathematician who never committed a crime but was remarkable in making a full recovery from schizophrenia after many decades of psychotic symptoms and inability to work effectively. His accomplishing this without medications or psychotherapy commands attention.

Hardly a day goes by that tragedies involving one person doing seemingly senseless and serious harm to another person or people are not in the news. Questions about why a person has committed such heinous acts are routinely puzzled over in the reporting. Commonly, explanations such as a traumatic childhood, severe mental illness, "bad seed," or, more recently, terrorism are invoked. People feel especially confused if the offender's family background appears relatively normal. Questions such as these often energize nature-nurture debates.

I investigated the cases in this part of the book because sufficient information is available about them in the public domain, such as in carefully researched books and articles, to draw reasonable conclusions about the emotional functioning of those involved. I have examined these situations through the lens of Bowen theory and have found that the theory enhances the understanding of what has unfolded. The theory is by no means a complete explanation—the complexity of the processes involved precludes that—but the lens of theory adds a great deal by revealing the hidden life of families and how it has affected their members. Journalists often describe these hidden processes but lack a conceptual framework to clarify their importance.

One other purpose for writing this part of the book is to emphasize the reductionism of psychiatric labels. Categorizing people based on the symptoms they manifest tells us very little about the present and past complex of forces driving their behaviors and overall life functioning.

CHAPTER NINETEEN

The Unabomber and His Family

Two months after FBI agents arrested Theodore John Kaczynski on the charge of being the Unabomber, a long article published in the *Washington Post* about the Unabomber and his family triggered my interest in the case (Kovaleski, 1996). (The FBI named the illusive perpetrator of a multiyear series of bombings the "Unabomber" because the intended victims were associated with universities or airlines.) The article contained many detailed descriptions of important family interactions that were consistent with Bowen theory. It is one of those not uncommon cases in which a normal-appearing family spawns a highly dysfunctional offspring.

Based on that newspaper article and other media sources, I began doing presentations about the family at professional conferences. I did one of those presentations in the Unabomber's hometown of Chicago, and it led to a chance to meet with Ted Kaczynski's mother, Wanda; his younger brother, David; and David's wife, Linda. That meeting occurred over a weekend in September 1997. I have not met Ted Kaczynski, but I corresponded with him a few times after he was incarcerated. Our letter exchanges included some of his ideas about his family life and my ideas about how Bowen theory could help explain the family patterns that he described.

Ted Kaczynski had refused to see any family member for several years before his apprehension and also since his capture. The family, of course, was shocked by the revelations about Ted and his alleged crimes. No one in the family had connected Ted with the bombings until the *Washington Post* and *New York Times* published the Unabomber Manifesto in the early fall of 1995. David's wife, Linda, read the manifesto and urged her husband to read it, believing that the overall theme and numerous passages sounded like things Ted would write or had already written in letters to the family. David agreed with Linda's assessment and, with his mother's agreement, notified the FBI of their suspicions. This was a difficult decision for the family to make because, despite the high level of family tension that had characterized their interactions with Ted since he was an adolescent and the considerable distance that had developed in recent years at Ted's insistence, he had remained a much beloved family member.

Between 1978 and 1995, using explosive devices that he had constructed and sent through the mail to the targeted victims, Ted killed three people and injured twenty-three others. I wanted to see if Bowen theory could help explain what drove him to do what he did and how family relationships (including the multigenerational family) may have unwittingly contributed to such a dire outcome. Bowen theory helped me explain my brother's severe dysfunction occurring in an outwardly normal-appearing family, and I thought I may be able to do the same for Ted's criminal actions. As I have emphasized before, family emotional process does not cause the problem, but it is important for increasing the vulnerability to dire outcomes.

The family's principal worry after Ted's arrest was that he would receive the death penalty. They hoped an insanity defense would mitigate Ted's responsibility for his actions. With his guilt being beyond question from the enormous volume of evidence that the FBI had collected, the family's best hope was that Ted would be sentenced to life in prison.

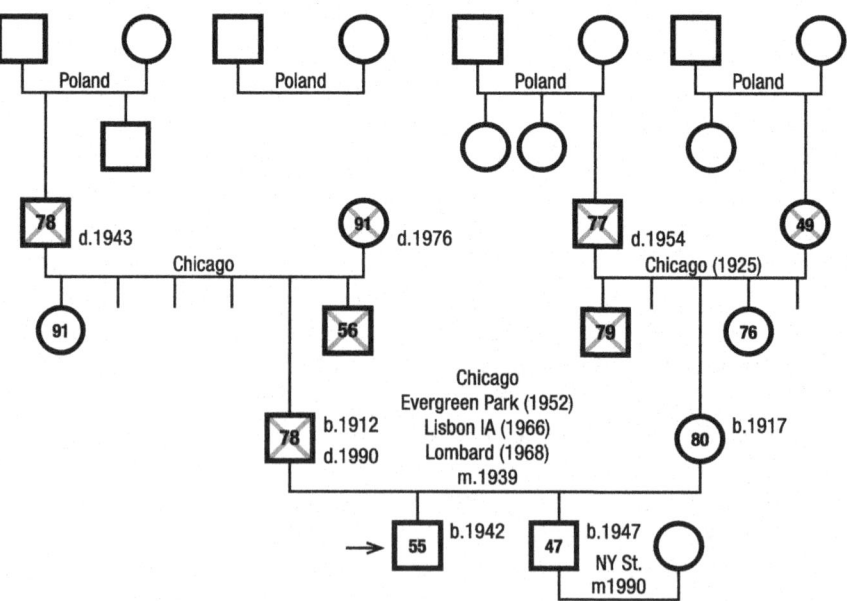

Figure 19.1 *Diagram of the Kaczynski-Dombek family about the time of the Unabomber's arrest.* The arrow at the bottom of the diagram points to Ted Kaczynski.

I begin discussion of the family with the incomplete diagram in Figure 19.1. The thick arrow at the bottom left points to Ted, born in 1942 and fifty-five years old as of 1997. His younger brother, David, was born nearly eight years later in 1949. The diagram includes David's 1990 marriage to Linda Patrik. They lived in Schenectady. David and Linda did not have children. David was a social worker and Linda was a philosophy professor at Union College. The boys' mother, Wanda Dombek Kaczynski, was born in 1917. She married Theodore Richard Kaczynski in 1939. They met in Chicago and spent almost their entire married life in the Chicago area. Ted Sr. killed himself a month after learning his body was riddled with cancer.

The most notable insight from examining data about the larger extended family systems pertains to Mrs. Kaczynski's family. She is the third of five children. Wanda's functioning position in the family system was strongly influenced by her mother's poor health and addiction problems. Much turmoil existed in the family, and even as a young girl, Wanda worked very hard to try to right the ship. Her mother died of a stroke when Wanda was seventeen years old.

Wanda's emotional programming in her functional oldest position contributed to an attitude that, when she had her own family, she would do absolutely everything she could to shape a family life that would make things turn out right for her children, one far removed from what she experienced growing up. This, of course, is not an unusual goal for a mother to have, but Wanda pursued it with unusually high energy and sense of purpose. With only limited data about the extended family, it is difficult to estimate the family's overall level of differentiation of self, but it appears to be in the low moderate range. The importance of at least an impression about differentiation in the multigenerational family is that Ted's very low level of "self" that I describe in this chapter did not appear out of nowhere. The intense anxious focus on Ted gave David the room to develop more of a "self" than his brother.

Both Wanda and her husband, Ted Sr., worked very hard to provide a solid family environment. Mr. Kaczynski managed a European-style sausage company, then worked at a few other jobs, and later worked as a manager in a foam-cutting factory. They had a comfortable home, first in Chicago and later in the Chicago suburb of Evergreen Park. Neighbors' impressions of the Kaczynski family in the 1950s were that they were extremely intellectual, productive, and civic-minded folks. The boys' father was gregarious and happy, loved the outdoors, and interested his sons in those activities. Wanda was a homemaker, doing only occasional part-time work until David was eleven, when she began having full-time jobs. She eventually completed teacher training and taught school for a short period. Both Ted and David entered college as sixteen-year-olds, Ted at Harvard and David at Columbia. Obviously, they benefited from their parents' dedication to their education.

As I describe Ted and his family through the lens of Bowen theory, I often refer to the timeline in Table 19.1, touching in more detail on some events than others. As I explain in the discussion of my own family in the epilogue, Bowen theory helps conceptualize how changes in social context over time correlate with changes in the emotional functioning of individual family members over time. I demonstrate that idea in the Kaczynski family as well.

TABLE 19.1
Timeline for Important Events for Ted Kaczynski and Family

DATE	EVENT
May 22, 1942	Theodore John Kaczynski is born.
March 1, 1943	Ted is admitted to pediatric isolation unit for six days.
October 3, 1949	David Richard Kaczynski is born.
June 1952	The family moves to Evergreen Park, outside of Chicago.
Fall 1953	Ted skips sixth grade at public elementary school.
Fall 1957	Ted skips the eleventh grade at public high school.
Fall 1958	Ted begins freshman year at Harvard on scholarship.
June 1962	Ted graduates from Harvard.
Fall 1962	Ted begins graduate work at the University of Michigan.
Spring 1967	Ted receives his Ph.D. in mathematics from Michigan.
September 1967	Ted becomes assistant professor in math at U.C. Berkeley
January 1969	Ted resigns from U.C. Berkeley
June 1969	Ted leaves Berkeley and moves in with parents in Lombard, IL.
June 1971	Ted and David buy a 1.4-acre lot in Montana. Ted builds cabin.
January 1972	Ted leaves Lombard and moves into cabin in Montana.
January 1973	Ted lives and works in Utah and Idaho.
June 1973	Ted returns to Montana cabin.
May 1978	Ted returns to Chicago area in search of work, lives with parents.
May 25, 1978	Ted's first bombing attempt at Northwestern University.
June 1978	Ted gets work where his father and brother work.
August 1978	Ted is fired from job.
September 1978	Ted gets another job in the Chicago area.
March 1979	Ted quits the job.
May 1979	Ted's second bombing attempt at Northwestern.
June 1979	Ted returns to cabin near Lincoln, MT.
November 1979 to April 1995	Twelve bombings occur between November 1979 and February 1987 resulting in one death. No bombings occur between February 1987 and June 1993. Four bombings occur between June 1993 and April 1995 resulting in two deaths.

July 1990	David and Linda Patrik marry.
September 1990	Ted's father diagnosed with metastatic lung cancer.
October 1990	Ted's father dies of self-inflicted gunshot wound to the head.
May 1988 to September 1991	Ted makes many attempts to find therapist, primarily wanting help with having a successful relationship with a woman.
September 1995	Unabomber Manifesto published.

The first significant event occurred very early in Ted's life: his hospitalization at the age of nine months. This event seems to have had a more lasting impact on his mother than on Ted. Ted had a severe allergic reaction manifesting in hives over much of his body and was confined for six days in a pediatric isolation unit in a hospital. This is obviously a difficult situation for any child to endure, but Mrs. Kaczynski believes to this day that Ted likely suffered lasting psychological trauma from that experience. She thinks it might be an important clue for why her son developed what she believes is a mental illness. She wanted desperately for him to have a normal life, but any signs of that not happening reinforced her speculation about the trauma notion. As a child, if Ted seemed angry or in some psychological pain, or if he withdrew, stopped speaking and making eye contact, for a period of time, the fear was reawakened in her. She later extended the trauma explanation to why he had so few friends and never a girlfriend. She would try to draw Ted out, wanting to know what was bothering him. The battle to understand Ted went on for years. She tried to lure neighborhood children to her home in the hope that Ted could begin to form some friendships. Wanda was fiercely dedicated to assuring Ted's emotional well-being. She was sometimes quite critical of him, particularly during his adolescence.

The information available about the family life indicates a powerful emotional fusion between Wanda and Ted that included very positive and very negative attitudes in each person about the other. This family projection process turned from largely positive to much more negative during Ted's adolescence. Unaware of its potential consequences, of course, Ted Sr. and David actively supported Wanda in the anxiety-driven child focus. Ted grew up feeling superior and special, like he was the most important member of the family, and in terms of impact on family emotional life, he was. Ted said in an interview after his capture that he got more attention from his parents than David did (Follett, 1999). Wanda read endlessly to Ted, including articles from *Scientific American* before he was even five years old. Ted's obvious brightness reinforced Wanda's dedication. She kept a meticulous journal about his life. It was an unmistakably intense child focus accompanied by a strong background anxiety in the form of fears that his social development was severely lagging. Wanda was quite involved with David as well, but her investment in him was less riddled with anxiety.

As I describe in the epilogue, the emotional process in the Kaczynski family had many parallels to my family of origin—it is one reason that I became so interested in the case. Each family produced one dysfunctional offspring and one or more seemingly normal offspring. The clinical outcomes were very different: my brother got a schizophrenia diagnosis and ultimately committed suicide, and Ted Kaczynski got a trial-generated schizophrenia diagnosis and killed other people. Bowen theory contributes new variables to predicting vulnerability to serious dysfunction in a life course, but it is difficult to predict the specific form the dysfunction will take. This seems to be the nature of complex systems, whether in the cosmos, life on Earth, or the human family.

One article suggested that life in the family was good until Ted was about age ten or eleven. Interestingly, an aunt (Wanda's sister) commented that about the time that David was born, Ted changed. She said he used to snuggle up to her, but afterward he became withdrawn. She speculated that maybe the family paid too much attention to the new baby (Thomas, 1996). Ted was about seven and a half when his brother was born.

From a Bowen theory perspective, the more intense a parent's emotional involvement with a child in the period before a sibling is born, the more reactive the child is, given the consequent intensely emotionally programmed need for attention, to the parent's attention being diverted to the new baby. Furthermore, the parent is anxious about being able to continue to meet the first child's needs because of the demands of the second child. It is not unusual for worry about adequately meeting the emotional needs of two children to delay a mother's decision to have a second child. Despite what may have been Ted's strong reaction to the addition of a second child, David became very important to Ted and grew to love his older brother dearly, following him "like a shadow" (Thomas, 1996).

A major downside to the anxiety about trauma that plagued Wanda about Ted is that, by being based on the idea that something bad happened in the past, a parent typically feels that the only recourse in the present is to shower the child with love and attention in the hope of countering the effects of the perceived trauma. Such an approach only further intensifies the fusion, further increases the child's need to rely on others to regulate any internal distress. The interactive process programs the child's needs for attention and acceptance far beyond what is adaptive in life.

From a Bowen theory perspective, it is this programming for a powerful need for acceptance and exquisite sensitivity to real or imagined rejection, not trauma, that made it difficult for Ted to have a long-term relationship with a woman. Ted was fiercely angry at his mother for not teaching him the necessary social skills to successfully form a romantic relationship. Interestingly, he described himself as unattached to his mother when, in fact, although he apparently felt unattached to her, it was an unresolved attachment that was the real problem. Many people who had very strong emotional fusions with their mother are not consciously aware of its impact on adult relationships. The extraordinary sensitivities in adult romantic relationships are undeniable, but the source of the sensitivities is a puzzle to them. Part of the problem is that people want to believe that they are more autonomous than they really are. Ted had to isolate himself to experience autonomy. He was easily unraveled in a potential romantic relationship with a woman and very much wished he could do otherwise.

As mentioned before, an unresolved emotional attachment unfolds in the parental triangle. Besides supporting Wanda's anxious focus on Ted and siding with her around major tensions during Ted's adolescence, one of the father's other contributions to the problem was his hypersensitivity to discomfort in Ted. For example, Ted Sr. would take his sons along when he hunted. When Ted's father killed a rabbit, Ted had such a violent reaction that Ted Sr. gave up the sport. As a young adult, Ted hated noise. Consequently, Ted Sr. gave up watching the television news when his son was home. Peace at any price is part of the problem, not part of the solution. The focused-on child's moods and behaviors can upset other family members to the point of rendering them increasingly passive in their responses. This taking the easy way out can program offspring to have unrealistic expectations about what others should do for them, holding others responsible for their happiness. Another way of expressing this process is that the family learned to normalize Ted's aberrant behaviors, to weave them into the family fabric. This is part of what keeps highly influential emotional processes hidden.

An emotional regression began in the family when Ted reached the age of eleven. No doubt a number of processes converged, ones that affected Ted directly and other family members directly. (Remember that the key to understanding emotional regression is recognizing not just the particular stresses individuals have in their lives but how family members interact in face of one another's anxiety.) The transition from elementary school to junior high school can be particularly difficult for children that feel socially insecure; the whole school routine changes in a way that can be overwhelming and isolating.

Ted dated the development of his anger back to that early adolescent period. In a letter to his mother in the summer of 1991, he claimed the many rejections, humiliations, and other painful influences during adolescence, at home and in school, caused his current difficulties (Kovaleski, 1997). Peer relationships clearly have a powerful impact on a developing young person, but the more intense the unresolved emotional fusion with the family, the greater the reactivity in peer interactions. Ted's anger was a product of the parental triangle, not of him as an individual. The inability of all three members of a triangle to maintain a "self" leads to anger that is felt primarily by one person. It is predictable that if a parent can change his or her part in the parental triangle by functioning with more "self," the teenager's anger will diminish.

Ted had tested in the genius IQ level and excelled through the fifth grade. The teachers recommended that he skip the sixth grade, which the parents approved. However, things seemed to change for him from seventh grade forward. During his adolescence, Ted spent much of his time in his attic bedroom, especially when company came to the house. David described Ted as having rigid and dogmatic opinions, even from an early age. The forensic psychiatrist who examined Ted in connection with the trial is quoted as saying, "By the time I left high school [at age sixteen, having skipped his junior year as well], I was definitely regarded as a freak by most students" (Chase, 2000, retrieved online). Ted left high school with low social esteem (he saw his social confidence as crushed in high school) but high self-esteem in other respects. He was confident in his ability to deal with things as opposed to people. He had no confidence in his ability to be accepted by people.

The change in family emotional processes during Ted's adolescence is symbolized in Figure 19.2. The diagram on the left symbolizes the Ted's preadolescence. Chronic anxiety was relatively low in the family system because it was bound in the triangles. The four lines between Wanda and Ted symbolize the intense emotional fusion in their relationship that was harmonious during this period. The three lines between Wanda and David symbolize a less intense emotional fusion that was also a harmonious. The lines between the boys' father and each of them with the plus sign indicate reasonable harmony in those relationships. The break in the line between the parents symbolizes emotional distance. Little information about the parents' marriage is available, but based on clinical experience, emotional distance always exists between the parents if there is significant anxiety-driven child focus. The parents much use some emotional distance to reduce the degree that their immaturities play out in their relationship. The distance may not be recognized by the parents or by other observers. A helpful way to grasp this is considering that the most fundamental aspect of the distance is the parents' anxieties and insecurities focused mainly on one or more children rather than on each other. I happen to like the term *immaturity*. It is not a criticism but a recognition of something in the human condition that is difficult to control. No one escapes it, but people differ in the degree it colors their emotional functioning.

The diagram on the right in Figure 19.2 symbolizes the adolescent period and the emotional regression in the family system. The fusion between Wanda and Ted now contained periods of friction, irritability, and conflict. More emotional distance existed between them as well (symbolized by break in fusion

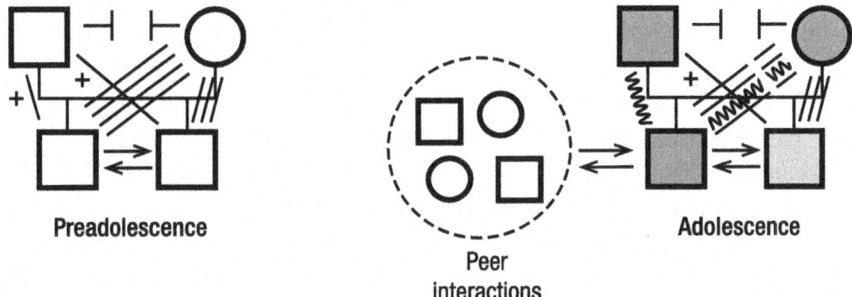

Figure 19.2 *This diagram symbolizes the difference in the Kaczynski nuclear family emotional process in Ted's preadolescent years versus adolescent years.* In the preadolescent period on the left, the four lines between Mrs. Kaczynski and Ted indicate an intense emotional fusion. The symbol between the parents indicates emotional distance. The three lines between younger brother David and his mother indicate a less intense emotional fusion. The father's relationships with each son and the sons' relationship with each other are stable and positive. The jagged line in the nuclear family diagram on the right (Ted's adolescence) between Ted and his mother symbolizes their relationship fusion being tense and often conflictual. The jagged line between the father and Ted also indicates conflict. The shading in all four family members indicates heightened chronic anxiety in the system. David is less anxious than the parents and Ted. David's relationship with Ted remains stable and largely conflict free. The four symbols with a dashed circle around them and reciprocating arrows with Ted symbolize peer relationships in which he often felt isolated and diminished.

lines). Considerable conflict between Ted Sr. and his older son had developed; he sided with his wife in blaming Ted for family upsets. Ted Sr., Wanda, and Ted Jr. are all more chronically anxious (symbolized by darker shading). Each individual's anxiety complicates interactions, and the problematic interactions increase each individual's anxiety; the intensity of the process ebbs and flows over time. Difficult interactions with peers that compounded the family problem are symbolized on the left of the adolescence diagram. David is symbolized (lighter shading) as being less reactive to the family process. Two sons were being raised in the same family but in different triangles. This commonly results in the siblings having very different perceptions of what family relationships were like.

Ted headed off to Harvard in the fall of 1958. He was sixteen years old. Serge F. Kovaleski and Lorraine Adam's 1996 *Washington Post* article reports that when Ted was accepted there, his parents' pride was tempered with apprehension—they feared he might not be able to cope with his erratic moods far from home. They seemingly recognized Ted's dependence on them to regulate his emotions. Ted had what his father described as a "melancholic shutdown" on a trip with his father to look at various schools, which would have reinforced their apprehension.

Ted would have had his own reservations about leaving for college. He likely had no definite object in going to college. He would have gone because his parents expected it and he did not know what else to do. His fantasies took him to faraway places to be alone. It was a lack of "self" that he was facing.

Nonetheless, Ted adapted reasonably well to Harvard. An article in the *Atlantic Monthly* quoted Sally Johnson, a forensic psychiatrist who did a pretrial examination of Ted, who described "his having intertwined his two belief systems, that society is bad and he should rebel against it, and his intense anger at his family's perceived injustices" (Chase, 2000, retrieved online). Johnson said this intertwining of belief systems began at Harvard. He had encountered among the Harvard faculty a vigorous polarized debate: on the one hand, science and technology is a threat to Western values and human survival; on the other hand, science was a liberator from superstition and an avenue to progress. Exposure to such attitudes in vulnerable people could help shape their later acting out of revenge on people involved in science and technology.

Ted graduated from Harvard in June of 1962 and that fall began graduate work at the University of Michigan. He received a Ph.D. in mathematics in the spring of 1967. It may have been at Michigan that he decided to deal with deep despair by deciding to kill people. The decision could also have come later, but he did not act on this idea until 1978. He was quoted by David Johnston (1998) in a *New York Times* article based on research done after Kaczynski's capture that committing the crimes made him feel better. He was still angry about the perceived injustices he had suffered, but the difference was that he was able to strike back, to a degree.

Ted became an assistant professor of mathematics at the University of California, Berkeley in September 1967. He resigned from that position in January 1969 and left Berkeley in June 1969. Apparently, he had become less enamored of mathematics and teaching it. Not surprisingly, he was not a popular teacher. His loss of interest in what he worked so hard to achieve is not surprising in that a limited "self" resulted in a life direction that was in reaction to others versus a clear, well-thought-out direction of his own. He isolated himself quite a bit during his time at Berkeley.

After Berkeley, Ted returned to the Chicago area and moved in with his parents. David would be returning to his senior year at Columbia that year. Ted returning to the roost for the next two years follows a pattern of an increasing number of young adults currently, only it was delayed until after he got his Ph.D. and a brief stint as an academic. Ted and his parents living together generated much anxiety in all of them. Ted spent lots of time alone, and his worried frustrated parents began pushing him to find work. He did get menial jobs but then quit them after a short time without telling his parents. Continuing his fantasy of wanting to live in a remote area, he filed an application to buy land in Canada, but it was turned down. He eventually left his parents' house quite abruptly and said nothing to them about going—no goodbyes. His mother pleaded with him to stay.

In June of 1971, David and Ted together bought a 1.4-acre lot in the Lincoln, Montana, area. Ted built a small cabin on the land and moved into it in January 1972. The cabin had no running water or electricity. He lived as a recluse and learned the survival skills to become self-sufficient. For nearly five years, he seems to have lived rather peacefully there. His parents and brother both sent money, which was his primary support. Kovaleski wrote the following in 1997 in the *Washington Post* based on reviewing a letter Kaczynski had written to his mother in 1991: He is always under stress whenever he is around people, except those he has known for a long time. The reason is that he doesn't feel that people will accept him. "This fear of rejection—based on bitter experience both at home and at school—has ruined my life, *except for the few years that I spent alone in the woods*, largely out of contact with people." He is referring to this period in the middle 1970s during which he experienced a reasonable degree of equanimity and exhibited fine survival skills.

His parents and brother visited him in Montana a few times in summers during that period. The contentment, however, did not last. Airplanes overhead, logging trucks and their roads, more people living nearby all congealed to incline him to give up on ever escaping the madness he saw being wreaked on society by science and technology. There seemed to be nowhere to run, nowhere to hide. This attitude and feeling state seem key in his deciding finally to seek revenge by killing people. In his mind, he was acting on principle in killing these people who were destroying civilization. In my opinion, one that Kaczynski might not agree with to this day, the dominant motivation was to express anger and hatred, to break free of moral constraints, and to exact revenge for the wrongs that had been done to him.

It was also about this time that Ted was increasing pressure on his family to send more money. The family insisted that he return to the Chicago area, get a job, and live with them. He did return to Chicago and eventually went to work in a factory managed by his father, with David as his immediate boss. His first bombing attempt, which was at Northwestern University and unsuccessful, occurred very soon after he returned to the Chicago area, where he remained for almost a year.

Working with his father and David lasted only a few months, curtailed by an incident that occurred with a woman who also worked at the company, which highlights Ted's core vulnerability. He went out on a few dates with this woman, but she decided not to date him anymore. Fueled by anger generated by his sensitivity to rejections and his default mode of blaming others, Ted posted many derogatory notes about this woman at the workplace. David had no choice but to fire his brother, and not surprisingly, Ted was furious at his brother for doing it. His second bombing attempt, which also failed, was a few months later and also at Northwestern University. In June of 1979, Ted returned to the cabin in Montana. Between November 1979 and April 1995, he conducted fourteen more bombings that resulted in three deaths. His mailed bombs had become more sophisticated. His parents and brother were unwittingly financing his crimes.

Little contact or communication occurred between Ted and his family in the 1980s. Then three important family events occurred: David married in 1990, Ted and David's father was diagnosed with metastatic lung cancer in September 1990, and a month later Ted Sr. died from a self-inflicted gunshot wound. Ted did not attend David's wedding or his father's funeral. David's marriage resulted in Ted distancing even more from David. During the late 1980s and into the 1990s, Ted's life as a hermit was becoming bleaker. He was very short on money, as there was little work for him, particularly during the winter. It is interesting that there were no bombing attempts during this period. Much of the information about Ted during this period comes from letters to a man he had befriended, someone David knew. Ted expressed much understanding and compassion for this man in his letters, illuminating another side of Ted. He sought therapy during this period, primarily wanting to find a way to connect successfully with a woman. None of the several therapy relationships he attempted to implement lasted very long, sometimes for lack of an available therapist.

Ted attempted no bombings between 1987 and 1993. I speculate that Ted may have been more despairing during that time. However, Ted resumed bombings in June 1993, with two attempts, and was planning another one at the time of his capture. The Unabomber Manifesto was published in September 1995, and he was arrested about six months later.

Ted's federal public defenders wanted to use an insanity defense at his impending trial, but Ted rejected that idea. At the court's request for an assessment, Sally Johnson diagnosed him as having paranoid schizophrenia, but Ted avoided a trial by pleading guilty in January 1998. He was sentenced to life in prison without the possibility of parole.

The principal take-home message in this case is that, from a Bowen theory perspective, Ted's low basic level of differentiation, related to an intense and unresolved attachment to his family, is the most significant factor that rendered him vulnerable to a severe emotional dysfunction that manifested in him becoming a serial killer. The two most obvious aspects of his life in which his lack of "self" manifested are his insecurity-driven inability to control the flood of emotional reactivity that interfered with him ever having a romantic relationship with a woman and his acting out murderous impulses on innocent people. His intense focus on a potential female partner, malignant level of reactivity to perceived signs of rejection, and blaming of others that disrupted his relationships with women all reflect the emotional programming created by the intense emotional fusion in which he developed. His intense anger and blaming of his parents and his failure to acknowledge his part in the process reflect the unresolved fusion.

The forensic psychiatrist Sally Johnson diagnosed him as having paranoid schizophrenia, but I fail to see that this adds anything to the understanding of Ted's dysfunction. I think her earlier-quoted statement about Ted intertwining two belief systems—society is bad and he should rebel against it, and a malignant level of anger at his family for perceived injustices—hit the nail squarely on the head. From the perspective of Bowen theory, such intertwining is not a disease but a condition that reflects an anxiety-driven fusion between his emotional and intellectual systems. The fusion of the two systems can result in irrational behaviors and other types of symptoms. It is hard to label Ted's beliefs as paranoid delusions, in the sense that many people agree with him that science and technology are having adverse if not disastrous effects on society and the planet. The coupling of rage with his beliefs is what made them dangerous. Rage was the fuel for seeking revenge; the beliefs selected the targets of that revenge. The principal point I am trying to make here is that the rage stemmed more from relationships with his family and others in nonfamily contexts than from the beliefs themselves.

Getting revenge by attempting to kill other people was his method of tempering anxiety-driven despair. It is very interesting that when he was able to reduce the threat of contact with others who could affect him adversely—referring here to that fairly calm period during the middle 1970s—he did not try to kill anyone. I suspect that even his impulses to kill were largely dormant during that time. Although the awareness that he could kill may have come far sooner than he acted on it, he did not act on it until he felt that no escape was possible from the societal events he rebelled against.

Could some sort of therapeutic intervention have occurred that would have prevented these serial killings? Wanda, David, and Linda were interviewed by Mike Wallace for CBS News 60 *Minutes* on January 11, 1998. Wallace asked Mrs. Kaczynski whether she saw any signs in Ted when he was growing up that indicated the seriousness of his problems. She answered, "Well, there was nothing gross." Her answer did not surprise me because families often go through fairly anxious periods believing that they can manage it themselves. Ted's withdrawal and conflicts with his parents had apparently not reached a level where they did not think they could handle them. The reader will learn in the epilogue about reasons my family did not seek help for my brother when he was growing up. One was similar to what Mrs. Kaczynski said: "There was nothing gross." Perhaps a more important reason is that my mother did not accept a recommendation that my brother have therapy when he was an early teen because she feared it would hurt his self-esteem. One could easily argue with the wisdom of Mother's attitude, but it illustrates that the feeling system can override objective judgments.

A point that family therapy might have been useful was when Ted resigned his position at Berkeley and came home. I saw no reports of their seeking help at that time, but had they sought help, a therapist's ability to help at least one of them to see that all three members of the triangle were highly anxious might have stabilized things somewhat. In such times, however, family members are so busy blaming one another for the family anxiety that it is difficult for any individual to see what to do to lower the anxiety. Any success depends on the therapist's ability to use systems thinking about the family process, to stay patient, and ask questions that help people divert their attention from focusing on what is wrong with others to figuring out what changes they needed to make in themselves. At this level of differentiation and with this level of chronic anxiety, feeling reactions so dominate that it is extremely difficult for anyone to gain objectivity. If the therapist can maintain emotional neutrality, that is attractive to the family and can keep them coming. Having consistent contact with a neutral party can in itself help lower family anxiety, even if family members have not grasped systems thinking.

CHAPTER TWENTY

Gary Gilmore and His Family

The psychotic thinks he's in contact with spirits from other worlds. He believes he is prey to the spirits of the dead. He's in terror. By his understanding he lives in a field of evil forces. The psychopath inhabits the same place. It is just that he feels stronger. The psychopath sees himself as a potent force in that field of forces. Sometimes he even believes he can go to war against them, and win. So if he really loses, he is close to collapse, and can be as ghost ridden as the psychotic. . . . [This is a possible] way to build a bridge from the psychopathic to the insane.
—John C. Woods, Utah State Hospital chief of forensic psychiatry, quoted in Norman Mailer's The Executioner's Song

The story of Gary Gilmore and his family could be considered a story of human nature in the raw, not so much financially raw—although that was the case for a time with the family—but emotionally raw. I first became interested in this case decades ago when I read Mikal Gilmore's book *Shot in the Heart* (1995), which was Mikal's effort to describe life growing up in the Gilmore family. There were four sons in the family; Gary was the second son, and Mikal was the youngest one. After reading Mikal's book, I immediately read Norman Mailer's *The Executioner's Song* (1979). Mailer's book concentrates on the last eight months of Gary's life and provides valuable detail about his relationship with Nicole. After reading both books, I had more than enough information to illustrate how Bowen theory could help explain Gary's murders. I began recommending both books as superb descriptions of family emotional process and its long-term impact on the offspring of a family. The repeated interactions in the parental triangle of Gary's father, his mother, and Gary fit with Murray Bowen's clinical observations that the parents of people who develop severe acting-out problems like Gary consistently convey a message to that offspring of "I love you no matter what you do" (Bowen, 1970). No matter how severe the punishments inflicted on the child, it does not dilute the basic message the parents deliver. From the perspective of Bowen theory, Mikal overly emphasizes the impact of the father over the mother in Gary's development, but the wealth of description of family relationships in the book lends itself to an alternative explanation by Bowen theory.

In reading Mailer's book, I was taken particularly by the quote by Dr. Woods that I used to introduce this chapter, about the suggestion of a possible bridge "from the psychopath to the insane." In reading both books again in preparation for writing this chapter, I began considering the question of whether people who fit the description of an extreme psychopath have any more control over their actions in committing a murder than people who are markedly psychotic when they commit a murder. People vulnerable to periods of psychosis or to antisocial acts both exist on a broad continuum in the degree of dysfunction that they manifest over their lifetimes. Gary was at the extreme dysfunctional end. Bowen theory views both extreme degrees of psychotic symptoms and antisocial actions as reflecting severe levels of emotional dysfunction. They are disorders of the emotional system, in Gary and in his family emotional system. Conceptualizing both as emotional system disorders provides one kind bridge from the psychopath to the insane that Woods speculates may be possible. Bowen theory holds that psychotic people internalize their anxiety in the form of delusions and hallucinations (which in some instances may direct them to kill someone), and socially acting-out people habitually externalize the anxiety into the relationship system (sometimes in the form of doing violence to others).

Exploring the question of degree of control is not an esoteric pursuit because the legal system currently views people who commit murder while in a psychotic state as less responsible for their actions than people deemed to be psychopaths and aware that their actions are morally wrong by socially accepted standards. During Gary Gilmore's murder trial, because he had no evidence of psychosis according to the psychiatrists who assessed him, he was considered fully responsible for his actions. However, the almost unfathomable intensity of emotional forces in this case makes me think that the dividing line here is not nearly as clear-cut as medicine and the legal system have assumed.

My discussion of this case begins with a family diagram of the Gilmore-Brown families (Figure 20.1). As this chapter proceeds I amplify some of the points that I make here about the diagram. Quite striking is Gary's father Frank Gilmore having had at least six brief marriages that ended in divorce before he met Bessie Brown, and there may have been more, symbolized by the question marks after his last known marriage before Bessie and the next to Frank's children (it is unknown if there were others). The first child Frank fathered was born out of wedlock (indicated by the dashed line), and Frank never saw or supported the child. His second marriage produced a son that Frank's mother raised. Frank left the mother of that child and took the child

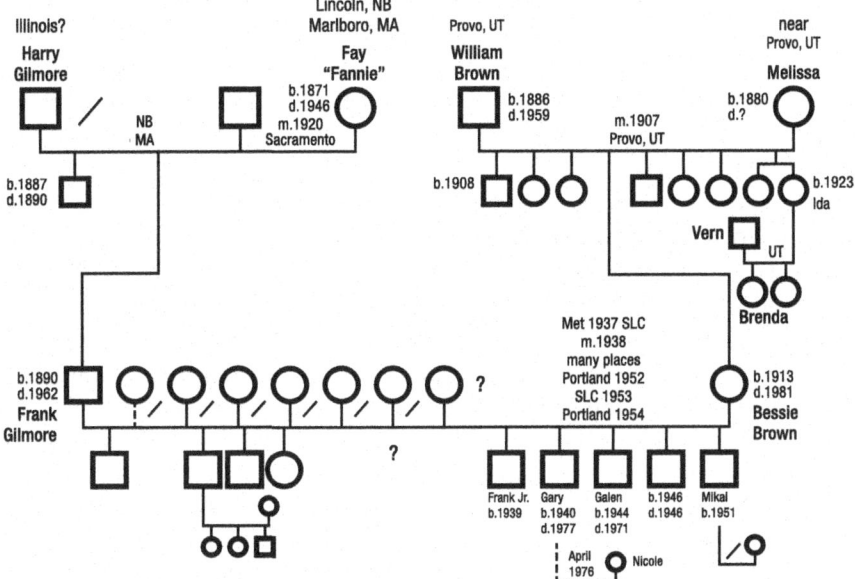

Figure 20.1 *Diagram of the Gilmore-Brown family.*

to his mother when he caught his wife in bed with another man. Frank then went eighteen years without seeing that son, Robert, or his own mother. In fact, apart from his mother, Frank had no extended family that were of any significance to him during his adult years. After leaving Robert's mother, he continued as a relationship nomad until he married Bessie in 1938. Despite horrendous conflict and abuse, that marriage lasted twenty-four years, until Frank's death in 1962. This information, combined with information about Bessie (described below), adds up to these being two poorly differentiated spouses. Bessie saw a little more of her extended family than Frank did, but the emotional cutoff with her family was also quite pronounced.

Another striking aspect of this family diagram is what Bowen theorist Roberta Holt (2011) referred to as a "family of extinction." The family of Frank and Bessie Gilmore has no descendants. (It is uncertain if Gary had a child, but he never saw the child or supported it if he did indeed have one.) In Holt's article, she cites Bowen (1976): "[Dying out families] referred to families that had patterns of low fertility, in the presence of extremely poor functioning, characterized by physical, social, and emotional dysfunctioning for many members of the family" (2011, p. 144). This description fits the Gilmore family. The theory assumes that the poor functioning is related to a low level of differentiation. The levels of "self" are so low and the emotional interdependence so extreme that most family relationships are woefully unstable and program far more undifferentiation than differentiation into the offspring. Mikal, the sibling that I assess to have developed the highest level of "self" in the group, has come closest to a productive life course, but he is the first to acknowledge his inability to have a sustained intimate relationship. The diagram in Figure 20.1 shows the one marriage he had, which lasted only a few years and produced no offspring.

Note also on the diagram that the last two of Bessie's siblings were twins. One was named Ida, whom Bessie felt especially close to. Ida's marriage to a man named Vern and their two daughters is shown. Most of Bessie's other siblings had children as well, but I show Ida and Vern's family because they were quite important in the Gary Gilmore story. Their older daughter, Brenda, with the strong support of her parents, worked to help get Gary paroled from prison in April 1976. Gary came to live with Ida and Vern and also lived some with Brenda and her husband in Provo, where his mother grew up. Gary wore out his welcome with that family in fairly short order.

The last person I point out on the diagram is Nicole Baker Barrett. Note the dashed line between Gary and her, which denotes their living together without being married. It was a wildly intense relationship that began some weeks after Gary was paroled. Gary moved into Nicole's rental house, but their relationship lasted only a little more than two months. Nicole began to feel threatened by Gary and left him. Mailer's description of the intensity and passion in their relationship is exceptionally vivid. The inevitable disruption of the relationship of two very needy people with unrealistic expectations of themselves and each other was the critical factor in triggering the murders Gary committed a week after she left him.

A useful place to start this story is with a summary of nodal events in Gary Gilmore's life. These events capture what a train wreck his life turned out to be:

- Gary was born December 7, 1940, in Texas under the name of his father's alias. The name was later changed at Bessie's insistence when the family left Texas.
- Gary's first serious behavioral acting out in society emerged when he was thirteen and the family was living in Salt Lake City.
- Gary's first time in jail was in 1953, for repeated petty thefts, when the family was back in Portland, Oregon.
- Gary was an exceptionally disruptive student in junior high school. He donned a greasy pompadour and a motorcycle jacket and was into smoking, drinking, skipping school, rumbles, and girls.
- Gary dropped out of school at age fourteen.
- Burglaries and car thefts resulted in Gary being sent to reform school

in 1954. During his fifteen months there, he escaped four times. He was released after he realized that behaving better will get him discharged. It was evident there that Gary had a high IQ and considerable artistic talent.
- He came out of reform school as an even more hardened criminal, wanting to be a mobster. He resumed house break-ins and stole guns especially. He was never free in his life more than eight months after reform school.
- Armed robbery and assault resulted in his being sent to Oregon State Correctional Institution (OSCI) in the fall of 1961. He was there for less than a year.
- After release from OSCI, driving without a license and with an open bottle of alcohol resulted in jail time at Rocky Butte jail in Portland, Oregon. He was released in 1962. News of his Dad's death in June 1962 resulted in him slashing his wrists while still in jail.
- After Rocky Butte, he was quickly back with the criminal element in Portland.
- Committing still more crimes resulted in a fifteen-year sentence to Oregon State Penitentiary in 1964. He was a warden's worst nightmare in his continual defiance of authority. He relished solitary confinement, often for very long periods. He was impressively calm and well behaved in solitary.
- The warden of Oregon State Penitentiary wanted to be rid of Gary Gilmore, so he was transferred to a federal prison in Marion, Illinois, in 1975. He exhibited good behavior there, and with the cooperation of Ida, Vern, and Brenda, this led to a parole in early April of 1976.
- His aunt and uncle paid his way to Provo, Utah, so he could live with them.
- Gary worked at his uncle's shoe repair shop for a few weeks but then at another job after he physically assaulted one of the other employees.
- By acting unstable and perpetually borrowing money from his uncle, Gary wore out his welcome with Ida, Vern, and Brenda. At that point he met Nicole Baker Barrett, about a month after getting out of prison. He quickly moved in with her at her rented house.
- Gary violated his parole and stole from stores routinely. Nicole was aware of it. The authorities tended to be lenient with him.
- After about two months, Nicole left a rapidly deteriorating relationship and made sure Gary could not find her. A week later, on consecutive nights in Orem, Utah, he killed Max Jensen and Ben Bushnell, without them being any threat to him, during burglaries of small amounts of cash.

- Gary was quickly arrested and charged with a capital offense. He was incarcerated at the Utah State Prison.
- Gary was found guilty on October 7, 1976, and given the death penalty. He chose a firing squad over hanging as the method.
- Nicole made contact with Gary again when he was in prison. Their intense relationship resumed—within the constraints of jail visits.
- Advocacy groups such as the ACLU attempted to delay Gary's execution, against Gary's wishes. In spite of Gary's opposition, several stays of execution did occur.
- Gary and Nicole made a suicide pact and attempted it at the same time on November 16, 1976. Both survived, but Nicole was hospitalized psychiatrically and was no longer able to visit Gary. They exchanged many letters.
- Gary made another suicide attempt on December 16 after a judge ruled for yet another stay of execution.
- Gary was finally executed on January 17, 1977.
- In a suicide note she never acted on, Nicole wrote that she wanted to be cremated and her ashes mixed with Gary's and scattered on a hillside.

As I provide a more thorough portrait of the Gilmore family in what follows, keep in mind that one principal reason for presenting the four cases in this part of the book is to emphasize that Bowen theory describes a unique conceptual framework of the forces that shape human development, unique because it is built on the discovery that families function as emotional units. Most mental health professionals are well schooled in the conventional thinking that trauma, abuse, and neglect during a child's development are principal causes of the vulnerabilities that increase the child's chances in adulthood of having psychological, behavioral, and physical illness problems. Most students of Bowen theory have been schooled by earlier training and the culture in this conventional view, and this makes it difficult to shift to a Bowen theory perspective that trauma, abuse, and neglect are common in poorly differentiated families, but lack of differentiation and the chronic anxiety it generates are most important in the development of clinical symptoms.

I describe the essentials of Bowen theory's understanding of development in Chapter 9. This understanding is anchored in the interplay of the counterbalancing life forces of differentiation and togetherness. The togetherness process, and the level of chronic anxiety driving it, manifests in a mix of communications and actions by family members that, on the one hand, function to restrict others and, on the other hand, are overly permissive. At the restrictive end of the spectrum, individuals are trying to manage their own anxiety by attempting to control what others say and do; at the permissive end of the spectrum, individuals are trying to control their own anxiety by attempting to meet others' unrealistic expectations of them. At the restrictive end, people adamantly believe that, if they can exert more control, they can make others function better; at the permissive end, people passionately believe that being more loving and understanding of others is what can fix them.

It is easy to lose sight of the profound emotional interdependence that is playing out in less differentiated families because of the whirlwind of anxiety-driven negative emotions and behaviors that spin off from it. We have all seen very loving people come to hate each other over time. Expressions of hate bury expressions of love. In sharp contrast, at the pinnacle of differentiation people's communications and actions reflect their ability to be closely connected to important others and yet remain calm and thoughtful enough not to try to control others or allow others to control them. The feeling of "emotional space" that differentiation fosters allows for good communication and cooperation and for the expression of positive emotions.

Now to a more thorough portrait of the main characters in this saga and their interactions, beginning with Gary's parents. Bessie Brown, fifth of nine children in a strict Mormon family living in Provo, Utah, was rebellious in her own right as an adolescent but not as extreme as two of her own sons would be. She routinely violated her parents' curfews and was often criticized for running around with the wrong crowd. She felt humiliated in her family, that damnation enwrapped her. She did not behave like Mormon-raised children should behave. Legacies for Bessie of her growing up years were a deep insecurity and much self-blame. A pattern of emotional cutoff surfaced between Bessie and her family, and it led to her leaving Provo in her early twenties to live in Salt Lake City. She also lived in California for a time. After a failed relationship there, she moved back to Salt Lake City and supported herself by cleaning houses and modeling jewelry. She felt the judgment and scorn of her family, especially when she returned home for brief visits.

Bessie was twenty-four years old when she met Frank Gilmore in Salt Lake City, and he was forty-seven. He claimed he was an advertising salesman for *Utah Magazine*. Bessie fell hard for him. He did not talk much, especially about his background, except when he was drinking. He had been a circus performer and movie stunt man earlier in his life. After just a few days, Frank told Bessie that he was getting married the next day, and they then lost track of each other for nearly a year. They met again by chance. Frank had just ended what turned out to be a very brief marriage. After being together just a few days, Frank told Bessie he wanted to marry her. Bessie accepted the proposal and went with Frank to Sacramento to meet his mother, whom he had not seen in eighteen years. Frank's mother, Fannie, was a licensed minister, besides being a psychic and fortune-teller, and she married Bessie and Frank.

Frank bought a house in Sacramento for Bessie and his mother to live in. He then abruptly left on business travel for several weeks. Abrupt and usually last-minute announcements of extended business travel would become a pattern for years in Frank and Bessie's relationship. Frank's son Robert, whom Fannie had raised, also lived in Sacramento, and Bessie got to know him—she later revealed to her sons that Robert was the father of her first child. During that first absence, Bessie learned a number of things about Frank that she had no clue about, such as his many previous marriages. Fannie realized that Bessie had married a man about whom she knew very little.

The next two years, compared to later years of their marriage, were good ones for their relationship, even though they moved often. Absent children, they cooperated well. Soon, however, Bessie realized that Frank made his money doing crooked deals. He was a scammer, selling magazine advertisements but then keeping all the money for himself. He had to keep moving and changing his name to avoid arrest. Bessie even participated in the scam by pretending to work for *Utah Magazine* and taking calls on a phone in their hotel room from potential clients.

Their relationship changed significantly when their first child, Frank Jr., was born. Frank Sr. had wanted kids, possibly more than Bessie did, and helped with the child care, but their relationship became much more tense and conflictual. Gary was born a little more than a year later, and family tensions escalated dramatically. Frank Sr. became wilder, and Bessie felt extremely isolated. Frank's drinking increased; he began beating Bessie and took less interest in the second child. Bessie blamed herself for the beatings. Frank did other strange things too numerous to itemize here. Most important, Gary was born into a highly anxious family system.

In December 1941, Frank was arrested in California and jailed for writing bad checks. Bessie went there with Frank Jr. and Gary in tow and attended the trial. During the trial, she learned about his long criminal record. He was convicted and sentenced to ten years in San Quentin Prison but was paroled for good behavior after two years. Bessie, feeling that Frank had already paid enough for his crimes, pitied him in those early years. The pity shifted to rage as the years wore on.

Rather than remain in California while Frank served his sentence there, Bessie took the kids and went back to Provo to live with her parents. Her parents had met Frank and strongly disliked him. She lived in cramped quarters in the backyard of her parents' home and experienced a growing rage at them and her situation. Interestingly, Bessie relied increasingly on Frank Jr. to help take care of Gary. This was a pattern that powerfully shaped the older boy's life. He would be the one that would take care of their mother until she died. Bessie felt so overwhelmed that she would sometimes rage at the kids. It reached a point that her mother threatened to take custody of the children, but that never happened. When Frank got paroled, he went to Provo. This was in July 1943. It did not go well, and Bessie's father finally kicked them out.

The war was on, and Frank was able to get legitimate work at shipyards and steel plants in California. When Frank's parole ended in 1945, however, he returned to petty crimes and the family continued a vagabond lifestyle. The couple's third son, Gaylen, was born in 1944. The family fell on financial hard times, often living in flophouses and relying on the Salvation Army. Frank continued his pattern of abrupt disappearances, and Bessie would soldier on with the three kids. She was clearly the mortar for the family bricks.

When Frank's mother died in 1946, his reaction was intense. He quit working, cried a lot, and binge drank—this was a man who had rarely expressed any caring and affection for his mother when she was alive. At that time, he learned he had developed significant liver damage and was told he must stop drinking. He did stop, but it was a mixed blessing. His rages became even more intense, and his beating of Bessie and the kids more violent and meaner.

The end of the drinking did herald a significant turning point for the family. Frank experienced less pressure to move, and they settled in Portland, Oregon, in 1948. Frank began legitimate work in putting together a book that was a guide to building codes in that area, and it included lucrative income from advertising. After that success, Frank made noises about moving once again, but Bessie said no. They bought a small house in Portland, and family life began to look more normal. Bessie had another baby, but it died after a few days. Their last child, Mikal, was born in February 1951. Bessie went through a period of feeling extremely overwhelmed and once tried to smother the new baby. Frank Sr. intervened, and things did improve.

Despite Bessie's objections, Frank insisted on another move in the early 1950s, this time to Salt Lake City. He continued the same type of legitimate endeavor there. Frank and Bessie also got lawfully married in Utah. They bought a house there, but Bessie came to believe it was haunted. Notably, Gary, now thirteen, began his first behavioral acting out in Salt Lake. He hung out with a rough crowd, stealing and committing other delinquent behaviors. Gary also had bad dreams that would wake him up, at which point he called out for his mother. Bessie wondered if there was a ghost in him. Gary did little with the stuff he stole—he stored it in the garage, but his father eventually found it and made Gary return all of it. Bessie became so upset about the house being haunted that she insisted they move. They went back to Portland and bought a house there.

Interestingly, Bessie feared years earlier that Gary would be executed someday. She said,

He had been a dear little guy, but she had lived with that fear since he was three years old. That was when he began to show a side that she could not go near. One time, near the end of the year that Frank Sr. was in jail (she was living with her parents in Provo), "She sat in her mother's house and watched Gary play in the yard. There was a mud puddle that she told him to stay away from. Two minutes after she went inside, he sat down in the middle of it. It sent a fear through Bessie. Would he always be so defiant?" (Executioner's Song, p. 514)

Bessie Gilmore did not see that she had any part in Gary being a defiant child. Some people believe that a child is born that way—it is in the genes, a "bad seed" notion. Learning the relevant facts about the Gilmore and Brown families shows that not following the rules is in the culture of these two not very well differentiated branches of family. Bowen theory does not dismiss the impact of the beatings Gary received at the hands of his father on the development of a character trait like defiance but attaches more importance to the overly involved and highly permissive parenting as interfering with Gary learning how to regulate his emotions adequately. From a Bowen theory perspective, the emotional programming that occurred in family interactions played the central role in his defiance and failure to develop a moral code. He was the subject of very intense child focus.

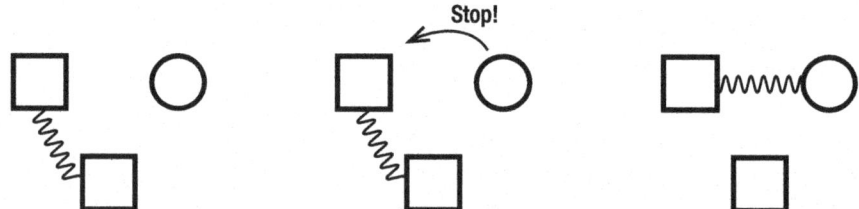

Figure 20.2 *This diagram illustrates a frequent pattern in the parental triangle of father, his mother, and Gary. The jagged lines indicate high anxiety-driven emotional conflict. The looped arrow in the middle diagram between Gary's mother and father symbolizes her pressuring the father to stop beating his son.*

Gary began school in Portland, but dropped out at age fourteen. He was now into stealing cars. The triangle of Frank Sr., Bessie, and Gary really heated up as Gary's behavior worsened. The most common pattern this took is shown in Figure 20.2. The diagram on the left symbolizes conflict erupting between Frank Sr. and Gary in response to some disobedient act. Frank strictly enforced discipline on the kids. He hated signs of willfulness in them. He would use a razor strap, belts, and fists when he beat them. Gary would yell, which only made the beatings worse. According to Frank Jr., Gary would feel outraged at the unfairness of it all. At some point Bessie would intervene, demanding Frank Sr. stop the beating. This is symbolized in the middle diagram. Frank Jr. noted that when Bessie intervened, the conflict would shift from between Gary and Frank Sr. to between the parents (Mailer, 1979), as symbolized by the diagram on the right. Frank Sr. would beat Bessie, who would scream and yell. Frank Jr. thought that the real problem was between his parents, each wanting the other's attention. This would be consistent with the intense level of emotional fusion between these warring parents.

The other interesting twist on these family scenarios is that, whenever Gary was arrested and charged, his father would hire lawyers to defend him vigorously. Frank's advice to Gary was, "Don't admit anything." The legal defense often got Gary off. Bessie supported her husband's efforts, with both delivering the message to Gary of "I love you no matter what you do"—permissiveness was punctuated by Frank Sr.'s harsh efforts to control Gary. This pattern prevailed through all of Gary's growing-up years.

As a teenager, Gary was involved with what was called the Broadway gang in Portland. This led to many arrests. In one instance, Gary was charged with throwing rocks at a school's windows and causing significant damage. Frank Sr. hired a private detective to prove his son was out of town at the time, and Gary got off. In May of 1954, Gary was arrested for car theft. Frank Sr. hired a lawyer that defended Gary as an unwitting accomplice. Frank Sr. strongly conveyed to the court that his son was not guilty. Gary was let off, but two weeks later he was charged with car theft again. The judge sentenced him to reform school this time. Frank Sr. cussed out that judge and was thrown out of the courtroom. The court's opinion was that Gary's parents refused to see him as he really was.

Reform school proved of no help to Gary. He identified with the criminal element there. Frank Sr. and Bessie argue that the family was not to blame for Gary and also thought he should be let go. Both parents viewed Gary as wrongfully punished. During one of Gary's escapes from reform school, Bessie lied to authorities to cover for him. Gary was eventually paroled from reform school and into his parents' custody. Not surprisingly, the family tensions dropped significantly during Gary's time in reform school. Bessie was the only family member looking forward to Gary's return. She referred to Gary as "my special son, the one I have to love the most." It is common for the offspring who becomes the most dysfunctional in a sibling group to be "special" to the mother. The mother perceives that child to need more of her love than the others.

The peace in the family lasted only a few days after Gary came home. Another interesting twist as to how the family peace would get disturbed is a variation in how the parental triangle with Gary played out. Frank Gilmore

Jr. told the following story that Mikal recounted in Shot in the Heart (1995). Bessie had made a scrumptious family dinner and Frank Sr., Bessie, Frank Jr., Gaylen, and Mikal were sitting at the table. The meal had been set out. At that point, Bessie said, "I wonder where Gary is at." He was expected for the meal. Frank Sr. visibly reacted to her comment, likely feeling he was supposed to fix the problem. When Gary finally did get there, Frank Sr. started yelling at him. It was very upsetting to Bessie and she and Frank Sr. got into a vicious fight. During the fight Bessie turned the dinner table over, spilling all the freshly made food onto the floor. This added twist illustrates Frank Sr.'s exquisite sensitivity to Bessie's upsets. Had he kept his cool and not jumped on Gary, the family might have derived some enjoyment from the meal. The point is that anxiety in any of the three members of the parental triangle can activate its escalation. People's sensitivities to each other are so great that it is often difficult to know where it starts. Frank Jr. lived in fear of these kinds of family meltdowns.

Gary returned quickly to his old criminal habits after his release from reform school. He was stealing, breaking into houses, smoking marijuana, partying, and womanizing. With each arrest, Frank Sr. hired yet more lawyers who get Gary off. As described in Chapter 14 on societal emotional process, the mid-1960s was during a time when Murray Bowen observed from a review of court records from the 1950s to the early 1970s that the courts were tending toward overly permissive decisions, similar to the decisions the parents of juvenile delinquents were also making.

Meanwhile, Gaylen's acting out was increasing as well, but it was relatively minor compared to Gary's. Gaylen was charming, funny, bright, and talented and subsequently managed to have affairs with many of his friends' wives. Gaylen's efforts to have long-term relationships never succeeded. Frank Sr. beat Gaylen as well as Gary. In an effort to prevent the beatings, Frank Jr. would do chores Gary had been supposed to do if Gary had not done them. The development of "self" for Frank Jr. was blocked by a functioning position in the family of taking care of others to the detriment of his own life moving forward. Through this period, Gary was jailed periodically when the lawyers Frank Sr. hired could not keep him out of prison. Frank Sr. even bought Gary a car in the hopes that would straighten him out—this of course had no effect.

Mikal's position in the family was different from the others'. He was beaten by his father only once, partly because Bessie protected him from Frank Sr. She forcefully told Frank that he was not going to beat this one. Mikal was a bit less caught in the family problem, but the legacy of his level of intense involvement manifested in the inability as an adult to sustain a relationship with a woman. Mikal's position in the family triangles programmed the type of reactivity into him that interfered with the success of a relationship.

In the late 1950s, Gary went to San Diego, California, and got into a heap of trouble. Like his father he changed his name; he took up with a former girlfriend living there and was arrested five times for various crimes. He was eventually charged with rape and sent home to Oregon. There he was sentenced to the Oregon State Correctional Institution (OSCI).

While Gary was serving his sentence, thanks to Frank Sr.'s newfound business success the family moved into a very nice new home in a desirable section of Portland. Bessie was obsessed with making the place into something very special, and she would get very upset if things did not develop the way she hoped. In such periods, she raged at her husband. Bessie's dream was that a fine and stable home would be good for Gary when he was released from OSCI and that he could turn his life around.

While Bessie was obsessing about matters related to their new home, Mikal was observing a change his father. He saw exhaustion in his face, resignation, weariness, and sadness. Mikal believed that Frank Sr. thought the new home would finally bring peace into the relationship with Bessie, but it was not happening. When she raged, he would give in and simply walk out of the house. His dad seemed helpless and drained. He yearned for a little concord, but Bessie's deep grief and anger were an obstacle. The marriage seemed to be dying. It was a portent of bad things to come.

Frank Sr. and Bessie were Gary's only regular visitors at OSCI. They continued to excuse, condone, and indulge Gary. His only plan after OSCI was to move back home and live off his parents. Gary was released from prison in time to be home for Christmas in 1961. Gary and his father got along remarkably well. Gary even told his father how much he appreciated all he had done to try to help him and that he loved him. Peace was short-lived, however.

In early 1962, Mikal's prescience and worry about his father's emotional state was born out. Frank Sr. discovered a lump in his neck, which led to a diagnosis of a widely metastatic colon cancer. Gary took the news very hard, but Bessie admitted that she had come to hate her husband.

Meanwhile, Gary got back into drugs heavily and demanded money from his father, which resulted in a bad shouting match. Gary raged at a now seemingly helpless Frank Sr. Frank Jr. even stepped into stop Gary from yelling at their father. The two brothers got into a fight. Bessie called the police, and Gary left. He later apologized to his brother but added, "I think I will have to go back to jail soon. I am a professional criminal." After being arrested in nearby Vancouver, Washington, Gary was back in jail in Portland. Frank Sr. turned his usual blind eye when he asked the police and courts, "Why are you always picking on my son?"

Frank Sr. died while Gary was still in jail. Gary reacted to the news by slashing his wrists but did not kill himself. Mikal was surprised at the strong reactions both Gary and Bessie had to Frank Sr.'s death. Mikal, reflecting on his parents' relationship, said, "Mother had delusions of grandeur, and Frank fed them." (Shot in the Heart, p. 241) Both were out of control in their own ways. One of Bessie's reflections was that she chose misery over leaving her husband.

Gary's criminal exploits continued. They culminated in March 1964 in a fifteen-year sentence in Oregon State Prison. His psychiatric assessment at that trial was sociopathy with occasional psychotic decompensation. Gaylen was in jail at that time, too. His were petty crimes, most of them involved with alcohol, and Bessie embarked on the same type of efforts to bail Gaylen out as she had done with Gary. I would estimate based on their life courses that Gary and Gaylen had fairly similar basic levels of differentiation, but their anxieties played out in different ways. Gaylen sought solace in alcohol and womanizing. He once said he was searching for a woman who could help him rise above himself. Gary sought solace in being a criminal. Neither of them were particularly proud of their actions, but emotions ruled. It is fair to say that none of the Gilmore boys felt particularly good about themselves.

While both Gary and Galen were in jail, Frank Jr. was drafted into the army. Mikal was in college in Portland and living on his own. This left Bessie living alone for the first time since before she was married. Not long into his service time, Frank Jr. was placed in the stockade for refusing orders on religious grounds. After some months, he was honorably discharged and returned to Portland to devote his time to his mother. He lived with her for the next seventeen years, until the day she died. At one point, Bessie's actions appeared to sabotage a potentially good relationship Frank had with a woman. Due in part to careless spending, Bessie eventually lost the house. She and Frank moved into a trailer. Galen died in surgery in 1971. He was being operated on for a stomach problem that had resulted from being badly beaten and stabbed by the husband of a woman with whom he was having an affair.

Gary's time at Oregon State Prison, as stated earlier, was a warden's nightmare. He spent considerable time in solitary confinement because of habitual misbehavior and rule violations. He had become such a headache to the prison that he was transferred in 1975 to the U.S. penitentiary in Marion, Illinois. For reasons unexplained, Gary was much less of a behavioral problem and rule breaker at Marion than he had been in Oregon. This, coupled with the help of his uncle and aunt, Vern and Ida, in Provo, along with their daughter Brenda, resulted in Gary being released from prison on the condition that he would go to live with them in early April 1976.

Vern, Ida, and Brenda cared deeply about Gary and believed he deserved a chance to turn a corner in his life. They felt he had paid his debt to society. It became evident fairly quickly that this hopeful threesome had taken on more than they could handle with Gary. From stories Gary told, they got a sense of how mean-spirited he could be. He was not a very responsible or talented worker in Vern's shoe repair store and was constantly leaning on Vern for handouts. He was very easily set off. His dark side increasingly came into view.

About the time it had become untenable for Gary to live either with Vern and Ida or with Brenda and her husband, he met Nicole Baker Barrett. She was in her early twenties, had divorced twice, was raising two small children, and lived in a rental house near Provo. Nicole's family lived nearby, although her parents separated about the time she met Gary. Gary moved in with her after knowing her just a few days. An exceptionally attractive woman, she had been quite promiscuous beginning in her early teenage years, even when she was married or living with someone. She described herself as tending to get involved with "losers," feeling sorry for the guys and wanting to help them. Nicole explained, "It is easier to let things happen in a relationship than to tell a guy to leave you alone" (Executioner's Song, p. 368). Brenda described Nicole as a "space cadet" (Executioner's Song, p. 67). Bowen theory would say that her lack of "self" was equal to Gary's. Gary tended to violate others' emotional boundaries; Nicole allowed others to violate her boundaries. Both acted out of their profound hunger for a romantic/sexual relationship to reinforce them.

Gary and Nicole were incredibly obsessed with one another. Gary's criminal tendencies and his nasty side became evident to Nicole early in their relationship. Yet, when Gary beat up a fellow employee at Vern's business and the victim threatened to file a lawsuit, which would have jeopardized Gary's parole, Nicole's link to Gary was so strong that she threatened to kill the man if he filed the lawsuit. He was certain she meant it. Cousin Brenda described Nicole as willing to do anything to please Gary. Gary was consuming large amounts of Fiorinal for his frequent migraine headaches and had huge problems sleeping. He also drank a lot of beer, which he regularly shoplifted. I would call him the poster child for a "tightly wound" human being.

Gary wanted a steady diet of sexual activity with Nicole. When she expressed distaste for some of the activities he wanted, he hit her in the face hard with a closed fist. Nicole described their relationship as them truly needing each other. Gary described it as follows: "Meeting Nicole, to each of us was like finding a part of us that had been lost and missing for a while" (Executioner's Song, p. 762). Lovers commonly say things like this, but these two people took this to the extreme. Gary had just two tattoos: "Mom" on his left shoulder and "Nicole" on his left forearm. Like Bessie passionately believed, Nicole believed that "the only way to help Gary is with love."

Over the two months or so that they lived together, the relationship became increasingly fraught with conflict, and Nicole began to have doubts about its viability. She was becoming afraid of Gary and what he might do. After several aborted attempts to leave Gary, she finally broke it off and located a place to live where he was unable to find her. Gary's reaction was intense. He said, "This is a pain I can't take," and added, "I never felt so terrible than I did the week before I was arrested. It hurt so bad, it was becoming physical. I could hardly walk, sleep, or eat. Booze did not dull it, and it was steadily getting worse. Every day grew into calm rage. I opened the gate and let it out. It would have gone on and on" (Executioner's Song, p. 717). He meant that he would have killed more people if he had not been arrested.

On the night of July 19, 1976, about a week after Nicole left, Gary walked into a gas station in Orem, Utah, held it up for a small amount of cash, and then told the lone worker there, Max Jensen, to lie face down on the floor. He then shot him twice in the back of the head, while saying, "One shot for me, one shot for Nicole" (Executioner's Song, p. 232). The following night, in Provo, he held up a motel and shot the lone man working there, Ben Bushnell. He was arrested fairly quickly after making some effort to elude capture.

He did not initially confess to the crimes but soon admitted his guilt. He made some interesting statements about it: "It is all real, and I know I did it . . . but I don't feel responsible. It's as if I had to do it, it was a compulsion. I wasn't planning anything, just going through the motions. I didn't know I was going to shoot him until I did it. I did not feel I had control of my actions. I didn't just kill for the money. It couldn't be stopped" (Executioner's Song, p. 397). His Uncle Vern suggested, "Gary doesn't like to be defeated, and when he is, he will not forget it. He is very revengeful." (Executioner's Song, p. 396) In a letter to Nicole from prison while awaiting execution, Gary wrote, "It has been a lifetime of lonely frustration. I have allowed weak habits to develop that have left me somewhat evil. I don't like being evil and I desire not to be evil anymore" (Executioner's Song, p. 493).

As mentioned in the list of events in Gary's life earlier in this chapter, Nicole contacted Gary after he was in jail. She visited him there and had face-to-face contact with him for a time. Other visitors included Vern, Ida, and Brenda, and also Frank Jr. and Mikal. Vern's and Ida's attitudes about Gary after the murders were that they were not mad at him and still wanted to help him. Vern opined that Gary really wanted to be loved by his family. It is notable that Brenda had drawn a firm line on how much she would help Gary elude capture when he requested she do that.

It was Nicole who smuggled into the jail the pills, which she had lied to doctors to get, that Gary took in his first suicide attempt, which Gary and Nicole agreed to do simultaneously. Both survived, but after recovering from her attempt Nicole was hospitalized psychiatrically and not permitted to see Gary again. They did exchange many passion-filled letters, significant portions of which are included in *The Executioner's Song*. The emotional fusion between them that the letters reflect is about as intense as it ever gets. In one of the letters, he characterizes his relationship with Bessie in the following way: "Mother always consistent in her love for me. Always a good relationship. We were also friends" (Mailer, 1979). Bowen theory assumes that the degrees of emotional fusion with Bessie and later Nicole were equal.

Another interesting comment by Gary, taken during an interview with him that was included in Mailer's book, poses an interesting question about the nature of emotion: "I was capable of murder. I can become totally devoid of feelings for others, unemotional. I know I am doing something wrong, but I still go ahead and do it" (Executioner's Song, p. 965). This statement suggests that Gary was capable of having feelings for others. Bowen theory would say that Gary's actions were emotionally driven, but feelings for the victims were absent. Brain researcher Paul MacLean (1990) suggested that the neocortex can act somewhat like a coldly reasoning, heartless computer. This is the kind of computer that makes it possible for monkeys to scheme their way like gangsters into another troop, murder the dominant male, and perform infanticide in the presence of the distressed mothers. Maybe neuroscience can one day offer an explanation for how this occurs, in monkeys and in people.

The "good" side of Gary while awaiting his execution was to donate his eyes for transplant surgery and his pineal gland to help his cousin Brenda's daughter. Given that Gary was to be the first person executed in the United States in over a decade, his refusal to appeal the sentence he had received, and the well-publicized relationship between Gary and Nicole, triggered a media circus leading up to the execution. Gary said he preferred death over spending any more time in prison. He dissuaded both Bessie and Mikal from filing for any stays of execution. They each came around to honoring that wish.

When Gary appeared before a pardoning board, he calmly told them that he sought nothing from them and that he did not deserve anything either. He wanted to die with dignity. His last words as he sat strapped into the chair awaiting the firing squad's execution, "Let's do it."

Bowen theory helps to explain Gary Gilmore and his family in some unique ways—it applies to this case in the way a mold fits perfectly over an object that was casted from it. The mold is a metaphor for the life forces and patterns of emotional functioning that Bowen theory describes. As I have discussed throughout this book, for observers to see the fit between the mold and the casted object they must shift from focusing on content to focusing on process, shift from individual, cause-and-effect thinking to systems thinking that permits seeing the family as an emotionally governed relationship system.

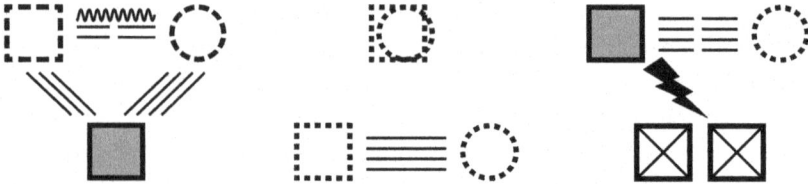

Figure 20.3 *The basic emotional processes in Gary's parental triangle, early relationship with Nicole, and the impact of the disrupted relationship with Nicole.* The dashed lines around all the male and female symbols in the diagram indicate very low levels of differentiation. On the left, the two broken lines and jagged line symbolize the fusion between the parents and associated conflict and abuse. The four lines between Bessie Gilmore and Gary symbolize a very high level of emotional fusion between them, and the three lines between Gary and his father indicate less emotional fusion between them—the father was most often in the outside position of the parental triangle. The dark shading in Gary's symbol indicates his extremely high vulnerability to escalations of chronic anxiety. The middle diagram symbolizes Gary's parents' intense interdependency in the period Gary was mostly out of the home and in prison. The lower part of the middle diagram denotes an extremely intense, positive emotional fusion between Gary and Nicole early in their relationship. The absence of shading in their symbols indicates the calming effect the relationship had on both people. The top diagram on the right symbolizes the disruption of Gary and Nicole's intensely fused relationship. The dark shading of the symbol for Gary symbolizes his intense level of distress in reaction to the split. The shaded jagged arrow from Gary toward the two males with Xs on them symbolizes Gary murdering the two men.

Figure 20.3 symbolizes the playing out of life forces and patterns of emotional functioning in the Gilmore family. The diagram on the left symbolizes the parental triangle in the Gilmore family that involved Gary. It shows the parents dealing with their undifferentiation (symbolized by the dashed lines or poor emotional boundaries for each parent) through the pattern of emotional conflict. The conflict pattern is a way for spouses to maintain both distance and contact. The two lines between Frank Sr. and Bessie that are interrupted in the middle symbolize the chronic anxiety related to their intense emotional fusion and the distance used to cope with it, and the jagged line between them at the top symbolizes the contact element of the conflict pattern. The symbol for Gary conveys that he has developed a level of "self" even lower than his parents' levels, meaning he has even more porous emotional boundaries than his parents and a consequent high average level of chronic anxiety generated in his real and imagined interactions with others. The four lines between Bessie and Gary symbolize their extreme degree of emotional fusion. Only three lines symbolize the fusion between Frank Sr. and Gary because other aspects of Frank's emotional fusion proclivities play out with Bessie.

Certainly Gary's parents were highly anxious too, but some of that anxiety was mitigated by their seeing the problem as in Gary rather than in themselves. Their view was that Gary caused the tension and anguish that they experienced. The triangle played out over time as it commonly does in families with acting-out offspring: Gary's anxiety spiked during adolescence as he moved out into the world armed primarily with pseudo-self and little solid self. His rebellious, defiant character was clearly a way to establish some sort of anxiety-relieving identity for himself. It is not differentiation but a reactive oppositional state.

I want to emphasize yet again that thinking in terms of patterns, forces, and the impact of the relationship system is impossible if observers are locked into individual, cause-and-effect thinking. If observers are explaining the decisions and actions of each member as reflecting that person's particular neurosis or character disorder, the patterns of relationships and how they regulate each person disappear from view. When it comes to seeing relationship patterns, cause-and-effect thinking creates a kind of fog, making it difficult to see what exactly is going on. The pattern of Gary and his parents was one involving three poorly defined people operating almost entirely in reaction to one another—no one person is to blame.

Gary's serious acting out continued to play out during his many years of confinement. The center diagram in Figure 20.3 symbolizes an intense emotional fusion or lack of differentiation between Gary and Nicole (overlapping square and circle at the top, four lines on the bottom). It was not until he met her and they developed an initially stable connection that Gary developed a strong sense of emotional well-being. He had gotten relief from the anxieties generated by his dealings with other human beings during periods of solitary in the prisons, but that nowhere near matched the contentment he derived from the relationship with Nicole.

Unfortunately, Gary and Nicole were unable to manage themselves in the relationship well enough to stabilize it, so it rather quickly deteriorated. Gary was extremely anxious about her being there for him, and Nicole lost her way by overly accommodating to Gary in the hope of relieving his anxiety and errant ways. In essence, he sought mothering and she tried to supply it. I suspect many people would primarily blame Gary for the problems in their relationship. The point is that a woman with more "self" than Nicole had would never have gotten involved with him in the first place or, if she had, would have ended it quickly.

The diagram at the right in Figure 20.3 symbolizes Gary's anxiety and distress going off the charts when Nicole left him (the intense shading). It also shows, as he described, that malignant level of emotional pain spilling out in his killing the two men. He externalized his anxiety into the relationship system. Gary had so little "self" that he could not function as a reasonably independent human being without going off the rails.

I conclude by posing the question of whether complex family life can indeed be reduced to two basic life forces and four patterns of emotional functioning. I have asked myself this repeatedly in my almost fifty years of studying Bowen theory. The many individual factors assembled by researchers over the decades that have been found to correlate with the development of various clinical conditions—such as smoking and cancer—are important to understand but do not provide a complete picture. The Gilmore family story is so transparently out of control that the powerful impact it had on each family member is impossible to ignore. The inclusion of variables that Bowen theory describes can help move our understanding of human problems toward a more complete picture.

Readers who are new to the ideas in this book may be wondering about the specifics of applying Bowen theory to their own families and other social networks. The difficulties people encounter in applying Bowen theory stem from emotions, often out of awareness, that strongly influence their attitudes and ways of interacting with other people. Jonathan Haidt (2012) refers to these as automatic responses that result from intuitions linked to emotions, a type of cognition that is different than reason. He adds that reasoning typically *follows* an emotionally linked judgment of others, a post hoc rationalization for one's attitude or action.

CHAPTER TWENTY-ONE

Adam Lanza and His Family

On December 14, 2012, twenty-year-old Adam Lanza entered Sandy Hook Elementary School in Newtown, Connecticut, and fatally shot twenty students and six adult staff members, wounded two other adults, and then shot and killed himself. Prior to driving to the school, he fatally shot his mother at their Newtown home. A November 2013 report issued by the Connecticut state attorney's office concluded that he acted alone and planned his actions, but there was no evidence as to why he did it.

Mass shootings began to be front and center in the American consciousness in 1966 when Charles Whitman climbed the tower at the University of Texas and began shooting at the people below. In most of the more than one hundred mass shootings since then, just as the Connecticut state attorney's office concluded, sufficient evidence about why the perpetrator did it has been found lacking. The course and outcome of any human being's life are always difficult, if not impossible, to explain. The myriad variables at play usually preclude assigning a specific cause to any outcome. Bowen family systems theory cannot answer the why question either, but it adds important variables to include in assembling a more complete explanation.

The emotional processes in the Lanza family are unusually transparent, because they were incredibly intense and a large amount of information was assembled by people interested in the case. I drew on many sources of information to tell this story through the lens of Bowen theory. The two most important sources were a book by Matthew Lysiak titled *Newtown* (2013) and an article by Andrew Solomon in the *New Yorker* titled "The Reckoning" (2014). Lysiak covered this story as a journalist for the New York *Daily News* beginning on the day of the murders. For purposes of his book, he moved to Newtown for several months to assemble a mountain of information from many sources. Solomon was the first person to interview Adam Lanza's father, Peter, at any length. Peter Lanza allowed Solomon to read and discuss with him hundreds of e-mails that were very revealing about the life of his family over many years.

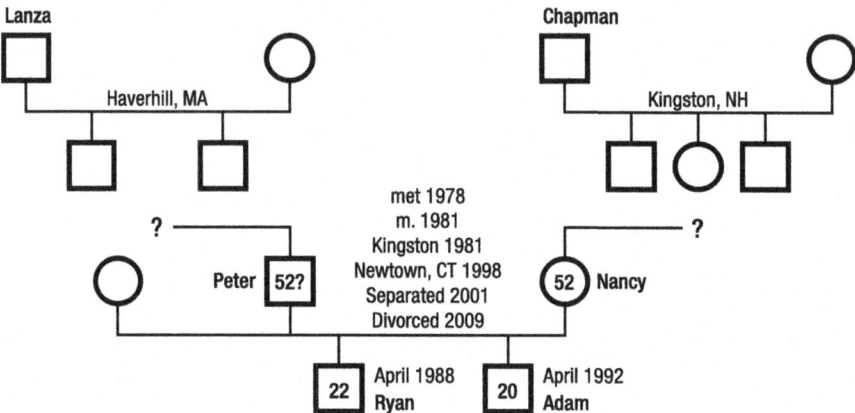

Figure 21.1 *Diagram of the Lanza-Chapman family. The question marks at the ends of the lines from Peter and Nancy toward their families of origin indicate that scant data is available about their families. The circle to the left of Adam Lanza's father denotes his second and current marriage.*

I conceive of this story as one about a relationship that died. It was an incredibly painful death and had the unspeakably tragic consequence of taking twenty-six other human beings with it. As with the other cases in this part of the book, I begin with the family diagram. Unfortunately, the information about Adam's parents' extended families is quite limited. Figure 21.1 is a diagram of the information I could find. The ages on the diagram are at the time of the shooting. Nancy Chapman Lanza is one of four siblings, but no information is reported about her sibling position. She grew up in Kingston, New Hampshire. Peter Lanza is one of three sons, but no information is reported about his sibling position either. He was born in Haverhill, Massachusetts, but later in his youth he lived in the Kingston area. Peter and Nancy met and began dating when they were in high school in Kingston. They married in 1981 and then for seventeen years lived in a home next door to her childhood home and near her extended family. The couple moved to Newtown, Connecticut, in 1998. Peter was a vice president working in finance at General Electric, which involved very long hours during the workweek. Nancy had worked as a stock broker at John Hancock until 1992, when Adam was born. She had planned to return to work after the baby was born, but it did not work out. Ryan is the older son by four years. The couple separated in 2001. They tried living together again but finally divorced in 2009. Nancy remained in the family home in Newtown. They had joint custody, but the children lived with Nancy. Peter maintained frequent contact and communication with Nancy and both of his sons until 2010, when Adam began refusing to see him. Peter remarried shortly after the divorce was final.

My discussion of the case begins with description of an incident described by Matthew Lysiak that captures the character of many interactions between Nancy and Adam over the years of his development. This one occurred when Adam was fourteen years old and in eighth grade at Newtown Middle School. He was having an anxiety attack early one morning and screaming at his mother. It was triggered by his not wanting to go to school. Apparently, he hated to face the din generated by the mass of students he typically encountered as he entered the school building. Nancy went through her usual attempts to plead with Adam, assuring him that everything would be okay, but Adam usually prevailed in this power struggle. He would stay home and play video games or use the computer. Her approach involved trying to understand what her son was up against. Adam had been diagnosed at age five to have Asperger's syndrome, and family stress was high after Peter and Nancy failed in yet another attempt to live together.

Andrew Solomon (2014) wrote the following about Nancy relevant to the encounter described above. I consider it a keen insight:

> All parenting involves choosing between the day (why have another argument at dinner?) and the years (a child must learn to eat vegetables). Nancy's error seems to have been that she always focused on the day, in a ceaseless quest to keep peace in the home she shared with her hypersensitive, controlling, increasingly hostile stranger who was her son. She thought she could keep the years at bay by making each day as good as possible, but her willingness to indulge his isolation may well have exacerbated the problems it was intended to ameliorate. (retrieved online)

I have repeatedly observed clinically what I think adds up to a kind of passivity about Nancy's mothering: the mother and other family members wind up in orbit around the child. The psychiatrist Robert King, who evaluated Adam when he was fourteen, described Nancy as being almost a prisoner in her own house as the result of the many strictures Adam imposed on her. Nancy's compliance to them reflects what I characterize as her passivity when it came to Adam. In contrast, she could be a tiger in pressuring teachers to orbit around Adam's idiosyncrasies as well.

As sibling variation in emotional functioning commonly occurs in families, not surprisingly older brother Ryan was socially well adjusted and a popular kid at Newtown High. During the period of Adam's temper tantrum described above, his parents had given Ryan a car, and he was spending more and more time away from home and hanging out with friends. He would soon graduate from high school and be off to a college not far from home but would be living on campus. This would leave Adam and Nancy living together at home.

On the particular morning of this outburst, Nancy judged the intensity of the outbursts trending toward more of an extreme. Adam began to hyperventilate, and it frightened Nancy. Fearing he was having a nervous breakdown, she got him into the car and took him to Danbury Hospital. She told the doctor there that something was very wrong with her son. When the doctor's level of concern about his mental health did not match hers, Nancy experienced what she had with previous school counselors, her family doctor, and other specialists: no one could give her an answer as to what was wrong, and worse, they did not seem to be taking her concerns seriously. She insisted to the doctor that Adam's behavior was not normal. Before leaving the emergency department, she asked the doctor for a note to give the school that would allow her to keep him at home for the remainder of the eighth-grade year. Nancy thought she could best nurture her son to prepare him for high school. The doctor was unwilling to do that.

Many readers may think that Nancy is a justifiably nervous mother, panicked about getting adequate help for a mentally disturbed son. Bowen theory asks the clinician to think about Nancy's anxiety getting focused on this son and this playing a key role in his anxiety and emotional functioning. The quote above from Andrew Solomon taps into one aspect of the relationship process between Adam and her that can transmit that anxiety. Her orbiting around Adam to alleviate his distress absolves Adam from having to learn how to manage his emotions. This makes his key relationships, such as with his mother, unusually important, and thus makes him hypersensitive to what is happening in those relationships. Therein lies the key source of his anxiety.

I conceive of three ways to think about the origin of a problem such as Adam's. One is that Adam was born with a biological predisposition to a mental illness that presents with his symptom picture, implying that biological processes within Adam fuel the symptoms. A second way to think about it is that family relationship processes and associated anxiety come to rest in Adam by virtue of an ongoing interactive process that activates biological and/or psychological vulnerabilities in him to certain types of symptoms. This implies that chronic anxiety related to the family environment fuels the symptoms. (Adam, of course, is part of that family environment.) A third way of thinking about it is that it is both a physical predisposition (pathology) in Adam and a family process that fuels the symptoms associated with that pathology.

This implies that pathology internal to Adam and family stress both drive the symptoms. It is difficult to prove which of these models comes closest to reality at this point in our knowledge. To clarify these three conceptions, the first model is a classic individual model, the second one is a systems or Bowen theory model, and the third one is a multicausal model. Of course, no family exists in a vacuum in that stressors in the extended families and other surrounding social networks affect the situation as well.

Adam was not typical in that he did not speak until he was three. He showed such hypersensitivity to physical touch that tags had to be removed from his clothing. In preschool and at Sandy Hook, he sometimes smelled things that were not there and washed his hands excessively. A doctor diagnosed sensory-integration disorder, and Adam underwent speech and occupational therapy in kindergarten and first grade. Certain predispositions in a person can become assets or liabilities, depending on the degree of family anxiety the person grows up in.

An aversion to social activities became apparent by age four. He did not enjoy playing with other children. He tagged along with his older brother when he went to Cub Scout meetings but would separate himself from the crowd there. He refused to engage in all group activities and would shrink away from them into the arms of his mother if another child touched him. Nancy was fiercely protective of Adam. If she ever sensed he might be in danger, that protective part of her personality would surface. As Solomon suggested in the quote above, this level of availability in a parent can inhibit the child's emotional growth. I suggest that Nancy was managing her own anxiety with this level of availability to Adam, as much as it helped Adam calm down. The mother does not see it as her own anxiety but as anxiety caused by an external source. The inability to discern the difference between her anxiety and Adam's anxiety is not Nancy's fault but part of her own emotional programming, a legacy of her childhood.

In sharp contrast, older brother Ryan was allowed to run and play by himself in the woods for long periods unsupervised. If Adam was out of her sight even briefly it was like a switch in her would flip. A long-time friend of Nancy's said that Adam was associated with the side of Nancy that was very intense, getting upset very quickly. Some part of her would become active if Adam was in distress, but not so with Ryan. Another friend described Nancy becoming hysterical and screaming when she could not immediately locate Adam at a basketball game. Nancy was having a panic attack. When the family moved to Newtown and Adam entered Sandy Hook, Nancy became a familiar face there due to her need to watch over her son.

By six years of age, Adam was perceived by Nancy to be getting worse. She was so overprotective of Adam that fellow parents began to experience her protective nature as extreme and overbearing. She was "paranoid" that other kids were bullying him, but other parents and classmates said that no one was bullying Adam. They tended to leave him be.

As Adam grew up, he seemed uninterested in developing any human relationships outside his immediate family. Even within the family home, the only person he felt truly comfortable around was his mother. He always wanted her near him, but also kept her at arm's length. It is an anxiety-driven punched-up example of the need for emotional closeness but the aversion to too much of it.

There is no lack of love here, no trauma, no abuse, and no neglect. It is an intense level of emotional fusion, an extremely poorly resolved symbiosis. One night when Adam had a fever, Nancy slept on the floor outside his closed bedroom door. Periodically he would call out, "Are you there? Are you there?" A friend of Nancy's said that Nancy told him that she was very upset that the teachers at school were not protecting him like a bodyguard. She increased her time monitoring the teachers.

Compared to later school experiences, Nancy was pleased overall with her son's progress at Sandy Hook Elementary. Adam attended Newtown's Read Intermediate School for fifth and sixth grades and then entered Newtown Middle School for seventh grade. He had much more emotional difficulty in middle school. This transition is difficult for many kids, but it was particularly difficult for Adam. He seemed quite fearful. One fellow student observed that Adam always looked terrified as he walked down the hall. His shoulders would slump and he would cling to the wall. "He would walk like he expected someone to hit him." Interestingly, Adam's father, Peter, viewed Adam as "always thinking differently, just a normal little weird kid." His view did change over time as Adam's behavior worsened. Adam's anxiety during middle school also spilled over into his home life. His outbursts there were more violent, and he became more resistant to going to school.

Peter was less anxious about Adam, but it was not helpful to Nancy. It seems that Peter did not view the situation with the same alarm as Nancy, but he consistently supported her efforts with him. I assume that he assumed, like many child-focused fathers, that she knew what she was doing, not that she was being an overly anxious mother. The father does not see the situation the same way the mother does, but he cannot usefully define a "self" to her. In a better differentiated marital relationship, spouses can view situations such as Adam's differently and communicate the differences in a constructive way. For example, rather than being blindly supportive of Nancy, he could say to her noncritically that he was less worried about Adam than she was. This may help a mother see the impact of anxiety on her decision-making about her son. Gary Gilmore's father was aggressive and authoritarian in an effort to straighten the child out. Peter was very different than Gary Gilmore's father

Frank, but I estimate that the degrees of emotional fusion between Bessie and Gary and between Nancy and Adam were very similar.

Nancy went the extra mile in trying to help Adam deal with what was referred to as his sensory overload problem. She spent many hours photocopying his textbooks in black and white because he found color graphics unbearable. In his early teen years he quit playing the saxophone, stopped climbing trees, avoided eye contact, and developed a stiff lumbering gait. His panic attacks at school sometimes necessitated Nancy coming to the school to quiet him. Adam's emotional functioning was declining, and his dependency on his mother was increasing. Even Peter began to believe that there was something truly wrong with Adam.

Nancy was so involved with Adam's schooling that she developed a reputation as "tightly wound, demanding, and with a flair for dramatics." She pulled Adam out of middle school when he was thirteen and enrolled him in the Catholic school in Newtown. She hoped the smaller classes would ensure Adam got the attention she felt he so desperately needed. It did not work very well and did not last very long. Besides his behavior problems, the teachers discovered a collection of disturbing graphics Adam had drawn. The pictures depicted people in various states of death. They were brought to the attention of school officials, who were concerned enough to bring Nancy in for a parent-teacher conference. She minimized the significance of the pictures by saying that Adam had Asperger's syndrome and was struggling to fit it.

About that time, Peter and Nancy took Adam for another psychiatric evaluation. The psychiatrist affirmed the diagnosis of Asperger's syndrome, but the now older Adam would not accept it. The psychiatrist recommended homeschooling for Adam. Nancy agreed. During his eighth-grade year, Nancy taught Adam the humanities and Peter, now living near Stamford, Connecticut, met with Adam twice a week to teach him sciences. It is important to note that, when Peter and Nancy were living together, although he worked very long hours during the week, Peter was very involved with both of his sons on the weekend. Son Ryan used to joke about how close Peter and Adam were. Expecting that Adam would eventually attend Newtown High School, Nancy coordinated the curriculum with the school so that he could graduate rather than just get a GED. Peter commented, "She made all such major decisions. I took the back seat."

Figure 21.2 symbolizes how the parental triangle played out for Nancy, Adam, and Peter. The diagram on the left symbolizes the poor emotional boundaries of each parent (dashed lines), with Nancy overlapping Peter and being, as Peter said, the dominant decision maker. Adam is symbolized as having even less "self" than his parents and deeply immersed in and being shaped by their anxiety-generating emotional fusion. The diagram on the right shows

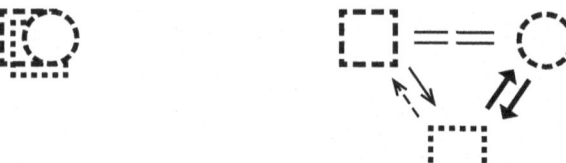

Figure 21.2 *This diagram symbolizes the most fundamental emotional processes in the Lanza family. On the left, the parents' dashed lines symbolize porous emotional boundaries consistent with people in the lower part of the middle range of differentiation. The overlapping with the symbol for their son Adam symbolizes intense emotional fusion in the triangle. The dots around the symbol for Adam indicate a level of differentiation in the lowest 20 percent on the differentiation of self continuum, less than his parents. The space between the lines between the parents in the diagram on the right indicates significant emotional distance between them. The heavy arrows between Adam and his mother symbolize a very high level of emotional/psychic energy each invests in the other. The father's emotional investment in Adam is less, but generally positive. The dashed line from Adam to his father symbolizes a low level of emotional investment in his father, the consistent outsider in the parental triangle.*

the emotional distance between the parents and a very tight, anxious focus of Nancy on Adam that Adam reciprocated. The diagram also shows Peter's significant emotional investment in Adam, but the dashed arrow from Adam to Peter indicates that Adam did not reciprocate. He was so involved with his mother that he was much less available to his dad. The parental triangle with Ryan would look very different: Ryan would have about the same connection with both parents and be less fused emotionally with them, benefiting from the strengths of his parents and less bathed in their weaknesses.

Andrew Solomon described Adam's very uneven relationship with his parents when he wrote about the period following the decision to homeschool Adam. Peter said he began to feel distanced by the intensity of Nancy's relationship with Adam but did not consider her involvement with him to be problematic. Peter's approach to parenting was as docile as Nancy's was accepting. Peter said that Nancy would indulge Adam's compulsions. "She would build the world around him and cushion it" (2014, retrieved online). For example, she had no idea that Adam could tie his own shoes until Peter observed him do it on a hiking trip that Peter and Adam took by themselves.

After Adam continued to have problems at the Catholic school, Nancy again sought out a mental health expert for advice. Matthew Lysiak quoted her response to that consultation: "If one more person tells me he is going to grow out of it, I think I am going to lose my mind. My son is sick, but no one seems to want to do anything about it" (2013, p. 39). Using individual theory, a mental health consultant can be vulnerable to taking sides: blaming the mother for being too protective or inadequately supportive of her child, or seeing the child as the primary problem. Systems theory helps a consultant see the role of the parent's anxiety in the functioning of the child and also appreciates that the child is failing to develop much of a "self." The child is not going to grow out of it in such an anxious fusion. Both parent and offspring contribute equally to the problem the parent wants fixed. Of course, even skilled Bowen-theory-trained therapists can be seen as not understanding if the therapist suggests to parents that the problem is as much in the them as in the child. Parents are often wanting the therapist's understanding of the problem to match their own understanding, meaning the problem is in the child, not them. It takes skill and solid theoretical thinking for a therapist not to sound judgmental, but some parents do not want to hear it and seek another therapist no matter how nonjudgmental therapist is. Being nonjudgmental is not a technique, it derives from a solid theoretical understanding of family process.

An interesting thing happened when the parents enrolled Adam in Newtown High School in 2006. A teacher/administrator there took Adam under his wing. He was impressed with Adam's brilliance and could also relate to Nancy in a way she trusted. His relationship with the family did not miraculously turn things around, but small signs of progress appeared. The teacher was calm and patient with Adam and believed Adam could function better. He would occasionally solicit Nancy's help if needed. Adam still needed the assurance that his mother was nearby. She would wait in an empty classroom next door to the class he was in. The teacher commented, "It's hard to imagine a more devoted mother, so involved in her son's life" (2013, p. 44). The teacher would sometimes encourage Nancy to leave, but it was difficult for her to let him out of her sight. The school mobilized considerable support to help Adam when needed. An escort would walk Adam through the halls, and many teachers had Nancy's phone number if they wanted her help. Adam was her full-time job.

The man who had taken Adam under his wing began to see Adam come out of his shell. Meanwhile, Adam had become interested in target shooting. Nancy had grown up around the safe use of guns and was comfortable around them. She began taking him to a gun range periodically, thinking she could better connect with him around a shared activity.

However, Adam's beginning changes at school were not matched at home. His panic and tantrums were getting worse, and he was making even more strange drawings. When Nancy would take him for haircuts every two months, the interactions at the barber shop were quite revealing. Nancy would walk into the shop, and Adam would be close behind. She then instructed him to sit in a chair and which one to sit in. He complied. The barber tried to converse with Adam but without success. At the end of the haircut, the barber would say, "You're all set, Adam." He would not get out of the chair, however, until Nancy instructed him to do it. This intense, puppet-on-a-string level of fusion between them was easy to observe. It is important to note, however, that the puppet was controlling the puppeteer as much as the other way around. Adam had no agency, no "self." When a shade of agency emerged later, it took the form of pure destruction of those around him and of himself. It was an abnegation.

Unfortunately, just as it appeared that Adam was beginning to slowly adjust to Newtown High School, right before the beginning of his junior year, the teacher who had been so important in his progress announced he was leaving the school for a job elsewhere. Nancy reacted by taking Adam out of school once again. The important teacher predicted her action would trigger a tailspin in Adam—and it did. He advised her not to do it, but Nancy trusted no one else at the school. She blamed the school for Adam's problems there. Adam did too.

Nancy then enrolled Adam at Western Connecticut State University. She hoped he would thrive in a more adult environment. He passed the GED test and did well academically at the university the semester he was there. As usual, Adam related little to the other students there.

Peter and Nancy's divorce was finalized in September 2009. Not only did Adam break off his relationship with Peter early the following year, but he also severed ties with Ryan and his uncle (Nancy's brother), a man Adam had been friends with as a child. The trend unfolding was increased isolation of the Nancy-Adam relationship.

Peter remarried in 2010, but Nancy remained largely unattached. She told a friend that she had no time for a serious relationship because she always had to be there for Adam. Meanwhile, Adam was becoming increasingly consumed by his computer, where he was researching weapons, wars, and the military. He had the fantasy of becoming a marine. Nancy continued to believe Adam could succeed, but not in the marines.

Adam developed a new online persona, an alias he created named "Kaynbred" that began to show his growing fixation with violence and mass murder. In the alternative universe he was creating, the skinny and frail teenager was an imposing muscle-bound soldier dressed in camouflage and other military attire. As these activities continued through 2010, he ceased having any desire for having academic activity and isolated himself more and more in the house. Nancy tried to pull him out of his isolation, but it seemed only to aggravate the situation.

Another very important development was that Nancy began to change her activities. She decided that she needed more time away from home. At the same time, she was considering taking Adam and moving to the Pacific Northwest, maybe enrolling him in a school out there. She even parted with her Red Sox tickets in anticipation of making a move. Neighbors noticed that Nancy's home was more quiet, private, and unknown to them. She began to lose confidence in her ability to help Adam. She made trips as far away as London, New Orleans, and New York City. She always invited Adam to come along, but he never wanted to. Before any departure, she prepared and froze all the meals Adam would need in her absence.

Her frequent travel continued through 2012. She went back home to New Hampshire for Thanksgiving that year. She was devoid of hope that he would consider going with her and left Adam at home with a frozen meal. She felt she had to put more energy into her own life. She had apparently been diagnosed with an autoimmune disease, and that worried her. In her fondest dreams, she hoped that by putting more energy into her own life, it would contribute to more independence for Adam.

However, Adam's behavior continued to deteriorate; he threw intense temper tantrums with any mention of his future. Any break from routine would make him hysterical. He would stomp and scream and not speak to Nancy for days. When Adam brought up the possibility of joining the marines, Nancy told Adam that he was not cut out to be a marine. Her comments were very upsetting to him. Adam rarely ventured outside anymore, playing video games all night and sleeping all day. Most were violent video games. Nancy found more violent drawings; one included a grassy field lined with the corpses of young children. Adam would no longer let Nancy touch him. Even more alarming is that a friend of Adam said that Adam thought his mother wanted him to leave, wanted to be rid of him. It is not clear how much her traveling and consideration of a move across country might have contributed to this attitude, but it would represent the ultimate in hopeless isolation if he felt this was true.

Nancy's last trip was for two nights at a luxury spa resort in New Hampshire. She returned home the evening of December 13, 2012. This was her second trip away from home in the past month and her fourteenth that year. She again invited Adam to come along, but he characteristically declined. Before leaving on the trip, she confided to a friend that she felt she was the only thing that anchored Adam to reality and that without her he would be gone. They had not spoken for three days before she left, and she did not see or talk to him the night she returned. Adam shot her the next morning as she lay in her bed and then proceeded to Sandy Hook Elementary. The guns that he used were in their home.

Adam may have feared that he was losing his mother, but that was the farthest thing from her mind. She told a friend that she anticipated living with Adam for a very long time. Peter thought that Nancy had no idea how dangerous their son had become. Nancy did feel that she was losing Adam, but she seemed to be thinking of this as withdrawal, not violence. Andrew Solomon suggested that Nancy was anxious about Adam but not afraid of him.

Peter told Andrew Solomon that he did not think Adam had any affection for him either, by that point in 2012: "With hindsight, I know Adam would have killed me in a heartbeat, if he'd had the chance. I don't question that for a minute. The reason he shot Nancy four times was one for each of us: one for Nancy; one for him; one for Ryan; one for me" (2014, retrieved online). A document found on Adam's computer gives an explanation of why females are inherently selfish. Solomon commented that he wrote this while one female was accomodating him in every possible way.

Ryan claimed his mother's remains a week after the shootings, and her body was cremated. The next day a small handful of friends and family members gathered at the family home in Kingston. Ryan spoke lovingly at the memorial service about his mother. She had never missed a school play and was usually in the first row of the auditorium to cheer him. She enriched his life with culture, taking him to museums in New York City and Washington, D.C. There were also many trips to Fenway Park to watch their beloved Red Sox. He said that his mother would make the two-hour drive from Newtown to Hoboken, New Jersey, where he lived and worked and sit with him for an hour's lunch before driving for the two hours back. She was always there. This seems a worthy tribute for an incredibly anxious, incredibly devoted, incredibly loving mother who went far more than the extra mile to do right by her sons. Intense emotional fusion creates a very thick fog, and she was lost in it. Peter was lost in it, too, but also tried his best to right the ship.

A goal in telling this story is to give the reader enough details to understand why I refer to the Nancy and Adam as being in a relationship that died. Adam's actions simply cannot be understood out of the context of his family relationship system, and most especially the relationship with his mother. Nancy reached a point of near hopelessness about her or anyone else being able to help Adam. However, her determination to stand by him never waned. At the same time, she was feeling increasingly overwhelmed by the situation and beginning to put more energy into taking care of herself.

The less easily explained change in the relationship was Adam's increasing withdrawal from the one person on whom his life was indeed dependent. Many relationships such as theirs endure for decades and decades, with the mother and child living out their lives together until the mother dies. It could be that Adam was indeed convinced that his mother wanted him out of the house. Adam was emotionally isolated in the extreme. Since not much information is available about what he said about his internal workings, I can only speculate about some of the emotions associated with his isolation. Peter Lanza's thoughts about why he shot Nancy four times may be the most informed. Somehow, referring to his actions as an abnegation rather than as rage and revenge seems closer to the truth. Of course, abnegation and rage are not mutually exclusive. He destroyed himself, his mother, and for reasons unexplained, the people at Sandy Hook. Again, one could speculate on what attitudes and emotions drove his killing all those people, but Bowen theory emphasizes the context in which Adam's actions occurred and critical changes in it, which is something that can be described with a little more certainty. Associated with those changes, Adam reached a point of no return.

CHAPTER TWENTY-TWO

John Nash

Correlating Clinical Course of Schizophrenia with Family and Social Contexts

The subject of this chapter John Nash described his psychotic delusions as reflecting an inability to reason. Nash's description is consistent with that of Eugen Bleuler, who named schizophrenia and considered it a thought disorder that interferes with reasonig to be its defining characteristic (Colman, 2001). A key and yet unanswered question—a question Bowen theory attempts to answer—is what processes shatter the ability to reason.

Bowen theory conceptualizes schizophrenia from two perspectives: an individual vantage point and a family vantage point. Looking at the symptomatic individual, the theory considers it to be an emotional dysfunction; looking at the family in which it occurs, the theory considers it to be an emotionally driven disorder of the family relationship system. Reasoning is clearly shattered in psychosis, but Bowen theory considers a sustained and high level of subcortically anchored emotional reactivity to be the force driving the symptoms. A person vulnerable to psychosis appears to have the same emotions that every human being has, but lacking a well-developed "self," the person has quite limited self-regulating ability. This significantly limits the ability to modulate periods of high emotional reactivity and associated physiological changes that can disrupt normal cognitive functioning.

Significant lack of "self" manifests in three prominent infantile yearnings in adulthood: to be taken care of (figuratively nursed), to be free of responsibility, and to have an all-loving, all-giving, nondemanding figure always alongside. Given the prolonged period most people spend being cared for by their parents, no one escapes these yearnings at times, but if unbridled they interfere with having a productive life direction. Viewing people who are vulnerable to psychosis as having the same emotions everyone has can contribute to reducing the stigma of mental illness. Viewing people as differing in degree and not kind thwarts compartmentalizing them.

Much of the information I have drawn on about John Forbes Nash comes from Sylvia Nasar's beautifully done, carefully researched, and thorough book *A Beautiful Mind* (1998). I have culled details from the book that illustrate how Bowen theory would explain the context of Nash's descent into and recovery from schizophrenia. Another valuable resource was the 2002 documentary about Nash titled "A Brilliant Madness." One other resource was an interview conducted by Mike Wallace for *60 Minutes* that included Nash, his wife, Alicia, and their son John Charles (CBS, 2002).

A primary reason of presenting John Nash's case is to illustrate why Bowen theory regards schizophrenia as a "functional dysfunction," a disorder of brain functioning as opposed to a disorder of brain structure. According to the theory, the driving force of a functional dysfunction is chronic anxiety. This sharply contrasts with the conventional view that brain pathology is the primary process driving the clinical symptoms. Inherited brain structural defects may have a role in rendering a person vulnerable to psychotic symptoms during periods of high chronic anxiety, but in a Bowen theory model, defects alone do not cause the symptoms. For most clinical dysfunctions, social context is the most important area to assess to explain the onset and course of the condition.

Figure 22.1 symbolizes impressions drawn from the facts of the Nash case viewed through the lens of Bowen theory. The fluctuations in the level of chronic anxiety shown on the graph reflect changes over time in the amount

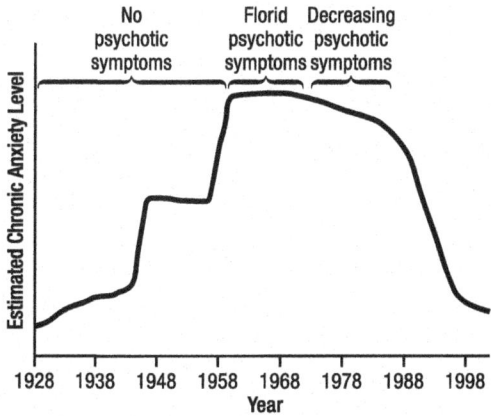

Figure 22.1 *This graph estimates of John Nash's level of chronic anxiety from birth through complete recovery from psychotic symptoms.* (Nash had no psychotic symptoms until the end of 1958; he had florid psychotic symptoms by the beginning of 1959 that persisted into the early 1970s; his psychotic symptoms started decreasing in the early 1970s and continued to decline until being barely present by the mid to late 1980s.)

of anxiety Nash absorbed (and helped create) from his most important disturbed relationship systems, especially the family system. What follows in this chapter is a description of the changing contexts to illustrate their impact on modulating or intensifying chronic anxiety over time.

Figure 22.1 symbolizes the following changes in estimated level of chronic anxiety: John Forbes Nash was born in 1928. He exhibited no psychotic symptoms until the winter of 1958–1959. All of his hospitalizations, use of psychoactive medications, and individual therapy occurred over the next decade. A gradual tapering off of symptoms began in the 1970s. He was much improved by the mid-1980s and quite rational by 1990. His level of behavioral agitation declined significantly in the early 1970s, but his "inability to reason" was slower to resolve.

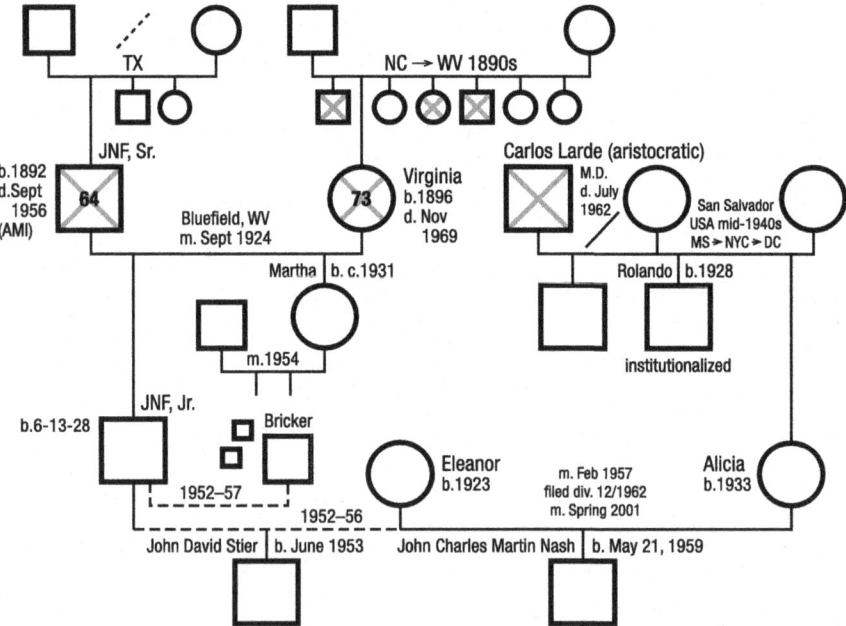

Figure 22.2 *Diagram of the Nash and Larde families.* The dashed lines between people in the same generation (Nash and Bricker, Nash and Eleanor) indicate people romantically involved with each other in the first case and living together unmarried in the second case. The dates above the dashed lines indicate when they were connected. The male symbol connected to the dashed line indicates that he was born out of wedlock. The slanted line between the marriage of John's paternal grandparents indicates that they were separated, but not divorced.

The family diagram for John Nash's family of origin is shown in Figure 22.2. John Forbes Nash Jr. (JFN, Jr. on the figure) was born on June 13, 1928, in Bluefield, West Virginia. The coal and rail industries built this town, which had about 20,000 inhabitants when John was growing up there. His father, John Forbes Nash Sr., was the oldest of three siblings from a Texas family and worked as an electrical engineer. That work brought him to Bluefield. His mother's family moved from North Carolina to Bluefield in the 1890s. Virginia, his mother, was the second of seven siblings and the firstborn daughter. She was a teacher. John's only sibling, Martha, is three years younger than John.

The most important people in John's personal life and some relevant dates up to 2001 are shown on the diagram. John formed very intense sexualized attachments to both men and women. He was involved with Eleanor Stier from 1952 to 1956. Eleanor got pregnant about two months after she and John met. John David Stier was born in June 1953. John Nash was romantically involved with a man named Bricker at the same time he was involved with Eleanor. The Bricker relationship spanned from 1952 to 1957. Bricker did not know about John's relationship with Eleanor until John told him just before his son was born. A lot of interaction between John, Eleanor, and Bricker followed. The two small squares just to the left and near the top of the Bricker symbol indicate other males with whom John had brief but intense romantic relationships.

The woman John married, Alicia Larde, and the son by their union are shown in the lower right of the diagram. They met when she was a student in John's advanced calculus class at MIT. They became romantically involved in 1956 and married in 1957. Alicia filed for divorce in December 1962, which was granted in May 1963. The couple remarried in the spring of 2001.

Alicia was from an aristocratic family in San Salvador. Her father was a physician who eventually moved to the United States. His first marriage ended in divorce and produced one son. The son came to live with his father and second wife. There was a firstborn son from that second marriage, and Alicia was the younger child by five years. Her full brother, Rolando, was in an institution of some type for reasons that I have not discovered.

John and Alicia Nash's story makes a case for how critically important that relationship was for John's sanity and lack thereof. This is a long and detailed story, but the details of his life prior to the onset of schizophrenia provide indications of his difficulty being a "self" prior to his symptoms emerging. The details of the periods of florid psychosis include John Nash's valuable insights into a psychotic state and how those insights helped preserve some degree of bodily homeostasis during a highly stressful time.

John was a healthy baby but a solitary and introverted little boy. He was bookish, socially awkward, and a daydreamer. Thanks to his talents and his mother's efforts, John learned to read by the time he was four years old. He liked to perform for his peers but, notably, formed no close companionships.

He did not date anyone all through high school. His parents were constantly trying to get him out in the world, but he resisted. He was an outstanding problem solver and with it had a sense of superiority. Virginia was much more anxiously focused on John than on his sister, Martha. His mother had him taking classes at a local college along with his high school studies. Virginia often sought Martha's help in getting John more socialized. She wanted Martha to include John in her social activities, something she, being somewhat embarrassed by her brother's oddities, was not keen on doing. The triangle involving Virginia, Martha, and John was very intense. John's father was a little more removed (outside position in the parental triangle), but quite available to John. Although the parents worried a lot about John, they never tried to involve him in any type of psychotherapy during his formative years.

John finished high school in Bluefield and headed off to Carnegie Institute of Technology in Pittsburgh in 1945. He entered there with a mind-set of becoming an electrical engineer like his father but soon switched over to mathematics. Because of the world war, the school offered a program to enable graduation in just three years, which John took advantage of, graduating in 1948.

Figure 22.1 symbolizes an increase in John's chronic anxiety after matriculating at Carnegie Tech. He was teased and ostracized there and formed few friendships. Notably, he exhibited a sexual attraction to other male students, which earned him the nickname "Homo." He was a star in academics but an outcast from the social group. He often voiced contempt for his fellow students, calling them "stupid fools." He was highly competitive academically and had very high expectations of himself. He craved recognition for his intellectual prowess. All of these traits and behaviors I just described I attribute to a fairly high level of chronic anxiety. I consider his same-sex attractions to be as much emotionally driven as sexually driven—lust is only one of the emotions involved in a romantic relationship. Many of John's actions indicate a strong need for someone to affirm and attend to him, a legacy of the fusion with his mother and other family members. The descriptions of his pursuit of males suggest frenzied ventures. His overall need for social affirmation in the form of being recognized for his brightness also betrays a significant level of chronic anxiety.

John began Ph.D. studies in mathematics at Princeton University in September 1948. He was cockier than the other graduate students and continued to want to be noticed for his "smartness." He was always in thought and fiercely independent intellectually. Many of the faculty did not like Nash's attitude, but others, in awe of his mathematical abilities, were more tolerant. Early in his studies at Princeton, he was interested in developing a systematic theory of rational behavior that would have an application to economics. His

Ph.D. thesis described what came to be known as the Nash equilibrium, for which he awarded the Nobel Prize in Economics in 1994.

During this period in his life, he appeared as if he felt nothing regarding love, friendship, or sympathy for others; he lived in his head. His primary pleasure in life came from his creative work rather than emotional closeness with others. He continued his intense pursuit of young males at Princeton, intrusively seeking their attention. His intense pursuit contributed to the relationships being unstable and short-lived. He was impractical, childish, and detached from everyday concerns. These traits were in sharp contrast to the way he conducted himself professionally. When involved in mathematics and in working with other mathematicians on problems, he acted more maturely. He was absorbed in his work, was not defensive or a whiner, and did not feel unappreciated. Bowen theory conceptualizes this work versus personal contrast as his having a higher functional level of differentiation in his work, consequent to more sureness and less chronic anxiety, than in more personal relationships. Like for Ted Kaczynski, Gary Gilmore, and Adam Lanza, social interactions were John's Achilles' heel.

While at Princeton and later at MIT, during the summers he worked as a mathematician at the Rand Corporation in Santa Monica. In the summer of 1954 he was arrested there for soliciting sex from a man in a restroom. This led to his losing his security clearance and being fired by Rand. He never told his family about this. Interestingly, Nash never regarded himself as a homosexual.

After completing his Ph.D. at Princeton, but not being appointed to its faculty consequent to many faculty members not wanting to deal with him, he was appointed as a mathematics instructor at MIT in 1951. He got along somewhat better in his relationships at MIT than he had at Princeton, but he was not a great teacher. His mother continued to send him money when he was in Boston, and she never let up on prodding him to be more social.

Nash met Eleanor Stier in 1952. She was a nurse in a hospital in Boston where he had some minor surgery. He met Bricker, a graduate student at MIT, at about the same time. Sylvia Nasar noted that the Bricker relationship helped Nash recognize for the first time the strong force that binds people together. He began to realize that, without special relationships like he had with Bricker, he felt incredibly lost in the world.

The relationship between John and Eleanor was in many ways a clear replication of the emotional fusion with his mother. He enforced a certain emotional distance with Eleanor. She had a soft heart—to the point of giving coats to strangers—and was extremely protective of John. She lacked self-confidence. John was highly critical of her, frequently putting her down. Nasar beautifully described the reciprocity in their relationship as John being egocentric and childish and Eleanor being self-abnegating and maternal. John never told his family about Eleanor, nor did he introduce her to his colleagues or even talk about her to them. When their child was born, their relationship deteriorated even further. John refused to marry her, would not put his name on the birth certificate, and provided no financial help. Eleanor went to a home for unwed mothers, and she later had to place her son in foster care for over five years. John pressured Eleanor to give their son up for adoption, but she refused. Despite John's attitude and Eleanor's distress, the relationship with Eleanor continued. She continued to make excuses for John and hoped for the best. She remained dazzled by his brilliance.

Figure 22.3 *The dashed lines around all four symbols indicate that the people have the same low basic levels of differentiation; the amount of overlap between them indicates the degree of emotional fusion; and part of the boundaries of one individual being obliterated by the figure in the foreground indicates that individual is the more adaptive (deferential) partner in the relationship.*

There were parallels in the Nash-Bricker relationship to that between John and Eleanor. Bricker was quite an insecure person himself and hero-worshiped John. He felt inadequate around him. John became increasingly critical of Bricker but was also very jealous of him. Bricker dropped out of graduate school and eventually ended the relationship with Nash.

Figure 22.3 symbolizes John's relationship with Eleanor (on the left) and with Bricker (on the right). The dashed lines around each symbol symbolize the fairly low levels of differentiation of the individuals involved. In both cases, John Nash is borrowing self in the relationship; Stier and Bricker are the deferential or adaptive ones and losing self. Nasar observed that, by not choosing either relationship, John minimized the dependence and demands on him in both relationships. When people close to Nash needed or wanted more from him, it was a huge strain on him. He hoped that people would be satisfied with his genius. It is tempting to blame Nash for being so selfish, but his partners' attitudes and behaviors were vigorously reinforcing his immaturities.

Alicia Larde and John Nash met in 1956. She was five years younger than him and a student in his advanced calculus class at MIT. Her parents had been living in the United States for a number of years at that point. Alicia's mother, a key player in this story, moved with her daughter to Boston when Alicia began her studies there. She was the primary emotional support for her daughter and also provided much help with child rearing in the early years of John's and Alicia's marriage. Her father remained in New York City. Alicia fell into the same hero worshipping of Nash that Eleanor and Bricker did. Although intelligent and determined herself, she was not a great student in college. She became preoccupied with Nash to a point that it adversely affected her studies. She chased after him initially. In Alicia, Nash found a more totally accepting figure than Eleanor. They began dating before the year was out.

From the beginning, Nash did not treat Alicia well. He launched into his being critical of his partner routine and never even paid for meals they had out together. They consummated the relationship within a few months. Both Bricker and Eleanor were still in Nash's life at that point. However, Eleanor discovered Nash's involvement with Alicia. The now spurned and very angry woman contacted Alicia, accusing her of stealing her man. She also told her about their son. When all this came to a head, Eleanor contacted John's parents and told them about the son she had had by John and the whole situation. Unsurprisingly, things became quite unsettled in Bluefield. John's father insisted that he marry Eleanor. Virginia wanted John to marry Eleanor too and to live a "normal" life. Possibly related, John's father's health deteriorated during 1956, and he died of a massive heart attack in September of that year. Virginia was angry at her son but blamed Eleanor for causing her husband's heart attack and death.

After John's father's death, John and Alicia went to Roanoke, Virginia, where his mother and John's married sister were now living, to meet them and celebrate Thanksgiving. John married Alicia in February 1957. They lived in New York City while John was on leave from MIT to spend a year at the Institute for Advanced Study in Princeton. Alicia also worked and helped pay the rent. They socialized as a couple a fair amount, but more distance existed in their relationship than Alicia wanted. Meanwhile, there were some signs that John was becoming more obsessed than usual with his math projects. It is likely that the level of chronic anxiety in the marital relationship was increasing (depicted in Figure 22.1) and was driving some of his obsessing. Alicia was totally dedicated to and supportive of John. The marriage was off to a decent start despite the tensions and emotional distance.

Nash experienced some disappointment in his professional work related to not gaining certain recognitions he sought. Additionally, he had not been given tenure at MIT, and like at Princeton, it was related to difficult relationships with some of the other faculty members. In the spring of 1958, now back at MIT, he became increasingly obsessed with trying to solve the Riemann hypothesis, which some considered the most important unsolved problem in mathematics. Since being married, he was also more worried about finances. When Nash ran into a mathematical problem he could not solve, despite his remarkable ability to persist, he could be very hard on himself. Many people have speculated that, among these disappointments and other weights on his shoulders, his mental obsession with solving the Riemann hypothesis may have contributed to a mental breakdown that came to fruition during the first months of 1959. Nash himself thought this might be the case. While his efforts on the Riemann problem could have had some impact, Bowen theory suggests more important relationship processes were at play.

In late July of 1958, John and Alicia traveled to Europe. While still in Europe in the early fall, Alicia discovered that she was pregnant. When they returned from Europe, they settled back in Cambridge, Massachusetts, and John returned to his duties at MIT. He met a male graduate student at MIT and began pursuing him as he had done with Bricker and others before his marriage. Alicia sensed there was something going on between these two men. She was also feeling ambivalent about the pregnancy. Her mood grew darker and more somber through that fall of 1958. She felt dispirited, anxious, and alone. She had hoped that the pregnancy would bring her and John closer together, but it did not happen. John grew even more cold and distant. Her emotional struggles deepened between returning from Europe in September and Thanksgiving. Figure 22.1 shows anxiety increasing during 1958, but still not enough to generate florid psychotic symptoms until near the end of 1958.

By Thanksgiving 1958, Alicia was seeing even more troubling changes in John. This led her to stop focusing on her own troubles and to shift her focus to John. Alicia feared John was having an affair, and John accused her of the same thing. Alicia wondered if the responsibility for the new baby was stressing John, or the state of their marriage, or worries about getting tenure.

John and Alicia attended a New Year's Eve costume party at one of his MIT colleague's home. John appeared in a diaper and with a baby bottle full of milk. He spent almost the whole evening in Alicia's lap. Many of his colleagues were alarmed by this behavior. In early January 1959, John made a trip to Roanoke to spend time with Virginia and Martha. They, too, were extremely alarmed by seeing John's unsettled emotional state.

Alicia tried to hide John's growing instability from his MIT colleagues. She found a job on campus so that she could watch John much of the time and keep him out of trouble. She picked him up after the workday, and they often went out to eat, but Alicia stopped inviting others to dine with them. The faculty at MIT were aware, however, of the deterioration in John's emotional state. Despite the impression that he was having a mental breakdown, John got tenure at MIT at the end of January. However, his department relieved him of all teaching responsibilities in the hope of reducing his stress level. John impulsively decided to drive to Washington, D.C., and deliver letters to embassies there. He wanted to tell various foreign dignitaries about his mission to form and head up a world government. He was convinced that military leaders around the globe were conspiring to take over the world and needed to be stopped. Alicia accompanied him on that trip to protect him.

Quite alarmed, Alicia made an appointment with a psychiatrist at MIT to discuss John's condition. Based on want she told the doctor, he recommended psychiatric hospitalization. He also speculated that John might need electroconvulsive therapy. Alicia feared John's mind could be damaged in some way from shock therapy, and felt that way about drugs, too. Alicia asked Virginia and Martha to come to Boston to help implement a plan of hospitalizing John. They committed him to McLean Hospital in nearby Belmont, Massachusetts, in early April 1959. John told the admitting doctors that he was the Prince of Peace, leader of a great movement for World Peace. He did not think he needed to be hospitalized and was fiercely angry at Alicia for doing it. He threatened to divorce her. Virginia was devastated when she visited her son at McLean, although he seemed fairly normal to some of his colleagues who visited him there.

The doctors diagnosed him to have paranoid schizophrenia and speculated that it might have been triggered by "fetus envy" or "latent homosexuality." These were popular ideas in psychiatry at the time. His psychosis disappeared in a matter of a few weeks, and he became a model patient on the ward. He told the doctors he was aware that he had been delusional. He continued with threats to divorce Alicia. He was discharged after a fifty-day stay, a week after his son's birth in May 1959. Alicia stayed fairly cool in the face of John's continued threats of divorce, even to hurt her, and to take all their money and go to Europe.

That clinical problems frequently arise in a variety of forms in one of the spouses during a pregnancy is a well-recognized phenomenon. If some type of clinical symptom develops in a husband, such as psychosis, an idea like fetus or womb envy is an attempt to explain what triggered the symptoms. The idea of womb envy comes from the feminist psychology work of Karen Horney (1942). She regarded the phenomenon as culturally or psychosocially driven, not something innate in a male. It describes the jealousy and resentment males can feel by not being able to perform the biological functions of the female sex.

In contrast, Bowen theory anchors the forces that propelled John Nash into schizophrenia in the emotional system, an innate system in human beings and other forms of life. An understanding of Bowen theory's way of conceptualizing symptom development during a spouse's pregnancy begins with one of the theoretical ideas described in Chapters 7 and 9: relationships function as if two counterbalancing life forces, individuality and togetherness, govern them. Both of these forces are anchored in the emotional system, and thus their roots are innate, not cultural. Culture may color the manifestations of these forces to some degree, but the forces are instinctually based.

Relationships vary along a continuum in the degree to which the togetherness force dominates. Relationships between people with low basic levels of differentiation are the most emotionally fused, most dominated by the togetherness force. In well-differentiated relationships at the other end of the continuum, individuality and togetherness operate more as a working team—neither force dominates; flexibility prevails. I estimate the emotional fusion between John and Alicia Nash to be at the very low end of the moderate range, slightly less fused than those in the lowest 20 percent of the continuum of differentiation of self.

It is important to keep in mind that marriages at all degrees of emotional fusion can be in balance. Balance typically prevails when people are courting or early in their marriage, when demands on the relationship tend to be low compared to when children and other responsibilities are added. Significant clinical symptoms are not unheard of during the early part of a relationship but are less common than later on.

Based on the information that I have presented, I assess the Nash relationship to have generated some chronic anxiety during courtship and the first eighteen months of their marriage. Nash seemed to become somewhat more obsessed with his math projects, which can be a form of emotional distancing, and Alicia was somewhat distraught by the distance she experienced between them. This level of anxiety was insufficient to generate clinical symptoms in either partner.

A palpable spike in chronic anxiety occurred after Alicia got pregnant. Two ways the spike manifested were in Nash's romantic interest in a third person and in Alicia feeling isolated and overwhelmed. The increase in chronic anxiety significantly disturbed the previously more comfortable balance in their relationship. As explained in Chapter 1, as the relationship changed each spouse changed, and as each spouse changed the relationship changed. This reciprocal interaction is key to escalation of chronic anxiety. Eventually, the level of chronic anxiety was sufficient to disturb Nash's functioning to the point of psychotic processes emerging. Based on how their marital relationship unfolded over time, despite her hero worship of her husband, Alicia became the more dominant partner. Nash's dependence on the significant female in his life became increasingly evident.

From a Bowen theory perspective, what was unfolding was not about a subjective concept like womb envy but about a first-order threat to the instinctual need for togetherness, a threat emerging from the disturbance in relationship balance with the pregnancy. Such threats are powerful in all of us, but as illustrated in my brother's suicide, the degree of threat experienced in an extremely interdependent or fused relationship can place one or both people in the relationship at very high risk. I was lucky to have a somewhat higher basic level of differentiation than my brother and never experienced the level of threat my brother did (or John Nash did), so I doubt that I adequately fathom the depth of the threat.

Clues for grasping the power of this threat may be provided by the research of affective neuroscientist Jaak Panksepp (2010). He has discovered discrete but closely interconnected emotional systems located in various primitive subcortical regions of the brain. The systems are anatomically, neurochemically, and functionally homologous in all mammals that have been studied. These systems are involved in generating emotional feelings (affects) that inform animals how they are faring in the quest for survival. At this point, the neural mechanisms that transform this subcortical activity into emotional feelings are unknown. Two emotional systems that integrate distress and despair related to emotional separation are overactivity of the PANIC/GRIEF system and diminished arousal of the SEEKING network. Panksepp calls these systems "ancestral tools for living." Their obvious importance for survival suggests that they likely play a key role in phenomena such as suicide and psychosis, two different ways of reacting to a major threat to survival. Given the powerful human need for emotional closeness, a real or imagined threat to a relationship on which a person is extremely dependent constitutes a threat to survival.

Returning to John Nash's case, Figure 22.4 symbolizes how Bowen theory conceptualizes the family process or context that rendered Nash vulnerable to psychosis. Diagram 1 symbolizes the courtship and early marriage period. The amount of emotional energy each spouse invests in the other is strong (symbolized by the dark shading and thickness in both arrows), and it shows the relationship as in balance. Some emotional distance and increased anxiety has emerged consequent to the marriage (symbolized by the break in the arrows and the light shading in each spouse symbol). At this stage, each person derives more comfort than unease from the relationship.

Diagram 2 symbolizes one emotional process that Bowen theory describes happening during a pregnancy, involving three changes that John and Alicia experienced: a significant increase in emotional distance in the marriage, Alicia making an emotional investment in the unborn child (arrow between her and the child), and John getting markedly anxious and manifesting symptoms (delusions and behavioral abnormalities). The arrow in Diagram 2 from Alicia to John contains anxiety and an indication of limits on her investment in him (symbolized by the absence of the solid black color). Her reduced investment is a fact insofar as part of her emotional investment in John is constrained by her investment in the unborn child. Depending on the level of differentiation, some expectant mothers are more vulnerable than others to feeling

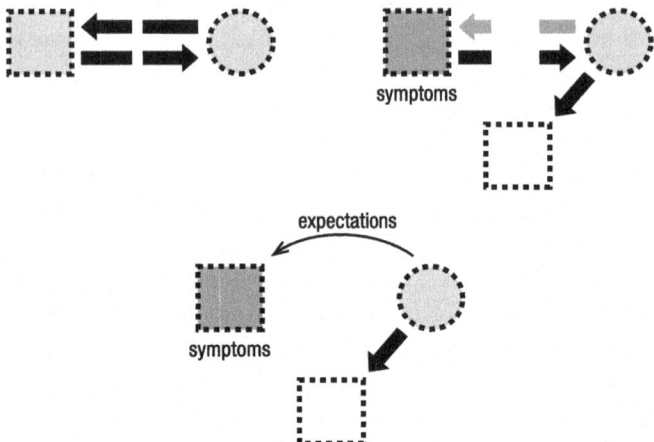

Figure 22.4 *This diagram symbolizes the emotional process that can destabilize a marriage following the birth of a child.* Diagram #1 indicates some emotional distance during the early part of the pregnancy and the light shading indicates some increase in chronic anxiety in each person. The dashed lines around the male and female symbols indicate a low basic level of differentiation. Diagram #2 indicates a marked increase in emotional distance between the spouses later in the pregnancy and after the baby son is born. The wife's emotional investment in the husband is less than his investment in her. (There is reality to less investment but there is also the husband's anxiety-driven perception of less investment.) The heavy black arrow from mother to baby son indicates more of her emotional energy directed at the baby son than at her husband. The dark shading in the symbol for the father indicates a sharp rise in his chronic anxiety related to the disturbance in relationship balance. The mother is more anxious too, but less than the father. The dashed lines around the infant indicate that he has not developed much of a "self" at this early point in life. Diagram #3 depicts another emotional process at work as well. The thick arrow from mother to husband indicates her increased expectations of him based on the new reality of the baby and her anxiety about becoming a mother.

overwhelmed about meeting the needs of two human beings who are very dependent on them. This can occur despite the mother's dedication to the father's well-being. For John, part of his experience of feeling less emotional investment from Alicia would also be intensified by his reactions, meaning he could be easily threatened by any real or imagined signs of her being less available to him. Both of these dynamics would be intensified by reciprocal interactions (reacting to each other's reactive behaviors) in their relationship.

Diagram 3 symbolizes another process that Bowen theory describes: the real and imagined level of expectations built into the increase in system complexity. Theory suggests that, for John, the infantile yearnings to be taken care of and to have no responsibility could be as powerful as the real and imagined perception of emotional isolation. His absorption of the chronic anxiety in the unstable system would eventually activate enough emotional disequilibrium and associated changes in physiology to seriously disturb reasoning processes. The same level of yearnings would operate in Alicia, but they are overcome by her overfunctioning position in their reciprocal interaction.

My assessment of the intense relationships with Eleanor and Bricker and the fact that Eleanor's pregnancy did not trigger psychosis in John is consistent with Sylvia Nasar's thought that John not committing fully to either relationship distanced him from their dependence on him and also his dependence on them. This offered emotional insulation from the changing contexts in those relationships, making it possible for him to adapt successfully (not go psychotic) to those emotional context changes.

After he was released from the hospital, John remained hugely angry at Alicia. He was able to go back to work. Virginia came to help with the baby but acted as if she needed to protect the baby from John. John thought that his colleagues at MIT had colluded in his hospital commitment, which was a factor in his abruptly resigning from MIT. The school resisted his resignation, but he insisted on it and withdraw all of his pension fund money from the university. He was already thinking about returning to Europe. Fairly quickly after being released from McLean, it was evident that John had not really recovered.

In July 1959, John sailed to Europe on the *Queen Mary*, with Alicia coming along, feeling she had to protect him. Alicia's mother took the baby with her to Washington, D.C., with a plan to bring the baby to Paris once John and Alicia were settled there. John was still clearly delusional. He wanted to give up his passport and become a citizen of the world. He tried unsuccessfully to do it and eventually destroyed the passport. Alicia suggested that John was trying to banish all aspects of his previous identity. A measure of the impact of John's decline on Virginia was that she was drinking heavily, and in September 1959 she was admitted to a psychiatric facility for a nervous breakdown.

John's delusions about his new mission in life kept him in high spirits. This highlights how a delusional state can lift despair and bind anxiety in that sense. The anxiety manifests in a delusion rather than a feeling of dread. He left Paris and went to Switzerland. At the same time, Alicia went to Italy to be with a cousin. The Swiss were not amused by John's odd behaviors and requests and began steps to deport him. Alicia went immediately to Geneva and retrieved her husband. The baby and Alicia's mother arrived in Paris in time for Christmas.

Nash's frenetic behavior and traveling around Europe continued. Alicia wanted to go back to the United States, but John resisted. Finally, with Virginia's financial support, the U.S. State Department arranged to bring John home in April 1960. Nash went to Princeton to live, and Alicia and their son went to Washington to live with her parents. They remained separated for a few more months, but Alicia finally succumbed to John's pleading that she come to Princeton. They lived together in an apartment, and Alicia resumed being very attentive to him. Nash continued to deteriorate. He grew a bushy beard, his gaze seemed almost dead, and he sometimes walked barefoot around town. He spent a lot of time on the Princeton campus. Despite often behaving bizarrely there, the university cut him a lot of slack. It helped that even though he was acting crazy he was not threatening anyone.

Alicia became depressed during this period and began consulting with a psychiatrist. The psychiatrist encouraged another commitment for John, this time to Trenton State Hospital. With Virginia's and Martha's help and support, John was committed there in January 1961. He was hospitalized for six months against his will. He was treated with insulin coma therapy and hated it, but the doctors judged it to be effective. He did improve in the hospital, even enough to work on a math paper. He eventually earned trips home from the hospital, seemed in remission, and was discharged in July 1961. Interestingly, John could describe the disappearance of his delusional hypotheses while he was in the hospital. Giving up his delusions, however, produced a sense of diminution and loss. He referred to the change as an enforced rationality. This dovetails with elevation of his mood in Paris with the help of viewing reality in a delusional way.

After being released from the hospital, through the efforts of his colleagues, John got a one-year research appointment at the Institute for Advanced Study (IAS) in Princeton. John did not see his son during all of 1961, but Alicia's mother finally brought the then two-year-old John Charles Nash to Princeton. Alicia's father came as well. The whole group was now living together. Alicia was working, and her mother took care of "Johnny." John recovered enough to produce a paper while working at the IAS that was published. He conducted himself reasonably well in one-to-one encounters with people and had a sense of humor. He agreed to see a psychiatrist regularly during that time.

However, big changes were on the horizon. John returned to France, this time without Alicia. By the latter half of 1961, their marriage was clearly on the rocks. John appeared woefully diminished in response to the prospect of losing Alicia. Despite being so angry at her for the hospitalizations, and their relationship having become cold and distant, he did not want to lose her. He reacted by becoming more angry, agitated, and restless. In June 1962, he once again took off for Europe. In July 1962 Alicia's father died. While overseas, John wrote a poignant letter to his sister, Martha, saying that he was a man all alone in a strange world.

John came back to Princeton later in the summer of 1962, but his functioning had not improved. Alicia allowed him to live with her and their son for a time but began divorce proceedings. The divorce became final in May 1963. The court awarded Alicia the custody of their son. John's colleagues saw his need for treatment and raised money for a long-term placement, maybe even two years at an institution in Michigan. Virginia contributed money to that effort as well. John was still routinely roaming the Princeton campus, writing cockeyed mathematical equations on blackboards in the classrooms. His relationships at IAS were deteriorating, but John firmly resisted attempts to persuade him to go to Michigan.

Finally, Virginia, Martha, and Alicia facilitated an involuntary commitment to the Carrier Clinic, a provider of psychiatric inpatient services near Princeton. Nash was again adamant about not needing treatment. He was adamant also about not having electroconvulsive therapy but was placed on a locked ward for five months. He took the antipsychotic medications that were prescribed and formed a relationship with a psychiatrist there that continued for the next two years. His psychotic symptoms improved quickly in the hospital. IAS again offered him a position upon discharge from Carrier.

John still yearned for a resolution with Alicia. That hunger is the defining characteristic of the entire 1960s decade for John. Alicia was definitely not interested. He rented a room in Princeton, kept a low profile, but felt very lonely. Alicia did agree to go with John to some social functions. Things were not great for her either during this period in the mid-1960s. She was having work issues and found her now five-year-old son difficult to manage. Her mother tried to help by taking Johnny with her to El Salvador for a few months, but Alicia missed the boy very much. She started seeing a psychiatrist regularly for her depression.

Her husband began to seem somewhat improved. He was still in outpatient psychiatric treatment and on medication, but the improvement did not last. His symptoms returned with a vengeance. Wanting to be back with Alicia dominated his mind-set. He took another trip to Europe, but the delusions, and voices were strong and his mood was dismal. When he returned home at the end of 1964, he was again committed to the Carrier Clinic. He was treated with antipsychotic drugs, and the the psychotic symptoms ameliorated, but his emotional pain was unresolved. He was discharged from Carrier in July 1965.

The next phase in the Nash odyssey took him to Boston. With the help of colleagues, he joined the mathematics department at Brandeis. He deeply missed his ex-wife and son, and his feelings of loneliness still dominated. He did manage to produce some published articles. He saw a psychiatrist weekly in Boston and took antipsychotic medications, albeit a low dose at his request. Eleanor and John David still lived in the Boston area, and John began to visit them regularly. Tensions arose fairly quickly, between both John and Eleanor and John and his son. Eleanor was not especially happy. John was highly critical of his son but encouraged him academically and offered to pay for college. This seemed to help David. They were among John's very few social contacts at that time. None of this diminished John's longing for reconciliation with Alicia, but at that point, Alicia was not inclined even to see John. Most of John's activities in Boston were solitary.

John began to feel a little more confident as time went on in that first year at Brandeis, and his colleagues found him "sane." He came across as less arrogant and aloof. Once again, it did not last. He began writing clearly delusional letters to Martha and by late 1966 was clearly paranoid. He meandered aimlessly around Harvard Square, much like he had done in Princeton. After a few impulsive sojourns, he went to Roanoke and lived with his mother in her apartment for over a year. His sister and her family lived nearby.

Given his poor emotional state, he feared that Virginia, Martha, and Alicia would again try to hospitalize him. The relationship with Virginia deteriorated. She died in November 1969, and John worried he had hastened her demise. After her death, John attempted to live with Martha, but she could not cope with that arrangement. After Christmas 1969 she decided to get John committed once again to a psychiatric ward in nearby Staunton, Virginia. He was hospitalized into February 1970. Furious with Martha for committing him, John broke off his relationship with her. Alicia had no role in this last commitment, having given up on the worth of yet another hospitalization. The Staunton hospitalization was John's last contact with hospitals, medications, or any other form of therapy for the rest of his life.

After leaving the hospital, John returned to Princeton. Reflecting later, he described delusions as desperate attempts to make sense out of chaos. Thoughtful statements to the contrary, John continued his old antics on the Princeton campus and its many blackboards. However, back in Princeton, a very important development in this story occurred. Alicia, worried about John further deteriorating, becoming homeless, and even dying, invited John to live indefinitely as a "boarder" in her home. Living with her and their son would prove to have a powerful impact in reducing his level of agitation. That drop in chronic anxiety in the early 1970s is noted on Figure 22.1. It is interesting that the agitation improved, but the irrational thinking continued. This was the beginning, however, of a gradual decrease in psychotic symptoms. It seems beyond question that Alicia's decision to take John in is what made the difference and eventually allowed for his full recovery. Princeton's tolerant policy toward John was also very important. It was a kind of therapeutic community for him. The mathematicians there, whether they liked him or not, were in awe of his math genius and wanted to preserve that "beautiful mind."

Alicia supported John fully and expected almost nothing in return. While still delusional, he was able to moderate his behavior. This enabled him to avoid hospitals and psychiatrists. He had developed a diffident, gentle, and shy demeanor. Nash stated that what he needed was safety, freedom, and friendship. Alicia credited her own postdivorce experience with depression as helping her be more understanding of John's plight. She endured a long period of work problems and had to rely on welfare and food stamps to get Johnny, John, and her through it. Her financial situation became dire enough that it forced the sale of her house in Princeton and a decision to buy a less expensive house in nearby Princeton Junction. John moved with her to the new house.

Another very important change in context was that Johnny was becoming increasingly unhappy as he moved into his teenage years. As Johnny's problems increased, John became increasingly important in helping with the parenting. He was "bad cop" with Johnny, and Alicia was the "softie." Fiercely protective of her son, she often defended him to her husband. She was the family leader. John did nothing without first consulting her.

During 1973, things began to look brighter for Alicia. She got a good job as a programmer, but it involved very long commutes. John's mother had left him some money, and he contributed it toward Johnny attending a nearby private preparatory school. Johnny had been getting difficult and moody at home but was an excellent student and had a talent for mathematics. His problems gradually got much worse, and it was now the seventeen-year-old son who was admitted to the Carrier Clinic. He was delusional and had been truant much of the previous school year. He had holed up in his room and became increasingly angry. He was reading the Bible obsessively, talking damnation and redemption, and also hearing voices. He fought treatment attempts more vigorously than his father had. John was oppositional, but not a rebel; Johnny was more of a rebel. He ran away frequently, once for as long as three weeks. At Carrier, Johnny was diagnosed as paranoid schizophrenic, but he improved quickly there. However, he would not return to school for three years. Like for her husband's mother, for Alicia her son was her "private sorrow," a situation she tried to hide from other people.

Despite lacking high school and college degrees, with the help of a mathematics professor at Rider College Johnny was admitted to a mathematics Ph.D. program at Rutgers and was awarded a Ph.D. in 1985. Interestingly, despite his success, Johnny had been ambivalent about his studies, arguing that he did not understand why he had to do anything. After all, his father did not do anything, and his mother was supporting him. Finishing his degree made things look hopeful for Johnny and the family. Johnny got an instructorship at Marshall University, and Alicia got a good job in Newark. John's functioning continued to improve, and so did his psychosis. He still had some paranoid thoughts and heard voices, but the "noise level" was way down. He could recognize the paranoid ideas and reject them intellectually.

Appearances were deceiving for Johnny, however. His year at Marshall was a disaster. He returned home and never left. He did not work and was hospitalized many times. He refused to take medication outside the hospital. Drugs could keep him out of the hospital, but they could not give him a life. This point again emphasizes an underlying lack of "self" as the core problem. Johnny gave up many of his past activities, such as playing chess and reading. He could get quite angry and violent at times, and his aberrant behaviors often terrorized John and Alicia. Much of John's life energy now focused on his son. From a Bowen theory perspective, the parental triangle with so much Johnny focus likely helped John improve his functioning, despite all of the anxiety that surrounded the situation.

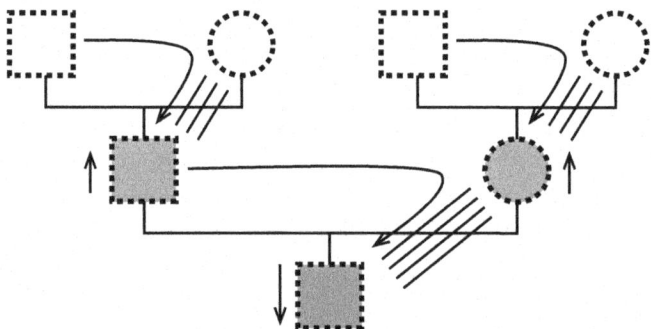

Figure 22.5 This diagram depicts an abbreviated (three generations) multigenerational transmission process leading to John and Alicia's son Johnny. The shading progressively increases in the second and third generations, indicating a greater vulnerability to escalations of chronic anxiety. The lines between the generations depict the increased amount of unresolved attachment in generation three compared to generation two. The curved lines from Johnny's paternal and maternal grandfathers indicates each of them supporting the projection process onto generation two. The arrows alongside the male female symbols indicate the overfunctioning-underfunctioning reciprocity between generations two and three.

Johnny's aforementioned infantile yearnings were even more in evidence than they were with his father. He returned to live with his parents after leaving Marshall and remained with them until they were both killed in a tragic automobile accident in May of 2015. Figure 22.5 symbolizes a small piece of the multigenerational transmission process and the decline in basic level of differentiation that left Johnny even more impaired than his father. The symbols of the two marriages at the top of the diagram are for John's parents on the left and Alicia's on the right. The dashed lines on each symbol symbolize a basic level of "self" just a little bit higher than that of their offspring. The male and female symbolized in the second generation are John and Alicia. Both of the abbreviated diagrams of their families of origin depict three fusion lines between mother and offspring that resulted in John and Alicia developing less "self" than their parents. Alicia as an adult was quite emotionally dependent on her mother and her mother overfunctioned with Alicia. Alicia was very anxiously invested in Johnny. The curved arrows from the fathers to their offspring symbolize their participation in the emotional fusion by supporting it and adding their own anxiety to it. By the third generation, Johnny is symbolized as being even more chronically anxious than his parents. Additionally, arrows in the John–Alicia–Johnny triangle symbolize the overfunctioning of each parent (arrows pointed up) and Johnny's underfunctioning (arrow pointed down).

A brief aside, before some concluding comments for this chapter, concerns Johnny's emotional functioning in the aftermath of his parents' sudden deaths from a car accident in May 2015. According to an article by Susan K. Livio (2017), who interviewed Johnny at his home two years after his parents' deaths), he had not been hospitalized since their deaths and functioned far better than most people who knew the family anticipated. The voices and visual hallucinations that he had since being a teenager had faded away. He had no psychiatric hospitalizations and continued to live in the house where he had lived since he was a teenager. He resumed playing chess. He had a treatment team that was very attentive to him, including getting him out for social activities. He also took psychoactive medications on a regular basis under the supervision of the team.

From the perspective of Bowen theory, Johnny's chronic anxiety decreased after his parents' deaths. (His improvement is reminiscent of my schizophrenic brother's significant improvements when our parents became dysfunctional.) Much of the chronic anxiety that fueled Johnny's long symptomatic period was generated in the parental triangle, with his parents anxiously focusing on him and overfunctioning and Johnny playing the opposite or dysfunctional side. Johnny's improvement represents an increase in functional, not basic, level of differentiation in response to the dramatically changed context with his parents' deaths. Livio noted that one of Alicia's greatest worries concerned the fate of her son after she and John died—they would have been pleased to know how well their son coped.

After considering it for several years, John and Alicia remarried in the spring of 2001. John was appointed to a senior research mathematician position at Princeton University and worked every day up until the end of his life. John also got back in contact with his sister, his older son, and many old colleagues with whom he had fallen out of touch. In 1994 John received the Nobel Prize and in 2015 the Abel Prize, awarded annually by the Norwegian government to an outstanding mathematician. John and Alicia were killed when they were traveling home after receiving the Abel award.

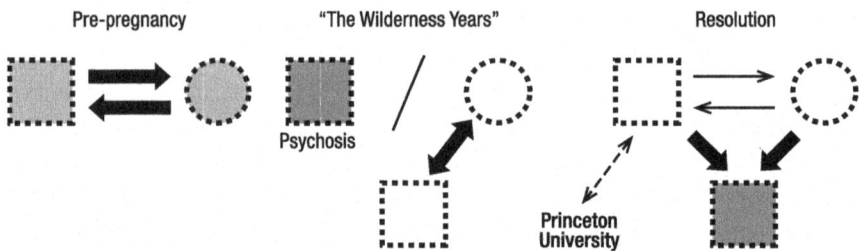

Figure 22.6 *This diagram summarizes the basic theme of this chapter.* The diagram at the left depicts low chronic anxiety and a reasonably comfortable, balanced early marriage. The slanted black line in the middle diagram depicts their marital separation and early years of their divorce. The shading in the symbol for John symbolizes his very high level of chronic anxiety. The thick dark reciprocal arrow between Alicia and son Johnny symbolizes an intense emotional fusion. The last diagram symbolizes the gradual impact of John again living with Alicia in an eventually balanced relationship that reduced his chronic anxiety, emotional isolation, and symptoms. The arrows from both parents toward their son indicate the extreme child focus that also reduced potential chronic anxiety generated in the marriage. The dashed reciprocal arrow between John and Princeton University symbolizes the importance of faculty and administration support for him.

Figure 22.6 illustrates the primary goal of this chapter, that a clinical problem such as schizophrenia is a chronic anxiety-driven functional dysfunction and that the level of chronic anxiety relates to the degree of disturbance in the symptomatic individual's important relationship systems, particularly the family. It describes in broad strokes the interplay between changing social contexts and clinical symptoms for John Nash. The diagram on the left depicts the context of the prepregnancy years of the courtship and marriage of John and Alicia. Some tensions exist in the relationship, but not enough to disturb seriously the individuality-togetherness balance of the relationship. Accordingly, the level of chronic anxiety in each partner is at a modest level (light shading).

The diagram in the center depicts the profound split that developed between John and Alicia after she got pregnant in the early fall of 1958, which I label "The Wilderness Years." Winston Churchill was out of power and out of favor for about ten years in the 1920s and 1930s, which many refer to as his "Wilderness Years." I thought about Churchill as I considered the ten years that John Nash experienced painful and debilitating isolation. He existed in the sea of humanity but, absent tethering to Alicia—something he often fought but needed desperately—he was in a wilderness. His psychotic symptoms and associated agitation were at a maximum during that period. That split lasted a little over a decade before Alicia initiated steps to bridge the gap.

The diagram on the right represents resolution. The term *resolution* refers not to resolving their emotional fusion but to the renewed tethering to Alicia that was profoundly calming for John. His psychotic symptoms began to gradually diminish after she allowed him to live as a "boarder" in her home. This part of the diagram symbolizes their relationship as in reasonably good balance and generating little chronic anxiety related to their dealings with each other. Their anxious focus on their increasingly dysfunctional son would have helped stabilize their relationship by helping confine their disagreements to how to deal with their son. John was already improving significantly by 1986 when their son's forward momentum came to a complete halt and he returned home. His presence generated much tension in the house, but Johnny was viewed as the primary source of any tensions between the parents. They cohered around trying to fix Johnny. Princeton University's important role in supporting John is also included in the diagram.

Many people are quick to assume that his second son genetically inherited the problem from his father. As I have stated several times in this book, Bowen theory does not rule out genetics as having a role in the transgenerational transmission of schizophrenia (and other clinical entities)—or some other not yet identified factor—but genes would be seen as perhaps having a role in whether the chronic anxiety plays out as schizophrenia rather than some other clinical dysfunction. Attaching this much importance to chronic anxiety is not far out of the mainstream. Many clinicians and researchers speculate that patients diagnosed with schizophrenia who experience remission as they get older do so because of a reduction in stress.

Arguments for genetics notwithstanding, the role of a multigenerational emotional transmission process is especially transparent in the Nash case. Alicia's relationship with her husband had many of the characteristics of an overfunctioning mother and an overly dependent, underfunctioning child. Alicia's relationship with their son Johnny was a more intense version of the same thing. The intense fusion between Alicia and their son was reinforced initially by her husband's absence during the 1960s and reinforced later by his very active overfunctioning with his son and reinforcement of the parental triangle during the period from the early 1970s until the parents' deaths in 2015.

One important clue for understanding Alicia's intense and overfunctioning mothering with her husband and son likely resides in the triangle involving her older and later institutionalized brother, her mother, and herself. She likely gained approval and attention from her mother by supporting her and tacitly agreeing that the cause of her brother's problem resided in him. Her father was likely on board with that view as well. I have no direct information about that triangle, but if I was the family therapist trying to help the Nash family, I would ask questions about Alicia's memory of that triangle. Some parents do not want to engage such questions, but some can. Helping them get a larger, multigenerational picture of what is unfolding can be quite useful for helping a mother be less blaming of herself and less convinced the primary problem rests in her offspring. I often refer to the calming effect of seeing and accepting one's part in a relationship problem as "the systems miracle."

PART IV

Special Applications

CHAPTER TWENTY-THREE

Unidisease

A Proposed New Concept in Bowen Theory

We all study the same disease.
—Peter Libby, *Inflammation and Atherosclerosis:*
A Translational Tale

This chapter describes many reports about scientific studies that are relevant to Bowen theory. Science is critically important for the future of the theory: given the difficulty people generally have in letting go of cause-and-effect thinking and applying natural systems thinking to human emotional functioning and behavior, facts from the social and biological sciences that are consistent with Bowen theory give it a credibility that helps people see the wisdom of making the transition to systems thinking.

The epigraph to this chapter from Peter Libby, a cardiologist and researcher studying atherosclerosis, is consistent with the idea of what I term a *unidisease* concept, which I propose be included in Bowen theory. Libby (2018) noted that the biological processes he observes in the pathogenesis of atherosclerosis occur time and again in all diseases. These processes, which interact with one another, include cellular proliferation (increases in cells), fibrosis (scarring), white blood cell recruitment (inflammation), and angiogenesis (growth of blood vessels), all of which are driven by inflammation's effects on the body's epithelial cells (line outer and inner surfaces) and mesenchymal cells (form connective tissue).

Bowen theory states that heightened chronic anxiety in a family is what triggers the development of physical, emotional, or social symptoms in a family member. According to the unidisease concept, many of these symptoms are caused by intensifying the biological processes that Libby lists to pathogenic levels. As a quick aside, I suggest that since anxiety-driven emotional reactivity is considered the driving force for each category of symptoms, a better term for the emotional symptom category would be "mind" or "mental" symptoms—the symptoms manifest in aberrant cerebral cortical processes, but the core of the symptom-generating force is the subcortical emotional system. Physical symptoms stem from disturbances occurring in organs such as the kidney, liver, bowel, or skin. Mental and physical symptoms reflect the internalization of chronic anxiety, but social symptoms reflect the externalization of anxiety into behaviors such as compulsive gambling, shoplifting, and substance abuse. Heightened chronic anxiety can also manifest in escalating family conflicts rather than symptoms.

Research by Kevin Struhl (2010) reveals that diverse diseases also have active gene networks in common. The common networks create what Struhl termed a "diseased cell state." The cells involved in all the different diseases all have the same active genes (*active* meaning they are producing a protein product). Different diseases also involve different active genes, depending on the cell type involved, such as liver cells versus kidney cells. For example, diabetes, atherosclerosis, and cancer express the same disease-cell-state genes, but they also express different genes depending on the tissues involved. The idea of a diseased cell state is consistent with the unidisease concept.

The unidisease concept is important because the physiological processes common to all diseases, rather than what is identified conventionally as the pathology, may be as important, if not more important, to treat. This means that, for a patient with rheumatoid arthritis, for example, family therapy that lowers chronic anxiety in the family may be helpful.

The unidisease concept does not address the question of why the similar pathology-generating biological processes target a specific organ. Answers to that question include such factors as genetics, potentially pathogenic microorganisms, and toxins. Use of the term *pathology* is meant only to describe the type of dysfunction playing out in a tissue, such as arthritis or a tumor; it is not to imply that the pathology is the cause or principal driving force for the symptoms. From a systems perspective, pathology is part of the process, not the cause of it. This perspective is unproven at present.

RESEARCH CONSISTENT WITH THE UNIDISEASE CONCEPT

Researchers have uncovered a common pathological mechanism for cancer and atherosclerosis. The research involves a physiological process that has received much attention in recent decades: chronic inflammation. Two studies and a commentary on them are consistent with the unidisease concept. Paul Ridker (2017a) at Brigham and Women's Hospital discovered that an anti-inflammatory medication given to patients who had suffered a recent heart attack significantly reduced their chance of another heart attack during a four-year follow-up period. Ridker, McFayden, J., Everett, B., Libby, P., Thoren, T., and on behalf of the CANTOS Trial Group, (2017b), also did a second study of patients with previous heart attacks who were also deemed free of a previously diagnosed lung cancer at the time the study began. The patients in the treatment cohort were placed on the same anti-inflammatory drug used in the first study. A three- to seven-year follow-up study found that the treated patients not only had fewer heart attacks but also had significantly lower cancer mortality than those in a placebo group. The authors suggested that treatment with anti-inflammatory drugs not only lowered the incidence of heart attacks but also reduced the mortality from the previously diagnosed lung cancer.

Siddhartha Mukherjee (2017), a Columbia University oncologist, wrote a commentary in the *New York Times* on Ridker et al.'s two studies and concluded that, because an anti-inflammatory drug significantly both reduced the incidence of a second heart attack and decreased cancer mortality, "the studies link disparate areas of medicine through a common pathological mechanism," namely, inflammation. This conclusion is exactly in line with the unidisease concept. The studies leave unanswered the question of what drives the inflammation. For many decades, it has been assumed that the inflammation occurs because the cancerous tumors make and secrete substances that trigger and sustain it. However, while it is true that cancers do release such substances, the unidisease concept suggests that the inflammation could also be significantly amplified by a patient's heightened chronic stress response.

The effort to link psychological factors, such as feeling isolated and overwhelmed, with the stress response was another important research step. Hans Seyle (1956) first described a nonspecific stress response, or general adaptation syndrome, in the 1930s. He focused on biological processes as the activators of the stress response (Gerson & Bishop, 2010). Research by endocrinologist John W. Mason, which demonstrated that psychological threats activate the stress response (Mason, 1959), is considered a crucial turning point in stress research. He established links between psychological threats, emotions, and the hypothalamic-pituitary-adrenal axis, a key link to the stress response.

Other research has established a link between psychological factors, the stress response, and inflammation. Cole, Hawkley, Arevalo, Sung, Rose, and Caccioppo (2007) compared a cohort of people assessed as being isolated and lonely to a cohort assessed as well integrated socially. His research team found more exaggerated endocrine and sympathetic nervous system activity (part of the stress response) in the people assessed as very isolated than in the people assessed as socially integrated. The increased stress response activity resulted in very different genes being expressed in the white blood cells (key players in the inflammatory response), which promoted inflammation. In contrast, the genes expressed or activated in the socially integrated cohort not only did not promote inflammation but also helped bodily organs and tissues resist viral infection through interferon production. This difference between the two cohorts rendered the isolated group more vulnerable than the socially integrated cohort to the many diseases that chronic inflammation can stimulate.

Research by Nicole Powell and colleagues (2013) presented in Chapter 15 showed that the mind's perception of a psychological threat can activate nervous system release of stress hormones that influence bone marrow to produce proinflammatory white blood cells. This is another link to explain Cole et al.'s findings. Combining Cole et al.'s and Powell et al.'s research with Bowen theory shows pathways by which emotionally significant relationships, whether soothing or stressful, can regulate genes to promote health or disease.

Research by Huang et al. (2011) implicates processes similar to those just described as being involved in infectious diseases as well. Most people are used to thinking of the immune system as protecting us from potentially pathogenic bacteria and viruses, but that turns out to be only part of the story. These researchers infected seventeen volunteers with the influenza virus. Nine of the people got sick, but the eight others reported only feeling under the weather and were without any clinically discernable symptoms. The ones who succumbed to illness were those whose inflammatory and stress responses were strongly activated prior to the symptoms appearing. Those who never developed clinical symptoms had a very different immune system response: they did not exhibit a stress response or inflammation but produced antioxidants and other compounds that took care of the problem. The researchers did not attempt to evaluate possible differences in the degree of stress members of the ill versus asymptomatic groups were under at the time they were exposed to the virus. They suggested that the differences in response by the two groups may be genetically based. The research is important because it demonstrates clearly that inflammation can make things worse, perhaps by triggering a virus's virulence factors. A quote from noted physician Lewis Thomas (1974) in an essay titled "Germs" is relevant to the findings of inflammation triggering disease: "Our arsenals for fighting off bacteria are so powerful, and involve so many different defense mechanisms, that we are more in danger from them than from the invaders. We live in the midst of explosive devices; we are mined" (p. 78).

A research team at Carnegie Mellon University led by Sheldon Cohen (2005) also studied a respiratory viral infection but came to a different conclusion than Huang et al. (2011) to explain variation in the strength of the symptom-generating inflammatory response. The Carnegie team concluded that a prolonged stressful event rendered an individual vulnerable to a strong inflammatory response. According to the researchers, the mechanism by which psychological stress can have a deregulatory effect involves the hormone cortisol. Normally, cortisol is produced by the stress response; besides helping the body adapt to adverse conditions, cortisol functions to suppress the immune system. Cohen argued that cortisol becomes unable to exert its normal regulation of the immune response because the immune cells become insensitive or resistant to its effects. Because of this resistance, runaway inflammation can occur that promotes disease.

Cohen's team used the common cold to test his theory that unregulated inflammatory activity triggers cold symptoms. The cold virus does not cause the symptoms of a common cold; the symptoms are a side effect of the inflammatory response. Over the years, I have developed a response to people suffering from a cold who notice that I may be developing a cold too and ask, "Oh, did I give you my cold?" I respond by saying, "No. I took it!" I cannot blame the virus for my immune system's strong reaction to its presence. Cohen found that the stronger one's inflammatory response, the greater the likelihood of experiencing cold symptoms.

Cohen found in his research that experiencing a prolonged stressful event was associated with immune cells developing a resistance to responding to cortisol's normally dampening effects on their activity. Cortisol resistance has implications for all the diseases in which chronic inflammation has a key role, such as cardiovascular diseases, asthma, autoimmune diseases, cancer, Alzheimer's disease, and perhaps schizophrenia and many others. My own clinical observations indicate that stress plays an important role in behavioral problems as well, such as compulsive gambling, antisocial acts, and excessive drinking. In the case of the cold virus, insensitivity to cortisol and the consequent runaway inflammation results in the release of high levels of proinflammatory cytokines by the immune cells that trigger the upper respiratory symptoms.

In terms of the contexts that trigger psychological threat, Cohen and his research team found that enduring (one month or longer) interpersonal problems with family and friends and enduring problems related to work, such as unemployment or being underemployed, were the most frequent threats. The longer the stressful life event or events lasted, the greater the risk of developing a clinical illness. The researchers also established that robust social networks and social support mitigate the perception of psychological threat and associated stress response.

Research by Ali Zahalka (2017) concerns another of the four biological processes Libby notes that occur frequently in the pathogenesis of all diseases, angiogenesis (the development of new blood vessels). In the mid-1950s, pathologists noticed cancer cells grow preferentially around blood vessels (Weinberg, 2007). Tumors located more than 0.2 mm away from blood vessels do not grow, and others farther away die. This is because oxygen cannot effectively diffuse through living tissue more than 0.2 mm. Normal cells in any tissue are never more than several cell diameters away from the nearest capillary. Developing vascularity through angiogenesis is critically important for the growth and survival of all types of tissue, normal and cancerous.

Nerves release neurotransmitters to regulate most physiological functions in the body. This research demonstrates that a variety of nerve-mediated signals control the development of cancers. Neurotransmitters affect both the cancer cells and the cells in the connective tissue that surrounds the cancer. The study found that noradrenaline (also called norepinephrine), which is associated with the stress response and is released from cancer-associated nerves, triggers angiogenesis and thus cancer progression: the endothelial cells that form blood vessels have many receptors for noradrenaline that trigger increased cell division and consequent blood vessel growth. The adrenergic stimulation also triggers metabolic changes that allow the endothelial cells to divide at a much higher rate than normal, to keep pace with the rapid growth of the cancer. These cancer-associated endothelial cells also release growth factors and cytokines that attract immune cells, which then participate in inflammation that also stimulates cancer growth.

Other ideas about the role of inflammation in how cancers develop came from Richmond Prehn and Harold Dvorak. Prehn (2007), whose research career was strongly devoted to understanding the interplay between the immune system and cancer, theorized that sublethal immune cell activity in a tissue stimulates cancer growth by interfering with communication between cells or between cells and connective tissue. Normally this communication is a major inhibitor of tumor growth by preventing normal cells from becoming cancerous. Dvorak (1986), an oncologist, observed that tumors and their surrounding tissue have the appearance of wounds that do not heal. Wound healing involves reactivating biological processes, including white blood cell activity, angiogenesis, cell proliferation, and cell migration, that are critically important in normal development of embryos. These processes become dormant when not needed but can be reactivated for wound healing. I suggest that the inflammation that is normally activated to heal wounds becomes chronic in tumors related to a chronic anxiety-driven chronic stress response, and stimulates the sublethal inflammatory activity that Prehn suggests.

This discussion of multisystem involvement in cancer supports a speculation by Candace Pert (1997) about a cancer's connection to the body as a whole. She suggested that a cancerous tumor is part of a network that permits an ongoing exchange of information between the tumor, the brain, and the immune system. These exchanges make it possible for these bodily systems to regulate, control, promote, or retard one another. One cannot explain the behavior of tumor cells without understanding how they are part of larger bodily systems—and Bowen theory would include family systems as well. Cancer is clearly a systemic disease.

Further support for regarding cancer as a systemic condition comes from research by Camilla Engblom (2017) that revealed a systemic cross-talk between lung tumors and bones that promotes growth of the cancer. A study of lung adenocarcinoma showed that the tumor secretes factors that mobilize a certain type of white blood cell from bone that fosters tumor growth by stimulating processes such as inflammation and angiogenesis in the tumor connective tissue. Bone homeostasis depends on the resorption of bone by osteoclasts being equally balanced by the formation of bone by osteoblasts. Imbalance of this tightly coupled process can cause diseases. The findings in this study show that when osteoblasts become overly active in relationship to osteoclasts, which is what the tumor-secreted factors promote, the osteoblasts stimulate production of the type of white blood cells that promote cancer growth. The unidisease concept suggests that this cross-talk is a reciprocal process: the cancer triggers the bone response and the bone response triggers the cancer. This does not occur when osteoblast-osteoclast homeostasis prevails. Stress may accentuate the bone's reaction to the cancer signals by inducing an overall disturbance in bodily homeostasis that manifests as a disturbance in bone homeostasis. This is conjecture at this point, but I describe the possibility to illustrate how the homeostasis concept could be applied. Just as anxiety is compartmentalized in a family system, stress-induced changes in the body, such a disturbance in homeostasis, could be compartmentalized in one part of the body.

The research interest in the relationship between stress and health has existed for a very long time. The examples cited in this chapter do not do justice to the long history of the field but are consistent with the importance Bowen theory places on chronic anxiety and make the unidisease concept seem plausible.

DEVELOPMENT OF THE UNIDISEASE CONCEPT

In the summer of 1976, I began a clinical study of families who had a member diagnosed with cancer. Over the next five years, I interviewed about 125 families, some for as long as two years, others as briefly as a few hours. My interest was in deciding whether emotional factors that operate within the patient and within the family influence the onset and clinical course of cancer.

Early in my study, I became interested in the biology of cancer as well as the emotional processes. I realized that conclusions about emotional factors could not conflict with biological facts about cancer. The idea of a unidisease concept gradually grew out of this effort. Rather than attempt to prove the accuracy of the concept, which seemed beyond reach, I looked for facts that were consistent with or contradicted the idea. I would characterize my effort over these many decades since 1976 as a "scientific inquiry."

My first inkling of the unidisease idea came with reading about the biology of cancer. I happened onto an article from 1913 by American pathologist Aldred Scott Warthin, who has been described as the father of cancer genetics. The finding that got my attention in that article was that some families showed the occurrence of carcinoma in successive generations and that the neoplasm had a tendency to develop at an earlier age in members of the youngest generations. Furthermore, when it develops at an earlier age than in previous generations, it often shows increased malignancy. Typically, these lines of family eventually went extinct.

Up to that point in my study, I had focused on emotional process in the nuclear family of the cancer patients I interviewed and had paid less attention to their multigenerational families. However, it struck me that if emotional process did play an important role in cancer, Warthin's findings might be consistent with the Bowen theory concept of a multigenerational emotional process. As described in Chapter 11, the concept states that, in certain multigenerational lines of a family, related to the family projection process intensifying down the generations, the level of "self" of individuals gradually decreases. Presuming that emotional factors were important in cancer, the heightened average level of chronic anxiety associated with lack of "self" struck me as consistent with cancers occurring at an earlier age and being more severe.

I wondered if what Warthin observed with cancer families might be present in families that had a high incidence of other diseases. By 1980, I had collected thirty-five to forty articles about families with a high incidence of a particular disease. These families exhibited the same multigenerational patterns of earlier age of onset, increased severity, and reduced fertility in certain generational lines that Warthin had described. This led me to the speculation that the multigenerational emotional process that Bowen had found in schizophrenia, namely, that it takes at least three generations, usually more, for emotional functioning to decrease from a fairly adaptive level to a level that rendered a person vulnerable to "hard-core" schizophrenia, occurred as well in a wide range of other physical, psychiatric, and behavioral conditions. Finding the same multigenerational patterns, no matter what disease was involved, contributed to formulating the unidisease idea.

The pattern of multigenerational changes that Warthin described with cancer and other researchers described with other diseases is termed *anticipation*. For a long time, the phenomenon was not considered a truly biological one. More recently, however, the phenomenon has been observed with genetic disorders, predominantly neurological ones, such as Huntington's disease (Dayalu, 2015). In Huntington's, a biological phenomenon termed *gene amplification* occurs in successive generations that results in the production of an abnormal amount of a deleterious protein, which is thought to contribute to these successive generations being increasingly vulnerable to earlier onset and increased severity of the disease.

Before describing how the phenomenon of anticipation could be a bridge between biology and emotional process, I want to state my conclusion from the interviews with the 125 families with cancer and describe the process of arriving at it. The conclusion is that basic level of differentiation and chronic anxiety are important factors in the onset and clinical course of many, maybe most cancers in these families. I arrived at that conclusion by reviewing the careful notes taken during my interviews with the families, constructing the types of family diagrams described in Chapter 11, diagramming my impressions of the patterns of emotional functioning in each nuclear family, and rating the number, intensity, and type of stressors each family encountered leading up to the cancer diagnosis. I also considered what the family members themselves thought about the role of stress in cancer. I then estimated the overall basic levels of differentiation for each family and compared the least differentiated 25 percent with the most differentiated 25 percent of the cases. I concluded that the cancers tended to occur earlier and to be more severe in the least differentiated families than in the most differentiated ones. I did not include childhood cancers in my assessment because I assessed only such thirteen families.

Returning to the biology of cancer, I am not convinced that gene amplification is a sufficient explanation of anticipation. The concept leaves unanswered the question of what drives the amplification process. It is possible that multigenerational emotional process fits into the picture as a driving force. Why I am holding out for a broader understanding that would include emotional process begins with Claude Bernard's concept of *milieu intérieur*, which he introduced in the second half of the 1800s (Bernard, 1974). Walter Cannon (1939) expanded on Bernard's idea, terming it *homeostasis*.

Bernard's and Canon's basic idea is that unicellular and multicellular organisms have physiological processes that maintain a constant balance or equilibrium regardless of changes in their external environment. Any tendency toward change in that constancy automatically meets with factors that resist the change. The adaptive capacities of unicellular and multicellular organisms attempt to preserve this state of equilibrium. The concept of homeostasis applies to the human body, and by viewing the family as a unit—an organism in its own right—it is possible to consider a family as a homeostatic system as well. For example, disturbances in the family relationship system trigger automatic emotional reactions to restore the balance. The fact that dysfunction in one family member reflects a disturbance in family homeostasis mirrors that dysfunction in a bodily organ often reflects a disturbance in bodily homeostasis. The unidisease concept suggests that disturbances in family homeostasis may affect bodily homeostasis and hence its related diseases. Gene amplification may reflect such a disturbance in bodily homeostasis.

An English radiation oncologist suggested more than fifty years ago that diseases reflect a disturbance in bodily homeostasis. Sir David Smithers published a paper in the *Lancet* emphasizing the need for what he termed a social science of the human body (1962). It would involve applying cybernetics, which its originator, Norbert Weiner, described as the scientific study of control and communication in the animal and the machine. Smithers suggested that most scientists understood that studying units of the body, such as individual cells, in isolation does not reliably demonstrate the behavior they manifest when they function in the context of the body. Scientists should recognize that the whole functioning of the human body is their concern. This viewpoint is at the heart of systems thinking. He suggested this approach was necessary to explain normal growth and differentiation but also disorders of those processes, such as cancer. I think Smithers described what I term a yet unformulated systems theory of the body. For example, a tumor growing somewhere in the body is a symptom of processes involving the functioning of the body as a whole. This is consistent with Candace Pert's view of cancer, along with Engblom's research on lung cancer, both mentioned earlier in this chapter.

Research by William Flavahan (2017) invokes the concept of homeostasis to explain the microscopic world of chromatin. Chromatin, which is located in the nucleus of a cell, is made up of DNA, histone proteins, and nonhistone proteins. The DNA double-helix strands that contain genes wrap around the histone proteins. The relationship between the histones and DNA strand varies over time, which regulates the activity (expression vs. nonexpression) of the genes. These are referred to as *epigenetic changes*, meaning that the genes are changing not structurally (genetic mutation) but in their activity levels. The histone-DNA interactions play a key role in stabilizing gene expression and cellular states and in facilitating appropriate responses to developmental and environmental cues. Most important for supporting the idea of unidisease is that inflammation is one of a number of factors that can disturb chromatin homeostasis, rendering the chromatin overly restrictive or overly permissive. These restrictive and permissive dysregulated states can promote cancer and other diseases.

Research presented earlier in this chapter establishes the fact that stress hormones such as noradrenaline, through changes in gene regulation, can shift white blood cells into a proinflammatory state. Flavahan's conclusion that inflammation can disturb chromatin homeostasis revealed yet another pathway by which stress can trigger disease. By linking the development of clinical dysfunctions to a local disturbance in homeostasis—in this case chromatin—it suggests that Smithers' conceptualization that disturbances in homeostasis underlie disease can be extended to conceptualize the nature of the disturbances playing out at multiple levels of the organism.

Another step toward formulating a unidisease concept occurred when I encountered an article by pathologist Earl Benditt (1977) in which he compared an atherosclerotic plaque to a benign tumor of smooth-muscle cells developing in an artery wall. Benditt suspected that the same kinds of agents and conditions that transform cells to initiate cancers might be involved in atherosclerosis. The processes driving smooth-muscle cell growth were unknown, but Benditt's conclusion that the pathogenesis of cancer and atherosclerosis have something in common gave support to the unidisease idea.

Research on psoriasis also supports the unidisease concept. In Chapter 15 I describe about some of my personal experiences with the condition and what it taught me about being aware of chronic anxiety. Like with studying cancer, in investigating links between psoriasis and chronic anxiety it was important to study the biology of the condition. A number of types of psoriasis exist, but plaque psoriasis has been the focus of my biological study. The skin lesions in plaque psoriasis are slightly raised, circumscribed red patches covered with silvery scales. The disease may involve the nails and joints as well as the skin. This discussion focuses on the skin manifestations to illustrate the biological processes that generate them. Genetics is a factor in being susceptible to psoriasis, but environmental factors trigger it. It is classified as an autoimmune disease and, like most all clinical conditions, exhibits wide variability in clinical manifestations and clinical course, ranging from mild with frequent remissions to severe and chronic. The biological processes that contribute to the pathogenesis of psoriasis have been increasingly well defined, but the forces driving those processes and accounting for clinical variation continue to be elusive. The phenomenon of anticipation occurs in psoriasis.

The skin is an epithelial tissue, one of four types of animal tissue that includes connective, muscle, and nervous tissues. Figure 23.1 diagrams the histology (study of bodily tissues) of normal skin, the changes associated with early psoriatic plaque formation (histopathology), and the histopathological changes typical of an advanced lesion. The diagram on the left depicts the dermal and epidermal layers of normal skin. The keratin layer on the surface of the skin is composed of cells that no longer have nuclei (are terminally differentiated) and are packed with the protein keratin. The epidermal layer below the keratin layer is made up of multiple layers of cells in various stages of differentiation: cells near the bottom of the layer are recently produced daughter cells that result from the division of epidermal stem cells, and cells near the top are ready to assume a place in the keratin layer. The stem cells

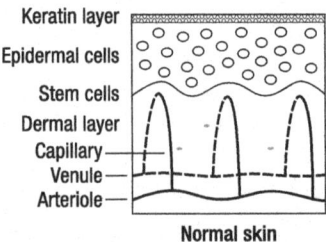 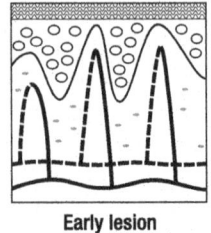 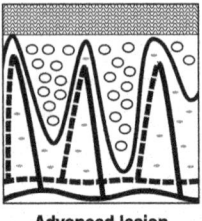

Figure 23.1 *This diagram depicts the transition from normal skin to an advanced psoriatic lesion that includes heightened cell proliferation, angiogenesis, and inflammation. The diagram on the left depicts a balance between cell division in the stem cell layer and the naturally occurring loss of cells from the surface of the skin. The diagram of early lesion formation depicts increased cell proliferation beyond what is necessary to replace natural losses, expanded arterial supply (angiogenesis), and the beginning buildup of inflammatory cells in the dermal layer of the skin. The keratin layer of skin has thickened. At the far right is an advanced lesion. The degree of angiogenesis has increased, along with more cell proliferation and inflammation.*

in the diagram are depicted as a gently undulating black line constituting the lowest segment of the epidermal layer, which consists of single cells lined up side by side. They are undifferentiated cells, meaning that they produce daughter cells from their periodic divisions, but the stem cells themselves do not differentiate. The dermal layer is below the epidermal layer. It contains arterioles bringing oxygenated blood and nutrients to the skin tissue, venules to carry off carbon dioxide and metabolic waste products, and capillary loops that exchange what the arteriole brings and what the venules remove. The dermal layer also contains hair follicles, nerves, and lymphatic capillaries, which are not depicted here.

Skin tissue normally exists in a state of homeostasis or equilibrium. The blood transport in and out and the rate of stem cell division match what is needed to generate new cells to replace keratin cells lost from normal wear and tear at the skin surface. This balance maintains a consistent and adaptive thickness of the skin.

The middle diagram in Figure 23.1 depicts three core processes involved in the pathogenesis of a psoriatic plaque lesion: angiogenesis, inflammation, and increased cell proliferation. A plaque lesion develops (in genetically vulnerable people) when normal homeostasis of the skin is disturbed by intensified activity of these three main processes. Psoriasis, like many other diseases, results from the exaggerated activity of normal processes. The early lesion differs from normal skin by developing thicker and longer arterioles and venules, a moderate influx of inflammatory cells (black dots in the dermal layer), and heightened stem cell proliferation. Note that the undulations of the stem cell layer have increased and the stem cell layer itself now contains more than one row of cells. This results from the daughter cell products of stem cells retaining their reproductive potential and dividing a number of times before differentiating. The increased undulations accommodate the increased number of stem cells. Consequent to this increased activity, the daughter cells not only increase but are pushed to the surface of the skin much faster. They arrive at the surface in a not fully differentiated state, thickening the keratin layer and populating it with immature keratin cells. This accounts for the abnormal appearance of the plaque lesion of psoriasis. The lesion is like an inflatable device floating on a sea of inflammation. The advanced lesion diagram to the right is more of the same, producing larger and thicker psoriatic plaques.

Studying the biology of a lesion such as a psoriatic plaque offers a valuable perspective that differs from thinking of the lesion as a pathology. It is actually an unsurprising outcome of excess normal activity of physiological systems. Yes, genes are involved, but their role may be to attract the inflammation to certain areas of the skin. Genes may help explain where chronic inflammation occurs but not what drives that inflammation. From a Bowen theory perspective, as I describe in what follows, a psoriatic lesion can be described as "bound anxiety," meaning chronic anxiety drives the biological processes that wind up expressing themselves visibly as a psoriatic plaque. This possibility is reinforced by the inability of researchers over many decades to identify a pathology in the epidermal or dermal layers of the skin that drives the process. What is clear is that a reciprocal interaction plays out between the epidermal and dermal layers of skin and that chronic inflammation, with the aid of other physiological systems, plays an important role in driving it. Elaborate communication systems exist between the two layers that support the reciprocity. Furthermore, psoriasis is definitely systemic—plaques usually occur in multiple areas of the skin at the same time.

Figure 23.2 summarizes Bowen theory variables and physiological processes that help explain how psoriatic skin lesions develop. Studying the biology of psoriasis along with other clinical conditions led me to formulate a "systems model of disease" during the 1980s, an idea that is at the core of the unidisease concept (Kerr, 1992):

> Although physical, psychiatric, and behavioral disorders are considered manifestations of family emotional forces, such forces are not held to be the "cause" of an illness. An understanding of any illness must include pertinent facts derived from all levels of investigation, intracellular to societal. The interplay among all of the factors must be examined, with no single factor or set of factors viewed as causal. A model that can incorporate all the facts and their interrelationship, without ascribing cause to any one fact, is a systems model of disease. (p. 102)

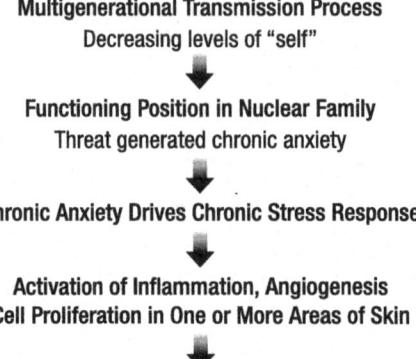

Figure 23.2 *This diagram summarizes Bowen theory variables and fundamental physiological processes that help explain how psoriatic skin lesions develop..*

The exceptions to a systems model would result from major biological disturbances, such as severe radiation poisoning, massive exposure to a pathogen, a major genetic abnormality, or some other circumstance that no one could adapt to.

Another disease example illustrates how the unidisease model deals with illnesses associated with potentially pathogenic microorganisms. Prior to the discovery by Marshall and Warren (1984) that the bacterium *Helicobacter pylori* has a central role in the development of peptic ulcers and gastritis, medicine had generally assumed that stress was an important factor in ulcers. However, the discovery of the bacterium's role relegated stress to a back seat. While discovery of the bacterium was important, it still leaves unexplained why a significant majority of human beings harbor *H. pylori* in their stomachs but do not develop ulcers. Nor does the presence of the bacterium explain remissions and exacerbations of the ulcers in those prone to developing them.

Based on an article on *H. pylori* by Lee (2005), I constructed some diagrams to illustrate how the unidisease concept addresses an infectious disease. Figure 23.3 is the first of four diagrams. It illustrates a stomach that *H. pylori* bacteria are inhabiting peacefully. The top of the diagram is the interior of the stomach, the lumen, where acidic gastric juice and water are present; the bottom is the serosa covering the outside surface of the stomach. The tiny empty circles on the surface of the serosa represent blood vessels. Starting from the bottom up, two muscle layers exist that are innervated (the four empty circles between the two layers). The next layer up is the submucosa, which contains nerves, blood vessels, and some white blood cells. The next layer, with a thin muscle layer between, is the mucosal layer. It consists of a certain

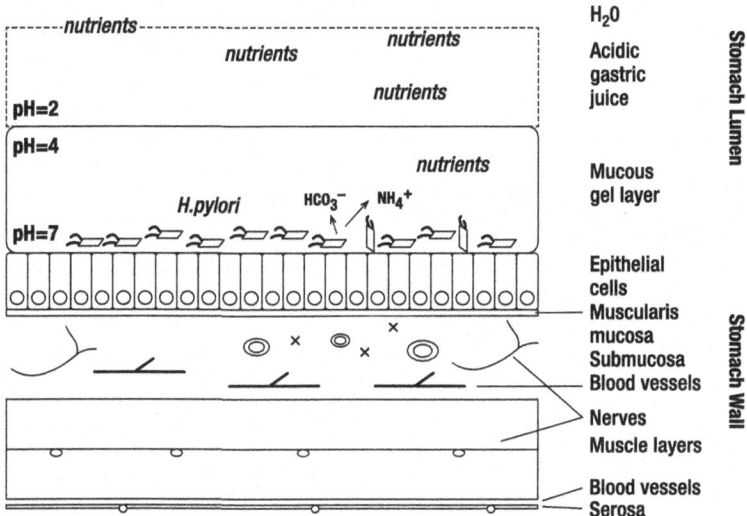

Figure 23.3 The information for this and the next three diagrams is drawn from the following: Lee, Y. (2005). *Korean J Gastroenterol.* 46:159-65. *This diagram depicts the key players and processes involved in the development of gastric ulcers.* The most important thing to note in this first of four diagrams is the presence of immune system cells (potentially able to launch an inflammatory response) in the submucosal layer of the stomach wall and a population of potentially virulent H.*pylori* bacteria in the mucous gel layer of the stomach lumen peacefully coexisting.

type of epithelial cell that forms deep pits in the stomach wall that, among other structures, are full of gastric glands that produce gastric juice containing hydrochloric acid and enzymes. The mucosal area is much more detailed than I have depicted it.

The *H. pylori* bacteria inhabit the area near the epithelial cells, sometimes even attaching to those cells, in a mucous gel layer. Note that near the bottom of the mucous gel area the pH is 7, which is neutral, not acidic. The bacteria produce and secrete substances that help neutralize the pH, enabling them to live there. Higher up in the lumen of the stomach, the pH is 2, very acidic. The acid does its job there in breaking down food nutrients for eventual digestion. As noted, some potentially inflammatory white blood cells are present in the submucosa, but this diagram depicts a state of détente between the bacterial and the white blood cells.

Figure 23.4 depicts a dramatic end to détente. War has broken out between the bacteria and the immune system, now in a state of vigorous inflammation, aided by that now familiar process of angiogenesis. The bacteria have transformed into a more virulent state, with release of virulence factors, such as CagA, LPS (lipopolysaccharide), and VacA.

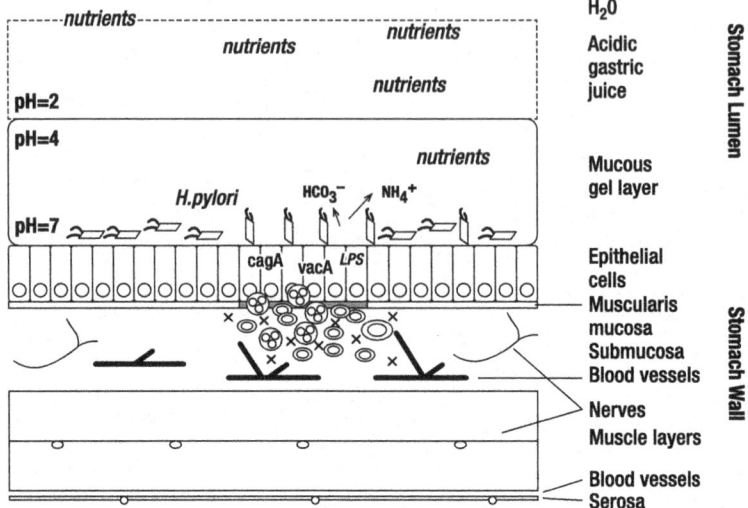

Figure 23.4 *This second in the series of slides depicts fierce conflict between the now highly virulent bacteria and inflammatory cells.*

It may be unknowable if this war was started by a stress-activated immune system or by the virulent bacteria triggering the immune system into defensive action. Traditionally, the bacteria have been blamed. Lewis Thomas (1974) pointed out, however, that bacteria gain nothing in an evolutionary sense by developing the capacity to cause illness. Furthermore, it is metabolically expensive for bacteria to activate virulence genes. He went on to say that "reasons not understood but probably related to immunologic reactions on our part" (p. 77) bring on the disease. When Thomas wrote these words in the early 1970s, much less was known about the role of stress in promoting inflammation. The unidisease concept fits here. It can help explain exacerbations and remissions of ulcers. Bacteria trigger the inflammatory response, but, as is evident from studies described in this chapter, a stress-driven inflammatory response also triggers the bacteria into a more virulent state.

Figure 23.5 shows the havoc this war inflicts on the wall of the stomach. The bacterial-inflammatory war sows the seeds of destruction of the stomach wall by killing endothelial cells and thus allowing hydrochloric acid to destroy a section of the mucosal layer, creating an ulcer.

Figure 23.6 shows the fourth of Peter Libby's biological processes, scarring or fibrosis. The black wiggly lines where the ulcer had existed can result from reactive or excessive wound healing. Stromal cells named fibroblasts produce the connective tissue of fibrosis. It is interesting that macrophages, which are

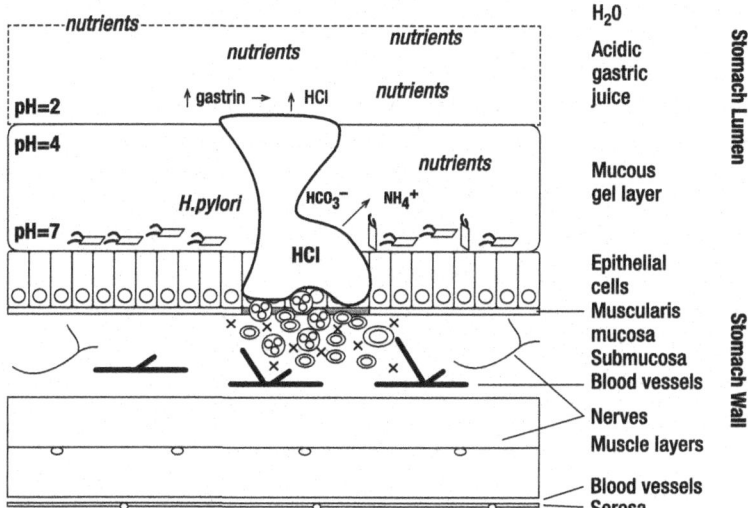

Figure 23.5 *This third diagram illustrates what could be termed the "collaterial damage" left by this battle: many epithelia cells of the gastric mucosa have been killed,* allowing hydrochloric acid and inflammatory cell hyperactivity to carve out the ulcer. Note the marked angiogenesis in the submucosal layer, which is constantly bringing in the increased supplies needed to sustain the battle.

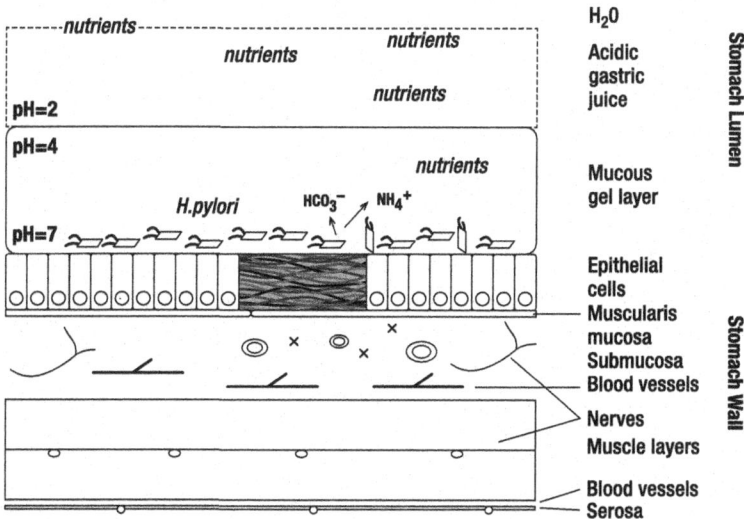

Figure 23.6 *This fourth diagram in the series depicts the end of the battle but with the remnant of permanent scaring (dark wavy lines in the ulcer crater).*

core immune system cells, stimulate and possibly overstimulate the fibroblasts to make the fibrous tissue.

I have a personal interest in the ulceration process, having developed an esophageal ulcer several years ago during a demanding transition in my life. I have no doubt that stress associated chronic anxiety played an important role in the ulcer, both in increasing hydrochloric acid production and in intensifying my immune system response. *H. pylori* is also associated with esophageal ulcers, so I assume I have a population of the bacteria living in my stomach to this day. I agreed to take a proton pump inhibitor to allow healing, and it worked beautifully. These drugs block the production of hydrochloric acid, without which an ulcer does not develop. Long after my ulcer recovery, I continue taking the drug—and will do so until this book is finished! Writing this book has been stressful at times, but it has not been the only source of stress. I mention this personal experience to emphasize that chronic anxiety may be a key component of unidisease—in this case peptic ulcer—but chronic anxiety is difficult to control in a world of responsibilities and uncertainties, and that needs to be respected. Using medication is preferable to potential perforation of the esophageal wall! Some level of chronic anxiety seems to be a fact of human existence.

Leaving clinical examples and returning to theoretical thinking and research, another subject relevant to unidisease is allostasis. Stress researcher Bruce McEwen (2002) has done much to develop this idea. Allostasis is related to the concept of homeostasis but differs from it in an important way. The essence of the homeostasis concept is that any change that threatens the constancy of an organism is met automatically by resistance to that change to preserve equilibrium or balance. Allostasis refers to organisms' ability to maintain stability (equilibrium) through change. For example, if you are sitting quietly in your living room in an easy chair, maintaining homeostasis is automatic. However, if you want to climb a flight of stairs to retrieve something, your body must adjust. As you are climbing, your heart rate increases and your heart pumps harder. You do not want automatic resistance reactions to keep your heart rate at the same level that it was while you were sitting in the chair. These adjustments are part of the acute stress response and can include activity of both the hypothalamic-pituitary-adrenal cortical axis and the autonomic nervous system. After climbing the stairs, your heart rate goes back to resting level and the heart stops pumping as hard. Acute stress responses are well tolerated by the body's organs and tissue. The adjustments are termed allostasis: short-term increase in physiological activity (heart rate and cardiac output) to maintain homeostasis.

The idea even more relevant to the unidisease concept is *allostatic load*, a term that refers to the wear and tear inflicted on the body due to repeated

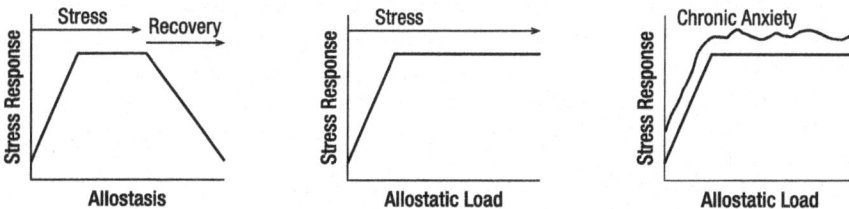

Figure 23.7 The y-axis on this diagram indicates activation of the stress response. The x-axis indicates the amount of time the stress response lasts before returning to base line. The diagram on the left indicates the stress response returning to baseline normally, a process that is termed allostasis. The middle diagram symbolizes a chronic stress response creating allostatic load. The curly arrow above the diagram on the far right indicates chronic anxiety as a possible key element in the stress response becoming chronic.

cycles of allostasis, such as occurs from repeated stresses or when the stress response system does not turn off when it should. Figure 23.7 illustrates allostasis and allostatic load over time. The stress response functions to preserve stability through change, and allostasis describes that phenomenon. A stress response is unnecessary for maintaining homeostasis under resting conditions, which is the reason for the separate terms. The graph on the left is the ideal scenario: the stress response persists as an adaptive response to the challenge; once the challenge ends, the response fairly quickly returns to baseline. Some variation in recovery time could exist among individuals due to genetics or development, but Bowen theory suggests that is not the whole story. The middle diagram depicts a high allostatic load, where the response persists. The diagram on the right suggests that chronic anxiety can be the major factor in how much allostatic load a person experiences over time. The challenges of life being what they are make allostasis a routine part of life. However, prolonged periods of allostasis are a "load" on the body's organs and tissues that can eventually impair their functioning.

A study by Daniel Belsky and colleagues (2015) concerning the pace of biological aging in people discovered something both interesting and possibly relevant to the unidisease concept and allostatic load. Biological aging refers to a declining integrity of multiple organ systems as people age. Belsky et al. studied a cohort of 954 New Zealanders who were all born in the same year. People in the cohort were thirty-eight years old at the time of this study, but their biological ages ranged from twenty-eight to sixty-one. The researchers assessed this by tracking eighteen health measures in each member of the cohort at three time points spanning the third and fourth decades of life. Biologically older participants were weaker, were less coordinated, had more rapidly declining IQs, and felt and looked older than their biologically younger counterparts.

From about the fifth decade of life on, the incidence of a wide range of chronic diseases such as cardiovascular diseases, type 2 diabetes, stroke, chronic respiratory disease, and neurological disorders begins to rise significantly. This study shows that the aging of physiological systems that contributes to those diseases begins before the diseases emerge. The thirty-eight-year-olds did not have chronic diseases at that point in time. However, the members of the cohort showing the least biological aging would be less vulnerable to chronic disease over time than those showing the most biological aging. The researchers did not investigate the reasons for the significant variation in biological aging.

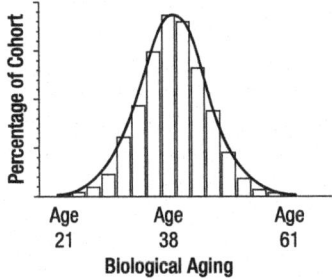
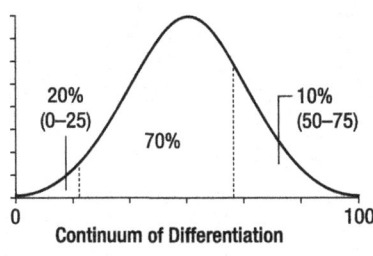

Figure 23.8 This diagram compares two bell curves. The diagram on the left is based on an article by Belsky, D., Caspi, A., Houts, R., Cohen, H., Corcoran, D., Danese, A., (. . .), Moffit, T. (2015). *PNAS*, 112, E4104-E4110. The diagram on the right is from Chapter 5. The data from the Belsky study on variation between individuals in rates of biological aging creating a Bell Curve and the Continuum of Differentiation estimated to be a Bell Curve.

A diagram in the article by Belsky et al. (2015) particularly caught my attention. It showed a bell-shaped curve in the cohort in terms of degrees of biological aging. Figure 23.8 represents the variation in the left diagram. On the right is the diagram from Figure 5.3, the estimate of what the continuum of differentiation looks like. There are limitations to comparing the distribution curve on the left, derived from hard data, to the one on the right, based on an estimate from extensive clinical experience and observations of society. I present this similarity because Bowen theory, unidisease, and allostatic load would have predicted Belsky et al.'s findings. The multigenerational transmission process generates a continuum of differentiation of self in every family. Those with the lowest levels of "self" are the most vulnerable to high average levels of chronic anxiety in their lifetimes. At the other end of the continuum, individuals tend to have the lowest average levels of chronic anxiety. Chronic anxiety drives a chronic stress response that presumably strongly contributes to a person's allostatic load over a lifetime. It seems logical that allostatic load accelerates biological aging: it is wear and tear on the body. Although this assertion has not been proven, as part of a scientific inquiry I present studies that are consistent with the idea of unidisease, such as Belsky et al.'s and McEwen's ideas.

The Bowen theory concept of emotional regression is another important part of the unidisease concept. I describe in Chapter 6 how this concept could be extended to other species. It appears that it can also be extended to help explain cancer. Two theoretical physicists, Paul Davies and Charles Lineweaver (2011), developed a controversial theory about cancer that I think is related to emotional regression. Their thesis is that cancer cells are cells that become dysregulated and default back to ancestral genetic pathways that drive their unregulated proliferation. Many of the same genes active in a cancer are also expressed in early embryogenesis and wound healing. These are not defective genes, the result of mutations, but perfectly normal ones. The authors described the genes as an "ancient cassette," meaning they are very old in evolutionary terms. The upregulating of these ancient genes in the early stages of embryogenesis is appropriate because the early stages are characterized by cell proliferation and migration. The same cell proliferation, migration, and other changes are required for wound healing. Davies and Lineweaver suggest that in cancer these genes are upregulated inappropriately. The authors refer to cancer as a not well-ordered rerun of embryogenesis.

A key part of Davies and Lineweaver's theorizing is the recognition that unicellular organisms exhibiting unregulated proliferation were the only life forms on the planet until about 600 million years ago, when the first multicellular (metazoan) creatures evolved. With the evolution of increasing complexity in metazoans, necessary cell differentiation and regulation systems emerged to coordinate the activities of a multicellular community. However, the evolution of these new systems did not mean that the 3.5-billion-year-old systems that support cellular proliferation disappeared. Their theory is that in cancer genetic mutations and epigenetic changes result in the more recently evolved regulatory capacities of multicellular organisms becoming weaker, allowing some of the body's cells to exhibit the uncontrolled cell proliferation typical of cancers. The authors refer to their model as *atavistic*, meaning a reversion to something ancient or ancestral. When cells transform into a cancerous state, they also revert to an ancient metabolic pathway to produce energy for the cells.

Bowen theory conceptualizes emotional regression as the loss of regulatory capacities and reversion to older, less complex ways of functioning, similar to what Davies and Lineweaver describe. The term *emotional* applies here because Bowen theory holds that an emotional system, in Bowen's sense, exists in single cells as well as in more complex organisms.

The research by Flavahan (2017) on chromatin, presented earlier in this chapter, suggests that a normal cell can transform into a cancer cell based solely on epigenetic changes. These changes unfold in the context of a disturbance in chromatin homeostasis, and one of the factors that can disturb it is inflammation. Research by Weinberg (2007), also presented above, implicates the stress hormone noradrenaline in promoting inflammation. Putting all this together using the unidisease concept suggests the following possible scenario: chronic stress triggers the increased release of noradrenaline, which disturbs chromatin homeostasis and triggers epigenetic changes that disable the regulatory systems that normally control cell proliferation, and a cancer results. This would represent a functional, not structural, change in a cancer cell that theoretically would be reversible. It is well established that cancers can remit spontaneously. As usual, this scenario based on the unidisease concept does not prove its accuracy, but it is not contradicted by the facts and theories about cancer that people like Davies and Lineweaver are discovering and putting forth.

One last component of the unidisease concept is an idea that I put forth at a conference on Bowen theory called the *family stress response*. I discussed all of its basic components at various places earlier in the book, so I summarize it briefly here. I then conclude this chapter with some discussion of the calm and connection system, a bodily system that helps counterbalance the stress response (Moberg, 2011).

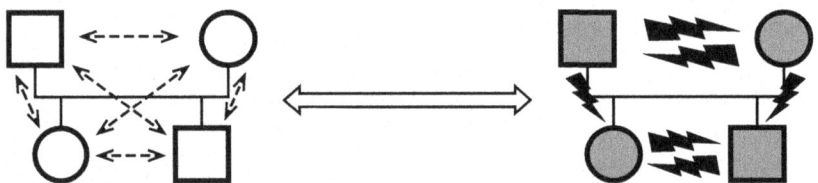

Figure 23.9 *This diagram depicts the family stress response. The family diagram on the left side with no shading in the male and female symbols and dashed lines between the members symbolize calm people interacting in a calm manner. The diagram on the right side with dark shading in all the family members and thick jagged shaded lines between them symbolizes highly anxious people interacting in highly anxious ways. The arrow between the two diagrams symbolizes the same family moving back-and-forth between states of calm and regression.*

The idea of a family stress response relates to the bodily stress response in that both responses are activated in an effort to restore homeostasis. Figure 23.9 diagrams how a family moves from a calm and well-functioning state to a chronically anxious and regressed state. The diagram on the left symbolizes a nuclear family of four fairly calm people (no shading) interacting with little tension in their relationships (dashed lines). The diagram on the right symbolizes four highly anxious family members (shading) with very tense interactions (jagged, dark symbols), heading into an emotional regression.

The potential for regression can begin with either an internal stressor (generated within the family unit) or an external stressor (generated outside the unit) affecting one or more family members. One stressed member can be sufficient for a disturbance to arise in the family unit as a whole. A series of stressors could also set the process in motion. The stressor triggers tensions in the family unit, not based on the stressor itself but based on how family members are dealing with each other in the face of the stressor(s). Whenever a system reacts with escalating anxiety to a stressor, it says more about the state of the system than about the stressor itself. The stressor does not cause the tensions in the family, but the family's lack of success in adapting to the stressor explains the escalation of chronic anxiety. The escalation of anxiety and relationship tension indicate a decline in functional level of differentiation in the family. Once an escalating process is set in motion, chronic anxiety generates disturbance in the balance of family relationships, and this disturbance generates its own chronic anxiety.

As described throughout this book, each family member's reactivity to attention, approval, expectations, and distress mediates the escalation. Family members also have the ability to self-regulate that reactivity through cognitive processes. The strength of the reactivity and ability to self-regulate vary with the basic levels of differentiation of the family members. The longer the chronic anxiety persists, the more likely self-regulation will be overwhelmed in all family members and for a regression to intensify.

Togetherness pressure increases in the family in response to anxiety in an attempt to restore system balance. If a comfortable balance is not restored, the patterns of emotional functioning come increasingly into play to compartmentalize the anxiety in one part of the system. These patterns can stabilize a system for a time. As a family's attempts to adapt fail, physical, mental, or social symptoms in one or more family members emerge or severe conflicts erupt. At that point, a family can stabilize somewhat around the presence of a symptom, which fosters it becoming chronic, or the regression can continue to get worse. In a best-case scenario, the appearance of a symptom can move a family (usually led by one member) into changing the way they are interacting.

The family stress response is similar to the body's stress response in that it can be acute, with balance restored quickly, or the togetherness pressure to make things better can make it worse. It is analogous to acute inflammation healing and chronic inflammation destroying. The family stress response and the individual family members' stress responses, as I have emphasized throughout, are interconnected, and this is often very hard for people to see and accept.

Because this chapter has focused entirely on chronic anxiety and its biological impact, I want to conclude by briefly describing a bodily system that helps counterbalance the stress response. Kerstin Uvnäs Moberg's (2011) research demonstrates that oxytocin, which interacts with the stress hormones, provides the body with a calm-and-connection system that can counterbalance fight-or-flight reactions. Moberg lists such factors as touch, warmth, fullness, sexual activity, social interaction, security, and certain medications as mobilizing the calm-and-connection system. People's perception of a relationship, the way they experience it, determines to what extent our fight-or-flight reaction is triggered or our calm-and-connection response is triggered. Bowen theory's concept of emotional objectivity is an example of how a change in one's perception of a relationship can activate the calm-and-connection system. The evaporation of experiencing a relationship as threatening reduces activation of the stress response, but the calm-and-connection system is likely also involved. Moberg's short book *The Oxytocin Factor* (2011) is well worth reading.

I conclude by summarizing the eight components that I have described as being part of the unidisease concept:

1. Biological processes that occur time and again in the pathogenesis of many diseases.
2. Multigenerational emotional process
3. Homeostasis
4. Allostasis and allostatic load
5. Biological aging
6. Emotional regression
7. Family stress response
8. The calm-and-connection and fight-or-flight systems

What does the future hold for the unidisease concept? Murray Bowen considered the theory he originated as work in progress. He did not add his name to the theory with the intention of constraining its future development. The important criterion for changing or extending the theory is that whatever change is proposed, it is based on facts alone and not personal opinion. As I stated in the introduction, I am proposing that the unidisease become a new concept in Bowen theory. As far as I know, no one has proposed a new concept for Bowen theory other than Bowen, so I am plowing new ground.

I first published my thinking that eventually led to the idea of a unidisease over thirty-five years ago (Kerr, 1980). It was a hypothesis. I talked about my thinking on this topic many times at conferences in the years that followed but did not publish anything referring specifically to the unidisease idea until my first book (Kerr & Bowen, 1988). I wrote the following in the book, "If physical and emotional illnesses are accurately conceptualized as symptoms of a more basic process, then all 'diseases' are rooted in one fundamental process, a *unidisease*." It remained a hypothesis in 1988, and it still is a hypothesis. However, as I tried to convey in this chapter, scientific support for the idea has strengthened significantly in the more than forty years I have been mulling over the idea. I think it is fair to say that over the last several decades science has powerfully challenged the dichotomy of mind and body. However, the toughest issue remains, which is proving the link between chronic anxiety in a family system and the psychological and physiological processes of individual family members. Theory says it is so but that does not make it so. It is very difficult to do the type of quantitative research on a complex family system that persuades scientists because of the multiple variables influencing the situation. I believe this problem will eventually be solved as systems thinking increasingly influences research.

In their heart of hearts, human beings know that family is important but do not recognize that the scientific thinking that has guided human beings to the Moon and back can be applied to families. A science of human behavior is possible. As the idea of a unidisease gains some traction in the public consciousness, the concept will have a useful impact by alerting clinicians and the public at large to a family-oriented approach being useful, whether the clinical symptoms are physical, mental, or behavioral. I do not expect this to happen in my lifetime. Paradigm shifts can occur rapidly when they finally happen but result from a slow building of a rationale over many years. If the unidisease becomes a concept in Bowen theory, science will make it happen.

CHAPTER TWENTY-FOUR

Toward a Systems Concept of Supernatural Phenomena

Science is about things. It is about rocks, stars, atoms, and living beings. It is about all those things that surround us and which used to be called Nature with a capital N.
—John Tyler Bonner, *The Scale of Nature*

On a strict level, I have not considered a theory to be valid unless it can somehow be synonymous with the universe, the earth, the tides, the seasons, the predictable cycles of life, and man as a reproductive, evolving form of life.
—Murray Bowen, "Subjectivity, *Homo sapiens* and Science"

I introduce this chapter with a quote about science by biologist John Bonner and a quote by Murray Bowen about determinants of the validity of a theory, because neither statement includes subjectivity. To quote Bowen, "When subjectivity creeps into theoretical postulations, the result is more chaotic and less scientific" (1997, p. 15). However, this chapter is about Bowen's thoughts on how to include supernatural phenomena in Bowen theory, which are phenomena by definition that are outside the laws of nature.

This chapter is a suitable companion piece for Chapter 23 because it discussed the potential healing impact of a changed context on a person's particular disease. Chapter 23 on the unidisease concept emphasizes how family and social context and its impact on the individual are essential to consider in explaining disease development. This chapter, in contrast, is very short, perhaps better labeled an addendum, because Bowen never developed his initial thinking about supernatural phenomena into a theoretical concept. Efforts by others since then to move that process along have fallen short of developing a concept.

Despite not being a concept in the theory, supernatural phenomena are discussed here for two reasons. The first pertains to misconceptions about what Bowen intended, and the second pertains to a historical issue. This potential concept has attracted considerable interest since Bowen first began talking about it in the late 1970s. The first and perhaps most pervasive misconception or misuse of the idea is people interpreting Bowen's consideration of supernatural phenomena as support for having faith in a supernatural realm. People do not generally express this directly, but it seems evident in that many discussions about the potential concept are associated with theology and religion. The possibility that Bowen theory's approach to human nature, along with explorations into including supernatural phenomena, could inform theology makes sense, but an agenda of somehow integrating Bowen theory with theology and the spiritual realm is a misinterpretation of Bowen's intent. The word *spiritual* is used in different ways, of course. When the term is intended to refer to that difficult to define but almost palpable human spirit, this seems close to what Bowen intended. When it refers to the assumption of a spiritual or supernatural realm, that takes it beyond Bowen's intention.

The second reason I include in this book what is only a potential concept in Bowen theory regarding supernatural phenomena is something I characterize as unfinished business from the Age of Enlightenment. The antecedents of the Enlightenment date back to the early seventeenth century. Sir Francis Bacon was an iconoclast in leading the charge to separate natural philosophy, which is the study of the world by natural human faculties to determine the nature of God's creation, from theological explanations (Kors, 1998). Bacon advocated studying the particulars of nature, forming tentative generalizations, testing the generalizations against nature itself, and then moving to higher levels of generalization. His ideas remain the basis of modern science. Alan Kors (1998) suggested that 1680–1715 was an unusually exciting time to be alive. Empiricism, quantification, naturalization, and induction guided studies of the Book of Nature. The thrust was to develop a "natural theology" that was devoid of supernatural explanations, God's providence in natural laws, miracles, and divine intervention. The Enlightenment ideas swept across Europe during the eighteenth century, creating the demarcation that Bacon had envisioned many years earlier.

Naturalistic explanations focused on the physics of bodies and the physiology of living things; spiritualistic explanations focused on the source of motion in the world and the nature of human behavior. What I consider the unfinished business of those heady times is that the natural philosophers failed to tackle human behavior. A few thinkers did, but too few to have a pervasive impact. The French philosopher Denis Diderot (1713–1784) and his philosopher-physician colleague Julien Offray de La Mettrie (1709–1751) argued for the idea that physical medicine could render spiritual explanations unnecessary and explain all aspects of human behavior. Clearly ahead of their time, they also held that a gradual transition from animal to human life (evolution) had occurred.

I propose that Bowen theory's effort to move toward science to understand human behavior addresses what the Age of Enlightenment failed to tackle. Bowen is not the first thinker to try to move human behavior into the realm of science, but his discovery of families functioning as emotional units and the application of natural systems thinking in studying those units were new. An additional dividend from Bowen's effort is considering a potential method for including supernatural phenomena. Subjectively based beliefs are powerful motivators of human behavior and are important to reckon with in any theory about behavior.

In a nutshell, the thrust of the supernatural concept is that *functional facts* exist about spiritualism, religion, ESP, black magic, voodoo, transcendental states, laying on the hands, and the entire range of "unseen forces." It is a functional fact that some people have died believing that a voodoo curse had been inflicted on them; it is a functional fact that people have gone to the Sanctuary of Our Lady of Lourdes in France and experienced dramatic remissions of an illness. Bowen emphasized that he was not talking about mysticism. A way to study such phenomena would be to assemble facts about religion, ESP, voodoo, and such, and those facts may eventually add up to something approaching the realm of science. Bowen's intent was not to prove or disprove supernatural causes but to pursue the phenomena in the way Bacon had championed: look to the Book of Nature.

The Roman Catholic Church has done incredibly detailed studies of people with serious illnesses who have made trips to Lourdes and experienced seemingly related complete and lasting remissions of their conditions without any medical explanation (Ferguson, 2014). As of 2014, there had been sixty-nine such cures that were judged to be miracles. Examples include a woman with an adrenal tumor that caused serious hypertension, whose hypertension disappeared; a person with a paralyzed arm that suddenly become functional; and a man with a pelvic bone tumor that disappeared and normal bone replaced it. It is a fact that these cures occurred. Regarding them as miracles, of course, does not preclude eventual scientific explanations for the processes that resulted in a cure.

It seems that a change in mind-set related to the Lourdes experience triggers emotion/feeling-associated physiological pathways that alter the body such that an illness remits. The physiological pathways involved possibly restore homeostasis in the diseased organ and tissue.

The considerable research that has been done on the placebo effect provides important insights about possible pathways. Pierre Rainville, Duncan, G., Price, D., Carrier, B., Bushnell, M. (1997) administered either a moderately painful or neutral stimulus to human research subjects and demonstrated that the sensory pain signal registered in the sensory cortex, but the perception of unpleasantness of pain was linked to anterior cingulate cortex (ACC) activity.

Prior to exposure to the pain stimulus, the subjects were hypnotized and given the hypnotic suggestion that the stimulus they would receive would either be painful or not painful. (This research is not specifically focused on the placebo effect but gets at the same idea.) This created a belief in the subject about what to expect. Rainville then demonstrated through functional magnetic resonance imaging that if the subjects received a hypnotic suggestion that the stimulus would be highly unpleasant, a corresponding increase in blood flow in the ACC occurred following the stimulus; if the hypnotic suggestion was that the stimulus would be minimally unpleasant, the ACC received low blood flow following the stimulus. Both subjects were receiving the identical pain stimulus that registered in the sensory cortex, but only the subjects that had the expectation (belief) that it would be quite painful exhibited increased blood flow to the ACC and an associated sensation of pain. Granted, the exact pathways through which a belief can lead to reduced blood flow to the ACC are still unknown, but it is a fact that it happened.

Another placebo-related research study has even more intriguing implications. R. Christopher DeCharms (2005) subjected research subjects to a noxious thermal stimulus while they were undergoing functional magnetic resonance imaging. During and between stimuli they were given visual feedback of activity in their rostral ACC, a brain region involved in pain perception and pain regulation. With the aid of the visual feedback, subjects could learn to control that specific brain region, and this was associated with significant diminution of perceived pain in response to the noxious stimuli. Furthermore, research subjects who had chronic pain before the study and learned to control the rostral ACC during the study reported decreased pain even after the study. This highlights a poorly understood phenomenon: when technology enables people to be consciously aware of objective data about ongoing physiological processes that they would normally be unaware of, they can learn to exert some control over them. This finding has parallels to what occurs in the process of differentiation of self. The lens of Bowen theory enables bringing previously unobserved automatic relationship processes into consciousness, which permits more control over them.

It seems very clear in the research just described, and in placebo research, that something does in fact change in the mind-set of the patient that ultimately makes a difference in the patient's symptoms; for example, "My doctor thinks this medication will relieve my pain, and I now do as well." At Lourdes something similar may be occurring. Lourdes apparently is an incredibly tranquil setting, a place where people report experiencing "spiritual relief." The sick who come there are treated as first and foremost in importance. A caring attitude, providing that sense of total acceptance without judgment, is something all human beings yearn for. A quote below by the physician Sir William

Osler, one of the founding professors of Johns Hopkins Hospital whom many consider to be the father of modern medicine, is relevant to the Lourdes discussion: "Faith in St. Johns Hopkins as we used to call him, an atmosphere of optimism and cheerful nurses, worked just the sort of cures as did Aesculapius at Epidaurus" (1910, p. 1471). Herbert Benson, a cardiologist and leading researcher in mind/body medicine, has been developing ideas quite similar to Bowen's but focusing more on the individual than on the relationship system. Like Bowen, Benson is not trying to prove or disprove the validity of a belief—whether God or supernatural phenomena exist—only trying to determine whether a patient's belief, particularly a spiritual belief, could promote health. One of Benson's studies tested the hypothesis that people who thought others were praying for them had more successful recoveries from cardiac bypass surgery than those who did not hold that belief (Benson, 2006). This particular study did not support his hypothesis but nicely exemplifies his attempt to bring spirituality into the realm of science. Benson had shown in earlier studies that the stronger a person's spiritual beliefs, the more impact they had on reducing the fight-or-flight stress response (Benson, 1975). It is interesting that Bowen and Benson were pursuing similar paths without being informed about each other's work.

Bowen theorist and wife Kathleen Kerr made some interesting observations about voodoo when she was in Tanzania some years ago (1996). A native Tanzanian cook where Kerr was living during her stay became convinced that a voodoo curse had been placed on her and suspected a particular person of doing it. Her boss was extremely understanding of what she was going through and eventually was able to persuade the cook that it was untrue. She was not bedridden, but her symptoms included nausea, vomiting, and hearing voices. Her functioning as a cook was significantly impaired for weeks, and she appeared to be going rapidly downhill and heading for death. She was dominated by fear and suspicion and could only very gradually let it go and fully recover.

A second case Kerr observed was of a young woman who had moved from her native village to marry a man who worked in a preserve some distance from where she grew up. Fairly soon after arriving, she became convinced that a curse had been placed on her. She expressed certainty that she would die. She took to bed and ate and drank little. When it looked like she was going to die, her boss sent for a witch doctor. The witch doctor performed certain rituals and provided a healing charm and some medicines. The young woman recovered.

Many people might write off a phenomenon like voodoo as something that people in primitive cultures believe. One value of this potential ninth concept in Bowen theory is that it can highlight the pervasiveness in the human species of beliefs that are unprovable but extremely influential. Belief in a supernatural realm is not a pathology but part of human nature. It is terribly difficult to realize that we think we know something that we do not and that we are frequently not the "rational animal" we believe ourselves to be.

The question of whether all types of illnesses can be stalled or cured (or triggered) by a change in belief or mind-set is unanswered. Discussions of a relationship between stress and illness commonly evoke comments about blaming patients for their illnesses, as if some sort of psychological weakness is implied. When I posed this question to one of the patients in my early studies of cancer, her reply was, "Don't people realize how powerful emotions are?" The implication of her comment was that just because emotions may play a role in triggering many diseases, it does not imply people should have or could have exerted control over the process. The idea that stress may not trigger an illness but could affect the clinical course is more easily accepted. That seems to be reflected in a growth in popularity of stress management techniques.

Bowen's initial interest in the function of belief as a way to incorporate subjectivity into his theory was sparked at a conference in March 1978 that included Gregory Bateson and himself. Bateson had been diagnosed with inoperable cancer of the lung not long before that conference. He had been visited by a faith healer, who told him, "The surgeons were too late, your cancer was already dying." He had refused palliative treatment, in part to devote all of his energy toward finishing a book. In June 1979, Bowen had occasion to meet up again with Bateson and learned that his lung cancer was in remission. Bowen wondered what went into that. In March 1979, Albert Scheflen, a researcher in the family movement well known for his work on nonverbal communication, had also been diagnosed with inoperable lung cancer. Then in March 1980, in a speech to the American Family Therapy Association, Bowen asserted, "Within 50 years systems theory could account scientifically for biological, psychological, and spiritual phenomena in a single frame of reference" (Bowen, 1980a). The idea of including spiritual phenomena in family theory had obviously germinated in Bowen's mind. A month later, Bowen was at another conference that included both Bateson and Scheflin. Each reported that their cancers were under control. Interestingly, Scheflin was also working on a book. On the trip back to Washington, D.C., Bowen envisioned that assessing the function of unproven beliefs rather than the validity of their content was the key to bringing supernatural phenomena into the realm of science. Beliefs can provide a sense of purpose and meaning in one's life.

Candace Pert (1997) was a pioneering researcher on neuropeptides, which are small protein-like molecules that enable communication between the cells of a multicellular organism. Based on her research, she proposed the existence of a new physiological system that she named the "psychosomatic information network." This neuropeptide-mediated system links psyche and soma through information exchange. Among the things that she discovered is that both brain and immune system cells produce neuropeptides. This meant that the information is going not only from mind to body but also from body to mind. I consider her idea relevant to Bowen's pondering that Bateson and Scheflin's strong determination to complete their books were factors in at least stalling the growth of their cancers. The complexities of mind-body interactions and our current level of knowledge about them make it difficult at present to prove the existence of a psychosomatic information network, but the following quote captures how Pert (1997) envisioned such a system operating:

> If I have a purpose, such as finding a cure for cancer, then every system in my body gets behind that intention and does what needs to be done, be it increasing my appetite for protein, mobilizing the gastrointestinal system to digest a protein better, sending blood flow into the digestive organs to produce necessary enzymes for maximum absorption, or whatever. There is a physiological integrity and directedness about this process that is the result of my clarity about my own intensions. When I am at cross-purposes, however, going through the motions but not really committed to my goal, saying one thing and doing another, then my emotions are confused, I suffer a lack of integrity, and my physiologic integrity is likewise altered. The result can be a weakened, disturbed psychosomatic network, leading to stress and eventually to illness. (p. 295)

Bowen gave his first formal presentation on this potential concept that could incorporate supernatural phenomena into Bowen theory in the fall of 1980 at the Annual Family Symposium sponsored by the Georgetown University Family Center. The presentation was titled *Towards a Systems Concept of Spiritual Phenomena* (Bowen, 1980b). This was followed in January 1981 by a videotaped interview in the Bowen-Kerr interview series (The Bowen-Kerr Interview Series is available at www.thebowencenter.org). titled *Towards a Systems Concept of Supernatural Phenomena* (Bowen, 1981)—he had substituted supernatural for spiritual. Even in his presentation the previous fall, he had said that he was considering replacing the term *spiritual* with *supernatural* because people were quick to assume that he was focusing on religion. He envisioned the idea to be much broader than religion.

In July 1987, a conference titled "Implications of Bowen Theory for Catholic Theology" was held in Silver Spring, Maryland, organized by Father Joseph Carolin, a Catholic priest. The potential for a concept about supernatural phenomena in Bowen theory inspired the conference. This was the first of many such conferences that followed, right up to the present time. The conferences are generally well attended, as many people interested in Bowen theory want this to become a well-developed concept. At that first conference, Murray Bowen did a presentation titled *The Theoretical Structure of the Catholic Church* (Bowen, 1987). The presentation did not elaborate on a potential supernatural concept as many attendees hoped it would, but one particular statement in Bowen's presentation merits repeating: "A major quality in the differentiation of self is complete selflessness in which doing for others replaces personal selfish goals. Jesus Christ has been a model for total selflessness." I say the statement merits repeating because this aspect of differentiation is often missing from discussions about it. I expressed this idea in a previous book as a high level of differentiation being reflected in the ability to act for self without being selfish and the ability to act for others without being selfless (Kerr & Bowen, 1988). Such actions are not devoid of emotion but are guided by principle. Principle-driven selflessness does not render people vulnerable to illness but seemingly does just the opposite—helping others seems to promote health.

A final point to make before ending this chapter is that while parallels exist between Bowen theory and Benson's work on the function of belief, Benson does not address specifically the phenomenon of how sharing beliefs supports emotional fusion between people (like attracts like), including large groups of people and, in turn, how the emotions that support the fusion process unconsciously dictate the content of the beliefs. These differences between groups reflect different levels of intensity of the togetherness life force. Propaganda is a prime example of triggering the togetherness process in a destructive way; religions generally trigger the togetherness force in a constructive way, supporting principles and ideals that people generally consider important but struggle to live by consistently.

I close this chapter with a quote by Steven Sloman and Philip Fernbach that is relevant to the togetherness process by suggesting the seeming necessity of human beings influencing one another's mental processes to the point of thinking we know certain things when really our knowledge of them is totally dependent on our social environment. We can firmly believe we understand things that we do not really understand at all. This phenomenon can be included under Bowen theory's concept of pseudo-self. Pseudo-self can enhance individual functioning and benefit the larger social group, but it can also be at the root of polarizing conflicts among individuals and groups.

Sloman and Fernbach argue for a distinction between cognitive science and neuroscience: "The mind stretches beyond the brain to include the body, the environment, and the people other than oneself, so the study of the mind cannot be reduced to the study of the brain. Cognitive science is not the same as neuroscience. We fail to draw an accurate line between what is inside and outside our heads" (2017, p. 15).

Epilogue

Applying Bowen Theory to My Own Family

I begin this concluding section with comments about schizophrenia because one of my brothers was diagnosed with that condition. I find it interesting and disquieting that many people assume that scientists and their brain research have proven that a brain disease *causes* schizophrenia. I consider that view reductionistic. Many brain changes have been discovered in actively psychotic people, and the major tranquilizers can calm patients and reduce psychotic symptoms, but there is more to schizophrenia than psychotic symptoms. Delusions and hallucinations are termed the "positive" symptoms of schizophrenia; blunted emotional expression and lack of motivation to live a productive and purposeful life are termed the "negative" symptoms. Psychoactive medications do little for the negative symptoms.

This is important because it is the negative symptoms in people with a diagnosis of schizophrenia that result in their remaining emotionally and financially dependent on their families or a community institution throughout their adult lives. The dependence often becomes a chronic source of family tensions. In many instances, the tensions precipitate a cutoff between schizophrenic people and their family.

Not all people diagnosed with schizophrenia are the same. Some have a psychotic episode at a critical juncture in their lives, such as leaving home for college or going into the military, and never have another episode. In others, it is a chronic condition with marked long-term impairments in functioning. It is clear that some people with schizophrenia have more psychological and emotional strengths than others, and those strengths or lack thereof affect the clinical course. Something exists underneath the psychotic symptoms that is important to understand. As I have discussed in detail in this book, Bowen theory refers to that something as *basic level of differentiation of self*. Some people that are diagnosed with schizophrenia, and their family members, have more "self" than others. The term *hard core* is sometimes used to describe the most impaired schizophrenic patients. From a Bowen theory perspective, these patients have very little "self."

My older brother was diagnosed to have schizophrenia at twenty-eight years of age, just before I began medical school at Georgetown University. He killed himself seven years later. Many people get diagnosed with schizophrenia in their late teens or early twenties. My brother's impairment was evident by age eighteen, but it manifested only in what are termed the negative symptoms, which can be summarized in one word, *avolition*, which refers to a lack of interest or engagement in goal-directed activities. In this epilogue, I describe my understanding of the family emotional processes that rendered my brother vulnerable to behaving in ways that led to his diagnosis and how later disturbances in emotional processes in the family contributed to his suicide. As I have emphasized several times in this book, Bowen theory does not assume that the family emotional environment *causes* schizophrenia but does consider it to be the most critical factor in triggering the various vulnerabilities that predispose an individual to that possibility. Commonly, the person becomes symptomatic during the period of attempting to leave home and transition into adult life. In some instances, the person manages to move out of the family home, forms an intimate relationship, but then develops symptoms if that relationship breaks down, which it often does.

When I began supervision of my clinical cases with Murray Bowen in May 1969 at Georgetown University School of Medicine, he emphasized to all of the psychiatric residents how important it was to understand our own family relationships better if we hoped to be useful clinically to others. I took his suggestion seriously, and Bowen "coached" me in the effort. That effort, along with many clinical observations of schizophrenic people and their families, gradually and radically changed how I thought about schizophrenia. A key change in my thinking about the family early on was realizing that the anxious and reactive functioning of family members presented as much of a problem for my schizophrenic brother as my schizophrenic brother's anxiety and reactivity presented for the family. This realization went a long way toward me no longer blaming my brother for the periodic family turmoil. It was like a breath of fresh air!

Bowen theory recognizes that psychological and biological processes are operating within the symptomatic person, but a systems view holds that family relationship system processes strongly regulate those psychological and biological processes and that the processes within the individual reciprocally affect the relationship system process.

The purpose of studying one's own family is more than about gaining more objectivity. It is also about *using* that knowledge to improve one's ability to function as more of a "self" in the family. In essence, being a "self" means being a more mature and responsible family member. It involves getting a more

EPILOGUE   333

factual picture of the family and being better able to distinguish fact from feeling. It is working out the relationships with one's parents and the family "organism" *in vivo*. It is a method of growing up that has been the cornerstone of training programs in Bowen theory for over half a century.

Murray Bowen set the trend of studying one's own family in motion during the 1960s when he began applying his family research and the theoretical ideas he had developed to his own family. He presented a seminal paper on work in his own family at a national meeting of family therapists in 1967 (Anonymous, 1972). The emphasis of his presentation was that it was absolutely essential to have a coherent family theory to guide efforts to manage oneself differently in the family.

A long-term disciplined effort to use the lens of Bowen theory to understand one's own family and one's part in the family system process, and to gradually apply that knowledge to alter constructively one's behavior in the family are key to making up one's own mind about whether the theory is indeed accurate. The effort boils down to using the lens of theory to think differently about family problems, acting based on that new way of thinking, and getting the predicted result. This is a way that people can gain more "self" than they had developed growing up.

FAMILY OF ORIGIN DIAGRAM

Students of Bowen theory are typically insistent on seeing a family diagram whenever someone presents a clinical case or talks about his or her family. If the presenter is talking about the family process involving parents and siblings or a clinical case, Bowen theorists want to make sense out what is playing out in the person's family of origin by looking at several generations. They have recognized that knowledge of the past is key to putting the present in perspective.

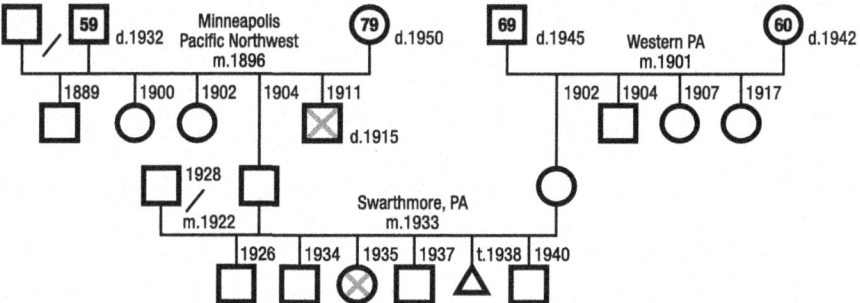

Figure E.1 *Diagram of my immediate family of origin and my parents' immediate families of origin.*

To orient the reader, I introduce this narrative about my family system process with a family diagram (Figure E.1). I have gathered much more information over the years than I present here, but I present enough to illustrate the difference between thinking about schizophrenia as a chronic disease, with a clinical course being largely determined by individual psychological or biological pathology, and thinking about the onset and fluctuations in clinical course as symptomatic of the ebb and flow of anxiety-generated fluctuations in the emotional functioning of the family system. This figure-ground shift from pathology driven to family context driven in reference to schizophrenia is not a new distinction in medicine. Louis Pasteur argued that microbes cause infectious disease, which is a pathology-driven model, but physiologist Claude Bernard (1974) argued that the microbe leads to a disease only if the body "terrain" is sufficiently disturbed, which is a context-driven model. Conventional medicine has long embraced the pathology model, despite Pasteur himself eventually coming around to the view that the terrain is, in fact, key for understanding disease. Family systems theory expands the terrain to include both the body as a whole and the family relationship system.

I will refer to the family diagram to aid the discussion of six factors that were part of the family emotional process that are possibly relevant in rendering my brother vulnerable to schizophrenia. As explained in Chapter 11, a family diagram typically includes data about the emotional functioning of each family member, very little of which is included on the diagram in this chapter—the most relevant data are described as the story unfolds. I say "possibly" relevant because in a complex system such as a family, it is difficult to assess how much weight or anxiety-generating potential each variable packs. To quickly orient the reader to the diagram, I am the youngest child of my parents' marriage, born in 1940. The first thing that stands out on the diagram is that three of my four grandparents died at relatively young ages. One of them, Dad's father, died less than two years before my parents' first child, Billy, was born in 1934. He was the one later diagnosed to have schizophrenia.

Theory predicts that early deaths of grandparents would be more common in less differentiated than in more differentiated families, with low differentiation increasing the vulnerability to some type of serious dysfunction. More important, Dad's father's death in 1932 likely had some impact on the level of chronic anxiety in the then nuclear family system of the new baby, my parents, and my mother's son Bob, from her first marriage. After my grandfather's death, Dad's mother and her older sister (not shown on the diagram) continued living with my parents and Bob, as they had been doing for nearly two years since moving to the East Coast. The death and consequent heightened chronic anxiety likely increased Mother's emotional investment in Billy. Thus, these unique circumstances at the time of Billy's birth may have been a factor in him taking on special significance as a support to our mother.

A second thing that stands out on the diagram is that my father, with two older sisters and a much older half-brother, was the youngest child in his family of origin, except for the brief period my paternal grandparents' last child was alive—he died very young of a nervous system disorder. My mother is a first-born, with a next younger brother and two younger sisters. Mother being an oldest and Dad being a youngest suggests likely aspects of the nature of their relationship, as discussed in Chapter 12 on sibling position.

Third, the diagram shows that Mother's first marriage lasted six years. She described not really wanting a child at the time Bob was born. She said that she gave in to pressure from her then husband to have a baby. She explained that she had married her first husband largely to get away from her family. When Billy was born, not only had the family context changed significantly with the death of Dad's father, but Mother now had a deep desire for a child. "Now, I'm ready!" she said. She loved and took excellent care of her first child, Bob, but his emotional significance to Mother was very different than that of my oldest full brother. This convergence of events would have promoted Mother being overly invested in Billy, and soon anxiously invested as she began to perceive him as a "fragile china doll" in need of more than average love and attention. A fourth thing to point out is that the early death of my parents' second child, a daughter, at age ten days of hyaline membrane disease, could have also had a strong impact on Mother's emotional investment in and worries about my oldest full brother. As best as I can determine from listening to family members and reviewing old family movies, Mother's perception of Billy being fragile was totally subjective, a feeling not a fact.

Turning to my parents' families of origin, two sets of family dynamics are a fifth thing to point out, which was particularly important in Dad's development. One dynamic revolved around my grandfather's drinking problem. (This information would normally be included on a family diagram.) He would sometimes disappear for more than a week at a time on an alcoholic binge. Naturally, there was a lot of tension in my grandparents' marriage around that issue. This likely contributed to my grandmother being unduly focused on all of her kids, meeting many of her needs for emotional closeness with them rather than with her husband. I mention this because it is evidence for the emotional processes my siblings and I grew up in having strong multigenerational roots. My grandfather invested heavily in his work life and also in the kids.

The other dynamic involved Dad's next older sister, Marie. I described something about this in Chapter 16 as playing a role in my mother having a an abortion in 1938 (shown on the diagram as a small triangular symbol). Growing up, Marie, the second daughter, assumed a lot of responsibility for doing something about the tensions in the family and was like a second mother to Dad. Protective of him, she unwittingly, along with other family members, programed him to be in the functioning position of a babied younger brother of two older sisters. All three of the women in the family (the two sisters and his mother) anxiously doted on my Dad.

Dad had the opportunity to go to college. He attended the University of Washington and Washington State but never graduated. (This information would normally appear on the diagram as well.) I mention this because such decisions are often related to lack of "self." In his mid-twenties he got a job as a salesman with a new company that became extremely successful. The company moved him to the Philadelphia area in the early 1930s. He met the woman who became my mother there. Dad had a fairly successful career with that company, working there until his early death in 1962. I describe the circumstances of his death later in the narrative.

To summarize the factors in my brother's vulnerability mentioned thus far: first was the early deaths of grandparents (which is more common in less differentiated families) the second was the sibling positions of my parents that fostered an overfunctioning-underfunctioning reciprocity in their marriage, the third was Mother welcoming the prospects of the first baby in her second marriage in contrast to the first time around, the fourth was the strong child focus in both parents' families of origin, and the fifth was Dad being a babied youngest child tending to go along with wherever Mother's anxieties guided her. The last factor I will mention is three sets of dynamics in my mother's family of origin that were particularly influential on her development. Her parents' marriage was fairly distant. My maternal grandfather supported the working-class family adequately but leaned on alcohol a good bit. My maternal grandmother was a hard worker as well. She is described as always doing something for somebody else and willing to take in family members in need, even when she was sick herself. Much of this rubbed off on my mother. While such attitudes are exemplary in many circumstances, they can be problematic if they unduly color a mother's relationship with a child.

Mother described herself as having a lot of guilt about her mother related to not being able to do more to relieve her mother's stress and "depression." This dynamic was more pronounced after her baby sister was born when Mother was thirteen. My grandmother was diagnosed as having cancer when Mother was a teenager. The evidence suggests that my grandmother felt significantly overwhelmed with the addition of the fourth child, ten years after the previous one.

A second key family dynamic was Mother responding to her mother's overwhelmed and distressed state by becoming like a second mother to her baby sister. My grandmother's strong caretaking characteristics were heavily transmitted to Mother through these first two sets of dynamics.

A third dynamic contributed as well. Mother's brother was anxiously focused on by his parents in the direction of being special. My mother was very tuned into her mother's worry about her brother and, like her mother, felt deeply protective of him. Her brother married and had three children but died quite young of a heart attack. The three dynamics added up to programming Mother to have a powerful need to be needed and a strong tendency to "feel the feelings of others," as she put it. People loved to talk to Mother about their difficulties in life, a fact she often found overwhelming. Murray Bowen once commented, "How come the mothers of schizophrenics are such nice people?" I don't know what percentage of mothers of schizophrenics that covers, but it certainly describes our mother.

Mother had a year of normal school and taught in elementary school for a short time. Her relationship with her father was often contentious. She was in a hurry to get away from home, marrying young to accomplish that. She left western Pennsylvania after the divorce from her first husband. She and her then very young son moved to Philadelphia. There was not a lot of contact with her ex-husband after the divorce.

I provide these details about Mother's family and the course of her early life because gathering such information helped me understand the many factors that promoted Mother's anxious overinvestment in Billy. It provided a path for me to become more neutral and realistic about the intense attachment between Mother and Billy. It just happens that way through a hidden emotional process (observational blindness), and it is nobody's fault. As I describe below, I did not arrive at this more neutral view soon enough to prevent some of my behaviors that destabilized the family situation.

Mother lived in Philadelphia for about two years before Dad and his "entourage" of father, mother, and aunt arrived from the West Coast. Mother had joined a favorite cousin when she moved to Philadelphia and attended a beautician school with her. Mother met Dad and his family in 1931. Dad's father died of cancer the following year. My parents married in April 1933 and moved out to the suburb of Swarthmore. At first they all lived together in a large apartment and then in a rental house. Mother got pregnant within a month after the marriage. Billy was born early in 1934. Very early in Billy's life, Mother viewed him as having the potential for problems. It seemed to be Mother's subjective response to Billy, not based on objective criteria, at least not initially. In a self-fulfilling prophecy fashion, things she worried about in Billy eventually became real in him. Mother thrived on being a mother and taking care of someone whom she believed especially needed her. Dad was busy with his new work responsibilities and also was beginning to drink heavily, a habit he retained the rest of his life. Throughout their marriage, Dad supported Mother's focus on the kids and generally deferred to her judgment on most things.

Had the baby girl born less than a year after Billy not died, it is possible that family life would have been easier for Mother through the years by having a daughter by her side. I note on the family diagram that Mother had an abortion between my second full brother's birth, Terry, and my own birth and in Chapter 16 explain the triangle of Dad, his sister, and his mother that contributed to that event.

Dad's distance, Mother's powerful caretaking tendencies, and the other factors mentioned earlier in this chapter were a setup for an intense level of energy investment by Mother in Billy, and a lot of worry to go with it. Her anxiety-filled emotional involvement extended throughout Billy's life. Mother's involvement with Billy bore many of the markings of her relationship with her mother, feeling guilty and responsible for distress in others, and of her relationship with her brother and baby sister.

Expectations for males in Mother's family were high but were coupled with a lot of fears about the male being able to handle the responsibility. Given the hidden nature of the family patterns and forces at work between family members during that period between 1934 and 1952, it is not surprising that family life looked good on the surface. The parental triangle that included my oldest full brother was poorly differentiated but was stable for eighteen years. Much of family anxiety was bound in the triangle. Gaining a more objective view of one's parents is the high road for getting beyond blaming them for our family life.

Some of Billy's elementary school teachers had expressed concern to my parents from time to time about Billy being shy, a bit anxious, and tending to fall behind in his schoolwork. He was likable and not a behavior problem. The sixth-grade teacher recommended a psychological evaluation for Billy. My parents took him for the assessment, but when they left the session my mother expressed strong reservations to my Dad about placing Billy in the counseling that the psychologist had recommended. Mother said, "I wouldn't want to do anything that could damage his self-esteem." I would later understand the depth of Mother's feeling for Billy. "If he seemed upset, I was upset," she said. They were like one person. She was quite protective of all of her children, but the loudest alarm bells went off with Billy.

As the youngest child, I was not consciously processing any of the family tensions at that point, but I no doubt got an early start in learning to worry about Mother and her distress. I became tuned into her attention and approval, worked to meet her expectations, and was responsive to her distress. My way of thinking about it now is that both Billy and I were very tuned into

Mother, but we differed in the degree of it. Mother focused less on me than on Billy, and consequently, I focused less on her than Billy did. This gave me a bit more room to develop a "self" than Billy had. All of the siblings were caught up in the emotionality of the family, but to different degrees, and each of us coped with it in somewhat different ways.

As was discussed in detail in Chapter 9, Bowen theory conceptualizes what I have described as happening between parents and their children as *emotional programming*. It involves cortical and subcortical processes. When a mother invests a lot in her kids in an anxious way, the kids focus back on her in a reactive way. This programs, for example, a heightened need for attention in the child. Parent and child become entangled in each other's emotions. The process may be subtle or obvious. The child may feel and act as if he or she is not getting adequate attention, but the child becomes addicted to attention and thus can be quick to feel inadequately attended to. A child's sense of emotional well-being becomes more dependent than it would otherwise have been on what the mother does and says. The child's well-being becomes excessively regulated by the relationship, and that process transfers into other relationships. The mother is key because she is usually the primary caretaker. However, as has been emphasized throughout the book, a mother-child relationship does not exist in a vacuum.

It may seem surprising, given what was to unfold later, but things continued to look fairly normal for the family until about 1951. Bob had a successful stint in the Navy during World War II and then went on to college, and he married a local girl in 1950. Dad advanced in his job success, which led to building a fine new house in a very nice part of town. Terry and I seemed to be thriving in our lives. My parents had many good friends, and there was some interaction with each of the extended families. However, after Mother's father died in 1945, tensions developed among the siblings about distribution of the estate. Mother thought they should all give their shares to their brother, who seemed most in need. This led to less contact with Mother's family for over ten years.

The family emotional climate changed dramatically during Billy's senior year of high school. He had struggled academically during high school but, with help from the school, managed to get through. He was smart enough but did not apply himself sufficiently to his studies. The big climate change was the buildup of anxiety in my parents about Billy going to college. Billy was anxious about it, and they were very anxious about it.

Billy, with a strong push and support from my parents, managed to do what was necessary to apply to college. I recall traveling with my parents and Billy to visit the Penn State campus and having to stop the car several times along the way so that Billy could get out and vomit. The anxiety was very high. Finally, with help from one of our neighbors, who was a professor at a local college, Billy was admitted there. He lived on campus the first semester, failed every course, drank soft drinks addictively, and gained a huge amount of weight. The school agreed to take him back for the second semester. This time Billy lived at home and made the short commute to school each day, but nothing changed. The school did not accept him back after a failed second semester.

In retrospect, it would have been easy to see this coming. Billy was highly dependent on Mother and the family, but living in that context, he managed to get by. The hurdle of moving on to the responsibilities of adult life was too high. Billy was incredibly anxious, and my parents were incredibly anxious, and they reinforced each other's anxieties.

Excessive emotional dependency, unwittingly fostered by the family, is best described as a condition, not a disease. However, the dependency can easily result in a failure to lift off into adult life. The anxiety that surrounds that failure, in the young adult and in the family, can be associated with many types of symptoms, such as drug abuse, physical illnesses, or psychotic episodes. Billy had no forward momentum. He froze in place and simultaneously gained an enormous amount of weight.

The next six or seven years were an anxious and regressed time for the family, manifesting primarily in the poor functioning of both of my parents and of Billy. Dad continued to meet work responsibilities, but periods of binge drinking resulted in his occasionally being unable to work for a few days. Mother was nervous and depressed and on a variety of anxiety medications, such as meprobamate. She also drank too much but continued to run the home adequately. Billy found no work that lasted and would periodically escape to Florida—at my parents' expense—to live at a retreat facility based in vegetarianism for sometimes weeks at a time to "purge his system." His life was going nowhere.

Brother Terry headed off to college out of town in 1955, departing with a comment to me, "How can you stand it here?" There were some very worried times for all of us, such as when Mother took medication overdoses and had to be hospitalized twice. These were more cries for help than serious suicide attempts. She was overwhelmed. These were my teenage years, but I was not in the direct line of fire. I went from being a B student in high school to an A student in college, so the process of being at home during high school may have taken some toll, but life in general for me felt fairly normal.

Bob, Terry, and I were by no means free of the emotional process, but we were freer than Billy. Years later when Mother died (Dad had died before Mother and a number of years before Billy's death), Bob and I, as coexecutors, met at a lawyer's office to review my parents' will, which neither Bob nor I knew anything about. It was not a huge estate, but it stated that if all four of their sons were alive when they had both died, all of the money would go to Billy. In the event that Billy had died, it would be divided equally between the three other sons. I turned to Bob in the lawyer's office and said, "Billy sure earned that money, didn't he?" Mother died in 1985, and that comment was influenced by what I had learned about Bowen theory by then.

A huge change in the family began in 1958, the year that I headed to the Midwest for my freshman year in college. Interestingly, Dad said he would buy me a convertible if I would continue to live at home and commute to a local college. I wanted to get away. I understood later that Dad's hope that I would stay home was a clue to my supportive "functioning position" in the family system, particularly for Mother, and that helped Dad out.

Another huge change was that Dad had talked Mother into selling the home in Swarthmore and moving down to the Eastern Shore of Maryland into a house on the water. Dad envisioned a gradual transitioning into retirement over about ten years with such a move. The Eastern Shore was part of Dad's territory in his work, and he loved the area. Mother was in tears at the closing for the sale of the home in Swarthmore, yet she signed it. She felt everyone wanted it, meaning Dad, Billy, and me. Why the family went through with it at that point is anyone's guess, but we did it. I was heading off to college, so Dad, Mother, and Billy would be the ones in Maryland full-time.

It was a disaster! Dad was now traveling part of every week, gone more than when he was in Swarthmore. He was drinking very heavily on the weekends, much more than before, although he mostly did all right during his travel workweeks. Mother went into a funk, a kind of infantile-like depression. Her drinking increased, too.

Who rose to the occasion to become the functional family member? Brother Billy! The change in Billy was beyond dramatic. He got a full-time job delivering prescriptions on his motorcycle for a local drugstore. He was pictured in an advertisement in the local newspaper. He bought groceries and the other necessities to keep the home fires burning and also ferried my mother around to doctors when she was too nervous to drive. When I came home for Christmas in my freshman year, Billy took me around town to meet a remarkably large number of people. I met his boss and fellow employees, all of whom were very positive about my brother. He had developed more of a social network than ever before. The pharmacist owner of the store was wonderful in the way he looked out for Billy. Billy, for his part, was a reliable and agreeable employee.

Such processes are not unique to my family—Bowen theory refers to what happened as a change in reciprocal functioning. Figure E.2 shows my parents shifting from being the overfunctioning ones and Billy the underfunctioning one to just the opposite.

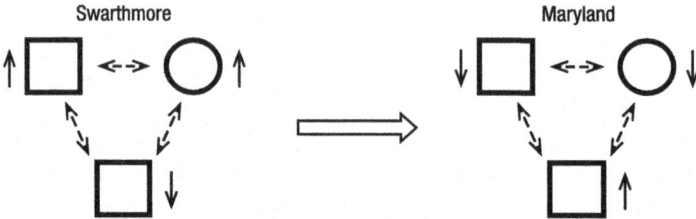

Figure E.2 *The purpose of this diagram is to symbolize the dramatic change in family emotional process in the triangle of our two parents and my schizophrenic brother. The move from my hometown in Swarthmore, Pennsylvania to Maryland's Eastern Shore. The black arrows next to each figure denote people who are overfunctioning and people who are underfunctioning.*

I was home in the summers, and that helped my parents some, but the improvements were not marked. Mother was in and out of the general hospital a number of times, but there were no life-threatening medical illnesses. She was commonly diagnosed as having cancer phobia, depression, and anxiety. Her doctor treated her with a variety of psychotropic medications, but they did little to improve things. When Mother got bad enough, we would drive her up to western Pennsylvania to her sister's house, where she would recuperate for a few weeks. She always improved there, but when she came back to Maryland she would deteriorate again. Half a dozen or more such trips occurred over the next three years. This sister in western Pennsylvania was the mother figure of her generation even though my mother was the older of the two.

Finally, in the spring of 1961 my parents decided to abandon the Eastern Shore venture and move back to Swarthmore. They sold the Maryland house and bought a house in Swarthmore, returning there in June. Billy did not want to leave the Eastern Shore. He rented a small apartment in town and continued with his job. My parents moved, feeling and hoping that Billy would make it. The next six months in Swarthmore were perhaps the happiest for my parents in years. They felt Billy was all right, and that gave them great comfort. Their six months of happiness provided a vivid portrait of the anguish that a fairly dysfunctional adult son or daughter creates in the parents. Mother's overinvolvement with Billy provided some stability for the family during his years from birth to eighteen—Mother felt needed by taking care of him, and her involvement mitigated tensions between my parents—but when he collapsed into serious dysfunction at age eighteen, the negatives of the situation far outweighed the positives.

Billy's functioning started to decline within a few months after our parents moved back to Swarthmore. About four or five months into his stay there, his boss phoned my parents and told them Billy was no longer coming to work and was mostly holed up in his apartment. He also seemed paranoid. The man recommended to my parents that they come down and get him, which they did in late December of 1961. Billy complied and moved into my parents' new home in Swarthmore.

I was in my senior year of college at that point and mostly through weekly calls home stayed in touch with the problems that developed around Billy's return. The situation between my parents and Billy after his return was malignantly anxious. The distress in all three was more magnified than ever. I dreaded calling home and gleaning the mood of the family, particularly Mother's upset. Unusually bad reports would be on my mind all week. I often prayed that if God would help my brother and my parents, I would devote my work in medicine (I was in a premed program at that point) to missionary work. Since I was not living in the midst of it, I do not think I fully fathomed the depth of emotional pain they were all experiencing.

By March 1962 my father had developed a stress-induced ulcer at the base of his esophagus. It caused him considerable pain. In May, Mother and my brother Bob, who lived in an adjoining town, got word from Bob's biological father that he was quite ill and needed help. Mother and Bob drove down to Washington, D.C., that weekend in May. In their absence Dad drank heavily, and Mother returned home to a blood-spattered bedroom, the result of my father vomiting blood. Mother and Bob rushed Dad to the hospital, but it was too late. The ulcer had perforated, peritonitis had set in, and Dad went into shock and died. It was a consequence of malignant levels of panic in the threesome of Dad, Mother, and Billy. I came home from school immediately. I still managed to graduate and attended the ceremony about a week after Dad died.

As we headed into that summer of 1962, Billy, Mother, and I were living together; Bob and his still young family of two boys were nearby. Mother was utterly devastated by Dad's death. Billy and Mother became increasingly reactive to each other. Billy would scream obscenities out the windows of the house, frightening people in the neighborhood. His behavior in the home was erratic and often bizarre. Mother was in increasing despair. My brother Terry was overseas in the military at this point. By mid-August, Bob and I were convinced something needed to happen or Mother likely would become ill due to the tensions. Billy was much out of control.

The father of my best friend in high school was a highly respected psychiatrist, and I had gotten to know him a little during my youth. I called him and described the malignantly tense situation in my family. He immediately invited us to meet with him at his home to discuss things. Bob, Mother, and I went. I don't think we thought we could get Billy to come with us.

After Bob, Mother, and I described the situation, my friend's father said to Bob, "You seem very angry at your brother." I will never forget the look on Bob's face. He was pale and taken aback. Years later I realized that Bob, who often tried to distance himself from tense family situations but still felt a deep responsibility to help, was angry at the incredibly adverse impact that Billy was having on our mother. I was, too, but presented more of an outward calm. I had a mix of feelings about Billy: wanting to help him, feeling sorry for him, feeling angry at him, and feeling guilty about his poor functioning.

After a little more discussion, during which Mother said little, my friend's father said, "I think your brother is mentally ill and should be hospitalized." He offered to take charge of the process. In retrospect, my friend's father was psychoanalytically trained and knew little about the family. Interest in families among the mental health disciplines had barely surfaced at that point in August 1962. Perhaps if he had understood families, he would have seen that we were all anxious and out of control, not just Billy. Our biggest fears were for Mother and her well-being. Perhaps a hospitalization could have been avoided, perhaps not. In any event, Bob and I arranged to get Billy to the hospital. We hired two off-duty policemen to be with us when we gave Billy the news, just in case Billy went off. I will not forget the look on Billy's face. He seemed incredulous that we would do this. It was an awful, guilt-producing experience for me. I hated to do this to my brother.

Once Billy was in the hospital, however, he calmed down remarkably fast. Mother, Bob, and I calmed down, too. It was a very positive experience in that sense. Billy spent ten days at the Institute of Pennsylvania Hospital. The doctors' conclusion was that Billy was suffering from "schizophrenia, simple type." Billy had had some paranoid thinking at that point but few other psychotic symptoms. They placed him on psychotropic medication. It was amazing to me how quickly Billy became the old Billy we knew and loved, once he calmed down. I do not remember their various follow-up treatment recommendations, but things in the family improved quickly following that experience.

I headed off to medical school at Georgetown in early September. Mother and I had a kind of unspoken pact that I would be there to support her now that Dad was gone. She had the fantasy that I would return home to live with Billy and her after finishing my medical training. My commitment to her stabilized her functioning and, as a consequence, improved the relationship between Billy and her. Bob was calmer, too, seeing that things were far less volatile between Mother and Billy. Billy was in a kind of subdued state, even after he stopped medication.

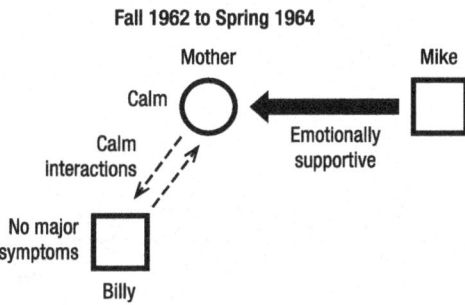

Figure E.3 *The diagram symbolizes what became a stable triangle that included Mother, my schizophrenic brother, and me during the first 18 months after my brother was diagnosed as having schizophrenia.* The dark black arrow pointing from me to Mother symbolizes my consistently emotionally supportive relationship with her during that time. The unshaded symbols for my Mother and brother and the reciprocal dashed arrows between them symbolize two fairly calm people with calm interactions. My schizophrenic brother was still quite dependent on mother but had no symptoms.

Since those days, I have sometimes thought that had I moved home and practiced medicine there, Billy's suicide would not have occurred seven years later. As I show in Figure E.3, I think my relationship with Mother was key to her functioning, and Mother's emotional state was key to Billy's stability. Bob was too reactive to Mother to fill that niche, and Terry was too far away. There was no hint of problems over the next eighteen months. The diagram depicts my full attention to Mother, her associated calmness, consequent calm interactions between Mother and Billy, and Billy manifesting none of the types of symptoms that had landed him in the hospital. This was not a shift based on a reversal of the overfunctioning-underfunctioning reciprocity that occurred during the period in Maryland, but a functional increase for both Mother and Billy based on the triangle reducing chronic anxiety.

During that period, Billy managed to work some, driving a taxi in nearby Chester. Mother's finances were not in great shape, but she got professional help to get herself on track. I was enjoying medical school, although I was sometimes disturbed by the descriptions by my psychiatry professors of "schizophrenogenic mothers" as people who are unloving or overly protective out of their repressed hostility toward the child. They were not describing the mother I knew.

I rarely dated the same girl twice during my first eighteen months in medical school. I was totally dedicated to the books. In the middle of January 1964, the medical curriculum shifted some from intensive classroom and laboratory studies to the first times working on the wards in the hospital. This took a little pressure off, which may have played a role in my dating a nursing student and then repeatedly asking her out. The relationship took very quickly. She has been my wife of over half a century.

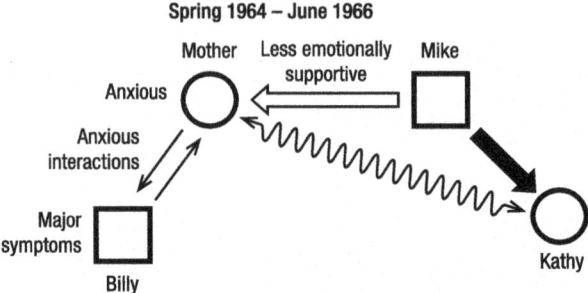

Figure E.4 *The diagram symbolizes the triangle of Mother, brother Billy, and me after I began a serious romantic relationship with my future wife Kathy. The thick dark arrow from me to Kathy denotes my investment of emotional energy in her. The unshaded thick arrow to my mother from me denotes less emotional investment in her. This change in my relationship with Mother significantly increased her anxiety, resulted in more anxiety filled interactions between Mother and my brother, and the recurrence of his schizophrenic symptoms accompanied by a series of psychiatric hospitalizations in him.*

What happened next, which I did not anticipate but easily could have in retrospect, is diagrammed in Figure E.4. Had I been a more mature (differentiated) person, I could have managed the relationships with two women more successfully. Part of me wanted to run from the expectation that I be there for Mother and Billy, meaning that distancing emotionally into a romantic relationship was appealing. However, I was not conscious of that dynamic at the time. It was evident to my mother that this was a serious relationship that could threaten my involvement with her. It was tense and sometimes conflictual between Mother and Kathy. The family system was now unstable, and that manifested in more tension between Mother and Billy and in more symptoms in Billy. He was hospitalized psychiatrically five or six times, usually for a few weeks at a time, between when Kathy and I started dating and when we married in June 1966. These hospitalizations were at nearby Haverford State Hospital.

Billy's symptoms were clearly related to stress, and the most important stressor was the serious disturbance in the relationship between Billy and Mother. Their relationship was in a meltdown. Mother got reactive to my involvement with Kathy. She felt, and was, the outsider in the triangle, and her anxiety escalated and infected her relationship with Billy. Billy was markedly sensitive to signs of distress in Mother—the look on her face, her body posture, and other cues. He would get anxious in the face of it, and Mother would get even more anxiously focused on his unsettledness. It was a vicious circle. As for my part, I got reactive to Mother's criticism and lack of acceptance of Kathy. Kathy got reactive to Mother, and Mother to her. Billy's symptoms were driven not by pathology but by chronic anxiety generated in a larger system process. At the time, I had no understanding of what was unfolding.

Kathy and I were married just as I began my year of medical internship at Georgetown University Hospital. Billy had gotten out of the psychiatric hospital just before the wedding. My wife had gotten through university partly on a Navy scholarship. She was stationed at Bethesda Naval Hospital, which meant we still saw a lot of both our families.

When tensions began to rise between Mother and Billy, my oldest brother, Bob, always got involved at Mother's pleading. Bob would call me in Washington to discuss whether it was time for Billy to go back into the hospital. This was usually when Mother was at her wit's end. The demands on Bob were a source of tension in his young family. I always supported Bob's position at that point, and he would arrange the hospitalization. This occurred about twice a year. Billy still managed to drive a taxi from time to time but was living with Mother, at least in a decent-sized apartment, and totally dependent on her financially and emotionally.

Billy would stay on psychotropic medications for a short time after each hospitalization but would eventually stop them. While he had some psychotic symptoms, most of the time he was socially isolated and lacking motivation. He seemed paranoid at times but did not talk about it much. Many people have suggested that if Billy had stayed on his medications that this revolving door of psychiatric hospitalizations might have stopped. However, many studies related to expressed emotion have shown that the presence of hostility, over-involvement (especially of the mother) with the patient, and relatives' critical comments significantly increase the chances of relapse even if the person is one medication. Mother was a wonderful and well-meaning person, but her worry and anxious focus could rise to toxic levels with Billy. His behaviors, of course, would trigger her focus as well. Absent the three emotionally valenced variables mentioned above, relapse is a much lower possibility even with patients not on any medications. An excellent article about what is termed "expressed emotion" is available at www.Houd.info. (Rabstejnek, 2014).

Mother and her next younger sister, Kitty, stayed in especially close contact during these years, as Kitty worried a lot about Mother, given the stress of dealing with Billy. I was getting more distant from the situation than I realized at the time. Terry was still overseas and now married with a child. Bob was distressed by Mother's distress, which he saw as the primary source of his ulcer.

He tried to insulate himself somewhat from the situation. Mother and Billy were becoming more isolated, although I did not recognize that as a problem at the time.

During my medical internship year, I would see Murray Bowen when he came through the hospital corridors on his way to and from the department of psychiatry. I recognized him because he had given a lecture to the medical students in my junior year in which he discussed his family systems perspective on schizophrenia. What stayed with me from that lecture was his nonjudgmental attitude about the mothers of schizophrenic people. He described my mother perfectly in her anxiety and total dedication to helping and protecting her dysfunctional adult offspring. He characterized overprotectiveness not as the product of repressed hostility but as "maternal instinct run amuck." That idea fit! Another point he made in reference to the intense interdependence especially between a mother and her adult dysfunctional son or daughter is that the degree of intensity is the outcome of a multigenerational transmission process. Overly involved mothers were dealing with stuff that they had never resolved with their own mothers, who in turn had never resolved with their own mothers. Whose fault is that? People were playing the hands they were dealt to the best of their ability.

It was all fascinating to me because it so matched my life experience. It was the opposite of what I was hearing from the rest of the department of psychiatry. I had decided to try a year of psychiatric residency after my internship rather than a residency in internal medicine, which had been my previous goal. This decision gave me occasional exposure to Murray Bowen in a few teaching conferences. I began to appreciate how radically different his viewpoint was from conventional psychiatry.

My clinical supervision by him, which began in May 1969, is the next chapter of this story. My brother's suicide occurred in November 1969. The suicide was not unrelated to my overly zealous efforts to change many generations of family emotional process in a matter of months. My part reflected a serious lack of understanding of what Bowen theory describes.

I launched into the project of trying to become a more differentiated person in my family with much excitement and energy. The early steps involved learning a lot more about my multigenerational family in an effort to gain perspective on the family emotional process as it existed currently. This involved gathering a multitude of facts from many sources, such as records and the remembrances of family members. I also sought closer contact with many members of both my maternal and paternal extended families.

Most relevant, I gained an appreciation of the intense tie between Mother and Billy and discovered how the rest of us supported that. We all saw Billy's functioning as the source of family anxiety. Until listening to Bowen, it had not dawned on me that my parents, my siblings, and I were as much a source of Billy's anxiety as he was of ours! Listening to Bowen's lectures about his theory, I also realized that I had tried to distance myself from the problematic situations in my family. I instantly made up my mind that I would no longer do that. My family was important to me. I loved them all dearly and wanted to be back in better contact with them. The understandings provided by Bowen theory gave me some confidence that I could do this without being overwhelmed by the family problems.

A huge problem or misconception that I developed early in my efforts with Bowen theory was that, while I could see what Bowen termed as the "unresolved symbiotic relationship" between Mother and Billy—a level of emotional involvement that is normal in the child's early years but resolves little as the child grows up—I was quite reactive about what I saw as the deleterious effects such a relationship was having on Mother and Billy. Failing to understand the forces in the relationship that worked against change, I made the error of assuming it should change and that I could somehow make it change.

A way my reactivity to the relationship between Mother and Billy played out was the following. I would often ask Mother to come down to Washington to visit with Kathy and me and our infant daughter. She made the trip once, and Billy came with her. Often, however, she was reluctant to come because Billy did not want to come with her. I was somewhat less sympathetic to Billy's situation now that I had a better understanding of his relationship with Mother, because I naively assumed that Mother's reluctance to leave Billy was not good for either of them. Consequently, I anxiously pressured Mother to come alone and was frustrated when she declined. It was arrogant for me to think I knew what was best for them.

On another front, I strongly encouraged her to be receptive to her sister, Kitty, and Kitty's husband, Dick, now both retired, and their many invitations to travel with them on car trips around the country to see family members who had moved away from western Pennsylvania. Mother's fear, of course, was that Billy would suffer if she left him for an extended period. Dick and Kitty had a six-week trip planned from late August 1969 until early October and wanted Mother to come along. The trip would include seeing Mother's lifelong close friend and first cousin in Miami. Mother expressed her ambivalence to me in several phone calls. I was thinking, again arrogantly, that Mother and Billy needed to be more separate from each other, and that attitude led me to prod her to go. Brother Bob would be nearby to help Billy if he needed anything. It surprised me, but Mother agreed to go.

Bob saw Billy a few times during that period but noticed nothing out of the ordinary. He seemed to be taking care of himself satisfactorily. When Mother returned in early October, however, Billy, by her description, was a wreck. He was extremely anxious and in need of her attention. I was a dunce not to have put two and two together at that point and realize that we were witnessing an intense reaction to Mother having been away. Mother was panicked about Billy in a way that I had never seen previously.

There were many phone calls between Mother and me over the next week or ten days. Mother involved Bob, and he thought Billy needed to go back into the hospital. I assumed that Billy would calm down eventually, but Bob wanted to go ahead with hospitalization and arranged it in late October. It was back to the nearby state hospital, where they medicated him and then released him to go back with Mother after a week.

During that week in early November 1969, things were not much better than in the weeks prior to his hospitalization. Even taking the medications that had been started in the hospital, Billy was unsettled. I did not realize the depth of the stress he was under, not appreciating the depth of his dependence on Mother and the degree of threat that had arisen in that relationship. Mother was desperately trying to reassure Billy, but it did not seem to help. Billy killed himself in Mother's apartment on November 13, 1969. He had cut his wrists, Mother found him, they rushed him to the hospital, but it was too late.

Bob called me that Friday night with the wrenching news. Kathy, my daughter, and I drove immediately to Swarthmore. Kitty and Dick managed to get there Friday night, too. The level of anguish need not be described. There was immediate finger pointing and expressions of "if only this or that had been done."

Later in the evening I called Murray Bowen in Washington. His wife, LeRoy, answered the phone. "Murray is in Philadelphia for a meeting of the Group for the Advancement of Psychiatry," she said. She told me where he was staying, and I called him there. He was shocked and offered immediately to meet with me in the morning at the hotel where he was staying.

We spent about an hour together the next morning, which gave me lots of time to describe the events of the previous two months. Bowen's response was pithy: "Mike, I think your mother pulled up and Billy suicided." Bowen meant she took a step toward functioning more independently of my brother. He even offered to come out to Swarthmore and meet with the family during the weekend.

It is hard to describe the impact of his comment. It was factual, it made sense out of things and, despite the tragedy of it all, was calming in a peculiar way. Yes, Mother leaving Billy was a manifestation of her putting some energy into her own life. I had not thought about it until then that she was also withdrawing some from Billy, but that was exactly what she had done. I don't know if I fully appreciated the profound depth of their emotional interdependence at that moment, but it eventually sank in.

I told Bowen that I did not think it was necessary for him to come out to meet with the family. I said that our discussion had given me the confidence to deal with things. Over the next several days before the funeral, I made it a point to talk with each member of my family individually. Kitty and Dick, Mother, and Bob were key, but I managed to have time with other family members and friends as well. Almost everyone emphasized the feeling of guilt that they had not done something to prevent this. We all, of course, felt that way.

I think my effort to meet with everyone helped the funeral be as good as it could be. We all came together in our sorrow, and the finger pointing had softened. Kitty and Dick wanted Mother to go back with them immediately to Sidman, where they still lived. I greatly admired Mother when she said, "No, I must go back to the apartment and deal with this." She did just that! In Chapter 16 I describe the family process during the six months after my brother's death. Reading that section again may be useful in light of learning about the emotional functioning of the family prior to my brother's suicide.

SUMMARY AND CONCLUSIONS

Figure E.5 graphs my estimates of my schizophrenic brother's functional level of differentiation from birth until death. This graph is similar to Figure 22.1, which graphs my estimates of John Nash's level of chronic anxiety over time. Functional level of differentiation reflects the same thing: when chronic anxiety goes up, functional level declines and symptoms emerge, and when chronic anxiety goes down, functional level increases and symptoms decline.

The period from A to D (1934–1952) depicts a slight and gradual change in functional level from Billy's birth until it being time to accept more adult responsibility in transitioning to college. A sharp decline occurs from D to E that lasts for about five years (1952–early 1959). That period was more about the negative symptoms of schizophrenia than the positive ones. Billy left my overfunctioning parents for only very short periods and fashioned no direction for his life. The sharp climb from E to F in his functioning was related to the move to Maryland and the parental triangle sort of turning upside down. The period from F to G represents what happened when my parents moved back to Swarthmore in 1961 and Billy's functional level plummeted. It culminated in Dad's death and Billy's first hospitalization in the late summer of 1962. The increase in functional level from G to H is the eighteen-month period when

352 EPILOGUE

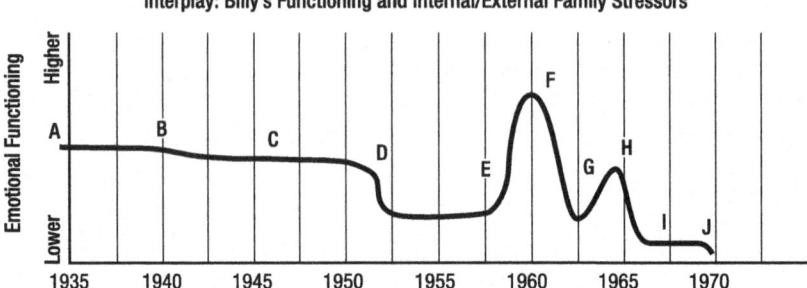

A – Billy's birth in 1934.
B – Billy enters school.
C – Transition to junior high school.
D – High school graduation and attempt at college.
E – Parents and Billy move to Maryland.
F – Parents return to Swarthmore.
G – Dad"s death and Billy's first hospitalization. Mike's attention is to mother and Billy.
H – Mike begins serious relationship with future wife.
I – Billy's serial psychiatric hospitalizations.
J – Mother's change and Billy's suicide in 1969.

Figure E.5 *This diagram* depicts my assessment of my schizophrenic brother's functional level of differentiation over the course of his life. Functional level is indicated on the y-axis and years of Billy's life on the x-axis. Letters A, B, C, and D denote milestones in his early life. His birth in 1935, beginning elementary school in 1940, the transition to junior high school in 1946, and his high school graduation and beginning college in in 1952. The decline in his functional level was gradual and not marked until the attempt to attend college. At point D, a rapid and marked drop in his functional level occurred. His functional level stayed about the same from 1952 until late 1958 while my parents and Billy were living together in Swarthmore. Point E is when my parents and Billy moved to Maryland and Billy's functional level soared. Point F is when my parents moved back to Swarthmore. Billy's functioning began to plummet. By the end of 1961 his dysfunction was at a lower point than ever before and that continued until his first psychiatric hospitalization. Point G marks the end of the period between Dad's sudden death in May 1962 and Billy's first psychiatric hospitalization in August 1962. An upswing in Billy's functional level occurred from the G to H period. This was the period diagrammed in Figure E.3. The period from H to I was described in Figure E.4. Billy's functional level remained very low over the next three years until his death by suicide in November 1969.

the triangle involving Mother, Billy, and I was fairly calm and stable; I to J depicts the decline in functional level and increasing symptoms after I met my wife-to-be and became less available to the triangle. My brother never really recovered from the change in context. Finally, J depicts Billy's suicide in reaction to Mother's change. Granted, much of it was Billy's perception that Mother was no longer there for him, but the stressor of her leaving him for six weeks was more than he could adapt to.

Bowen theory's conceptualization that changes in a relationship can either increase or decrease the chronic anxiety that one member absorbs from the system, and that those changes either ameliorate or exacerbate clinical symptoms, is truly a figure-ground shift in thinking from the medical model of a pathology-driven process. Billy was the canary in the coal mine.

An important point is that stressors, such as trying to go to college or an offspring's meeting his future wife, are only *potential* triggers for the escalation of chronic anxiety in a family system. It is how people deal with each other in face of the stressors that leads to the escalation of chronic anxiety, if the family unit is adapting unsuccessfully to the challenge at hand. The magnitude of the stressor is important, but differentiation of self is the key variable governing a family's ability to adapt. Many stressors are inevitable, but people can learn to manage themselves more successfully in the face of the buildup of chronic anxiety in the system and thus reverse regressions and reduce the associated symptoms.

I know that I unwittingly played a part in my brother's suicide, but I did not cause it. The suicide was the outcome of a system process that was generations in the making. Saying that a multigenerational emotional process was involved is not about shirking responsibility for one's actions or inactions but about being more objective in one's assessment of the total situation: the level of family interdependency that had been building to increasingly inflexible levels (loss of adaptive capacity) for at least several generations. That became clear as I got to know more about my father's and my mother's multigenerational families.

A fitting end for this epilogue, which describes an attempt to see things more as they really are, is a quote from the French philosopher and prominent figure during the Enlightenment, Denis Diderot: "Nothing is more dangerous than to deceive ourselves about the world in which we find ourselves. We need an ethic of truth to coexist with nature" (Kors, 1998). Which is more of a deception, the individual, cause-and effect model or the systems model? Each of us has to make up our own mind about that. For me, the cause-and-effect model is useful, accurate, and important in narrow circumstances but is inadequate for addressing the complexity of a family system and, more obviously, the human body as a whole.

I conclude this book by stating my belief that, when Bowen theory finally enters the public consciousness—it could be a century from now or it could be less—and human beings come to understand and truly accept how little emotional autonomy we have, both in mind and body, it will have a constructive impact on human interactions. I believe this because of my observations of slightly increasing one's basic level of differentiation at a personal level. The objectivity and neutrality that flow from applying systems thinking to human behavior facilitates people living more in harmony with one another and with the natural world.

References

Ackerman, D. (1991). *The moon by whalelight.* New York, NY: Vintage Books.
Ackerman, D. (2012, March 25). Opinion: The brain on love. *New York Times.*
Anonymous. (1972). Toward the differentiation of self in one's own family. In J. Framo (Ed.), *Family interaction: A dialogue between family researchers and family therapists* (pp. 111-173). New York, NY: Springer.
Barzun, J. (2000). *From dawn to decadence: Five hundred years of Western cultural life, 1500 to the present.* New York, NY: HarperCollins.
Belsky, D., Caspi, A., Houts, R., Cohen, H., Corcoran, D., Danese, A., (. . .), Moffitt, T. (2015). Quantification of biological aging in young adults. *Proceedings of the National Academy of Sciences of the United States of America, 112,* E4104–E4110.
Benditt, E. (1977). The origin of atherosclerosis. *Scientific American. 236,* 74–84.
Benson, H. (1975). *The relaxation response.* Harper Collins, New York, NY.
Benson, H. (2006). Study of therapeutic effects of intercessory prayer in cardiac by-pass patients. *American Heart Journal, 151,* 934–942.
Bernard, C. (1974). *Lectures on the phenomena common to animals and plants.* (H. Hoff, R. Guillemin, & L. Guillemin, Trans.). Springfield, IL: Charles C. Thomas.
Bertalanffy, L. (1968). *General system theory: Foundations, Development, Applications.* New York, George Braziller.
Bonner, J. T. (1969). *The Scale of nature.* New York, NY: Harper & Row.
Bowen, M. (1966). The use of family theory in clinical practice. *Comprehensive Psychiatry, 7,* 345-374.
Bowen, M. (1971). Family therapy and family group therapy. In H. Kaplan and B. Sadock (Eds.), *Comprehensive group psychotherapy* (pp. 384-421). Baltimore, MD: Williams & Wilkins.
Bowen, M. (1976). Theory in the practice of psychotherapy. In P. Guerin (Ed.), *Family therapy* (pp. 42-90). New York, NY: Gardner.
Bowen, M. (1978). *Family therapy in clinical practice.* New York, NY: Jason Aronson.
Bowen, M. (1980a). Paper presented at the American Family Therapy Association Conference, March 14, New York.
Bowen, M. (1980b). *Towards a systems concept of spiritual phenomena.* Paper presented at the Georgetown University Annual Family Symposium on FamilyTheory and Family Psychotherapy on November 9 in Washington, D.C.

Bowen, M. (1981). *Towards a systems concept of supernatural phenomena.* Bowen-Kerr videotaped interview series, January 1981.
Bowen, M. (1987, July). *The theoretical structure of the Catholic Church.* Paper presented at the conference "Implications of Bowen Theory for Catholic Theology," Silver Spring, MD.
Bowen, M. (1997). Subjectivity, Homo sapiens and science. In R. Sagar (Ed.), *Bowen theory and practice* (pp. 15-21). Washington, DC: Georgetown Family Center.
Bowen, M. (2013). *The origins of family psychotherapy: The NIMH Family Study Project* (2nd ed.). J. Butler (Ed.). New York, NY: Jason Aronson.
Bowen, M. (1970). *Symptom development in the nuclear family.* Videotaped lecture by Murray Bowen. Retrieved, from http://www.thebowencenter.org/. , September 2017, The Bowen Center, 4400 MacArthur Blvd., Suite 103, Washington, DC 20007.
Bowen, M. & Kerr, M. (1985) *The Best of Family Therapy. Videotaped interview.* Retrieved, from http://www.thebowencenter.org/., September 2017.
Bowlby, J. (1950). *Maternal care and mental health.* World Health Organization Monograph no. 3. Geneva: World Health Organization.
Bowlby, J. (1969). *Attachment.* New York, NY: Basic Books
Bowlby, J. (1988). *A secure base: Parent-child attachment and healthy human development.* London: Routledge.
Boysen, S., Berntson, G., Hannan, M., & Cacioppo, J. (1996). Quantity-based interference and symbolic representations in chimpanzees. *Journal of Experimental Psychology: Animal Behavior Processes, 22,* 76–86.
Cannon, W. (1939). *The wisdom of the body* (2nd ed.). New York, NY: Norton.
CBS News 60 Minutes (1998). Ted Kaczynski's Family, Retrieved videotape of January 11, 1998.
Chase, A. (2000). Harvard and the making of the Unabomber. *Atlantic Monthly, 285,* 41–65.
Cohen, S. (2005). The Pittsburg common cold studies: Psychosocial predictors of susceptibility to respiratory infectious illness. *International Journal of Behavioral Medicine, 12,* 123–131.
Cole, S., Hawkley, L., Arevalo, J., Sung, C., Rose, R., Cacioppo, J (2007). Social regulation of gene expression in human leukocytes. *Genome Biology, 8,* R189.
Collins, M. (2002). *Without a trace.* New York, NY: St. Martin's.
Colman, A. M. (2001). *Oxford dictionary of psychology.* Oxford, UK: Oxford University Press.
Conley, D. (2004). *The pecking order: Which siblings succeed and why.* New York, NY: Random House.
Damasio, A. (2010). *Self comes to mind.* New York, NY: Pantheon.
Damasio, A., & Brooks, D. (2009). *This time with feeling: David Brooks and Antonio Damasio.* Interview recorded at the Aspen Ideas Festival, posted January 29, 2015, at Aspen Institute.
Davies, P., & Lineweaver, C. (2011). Cancer tumors as metazoa 1.0: Tapping genes of ancient ancestors. *Physical Biology, 8*(1), 015001.
Dayalu, P. (2015). Huntington disease: Pathogenesis and treatment. *Neurologic Clinics, 33,* 101–114.
deCharms, R. (2005). Control over brain activation and pain learned by using real-time functional MRI. *Proceedings of the National Academy of Sciences of the United States of America, 102,* 18626.

DePisapia, N., Bornstein, M. H., Rigo, P., Esposito, G., DeFalco, S., Venuti, P. (2013). Sex differences in directional brain responses to infant hunger cries. *NeuroReport, 24,* 101–159.
De Waal, F. (1996). *Good natured.* Cambridge, MA: Harvard University Press.
De Waal, F. (2007). *Chimpanzee politics: Power and sex among apes.* Baltimore, MD: John Hopkins University Press.
Eagleman, D. (2015). *The brain.* New York, NY: Pantheon.
Engblom, C., Pfirschke, C., Zillionis, R., Da Silva Martin, J., Bos, S, (. . .). Pittet, M. (2017). Osteoblasts remotely supply lung tumors with cancer-promoting siglecf^{high} neutrophils. *Science, 358,* 1147.
Federal Reserve. (2015, April 6). *FEDS Notes:* Deleverging and recnt trends in household debt Retrieved April 2015, from http://federalreserve.gov/. https://doi.org/1017016/2380 -7172, 1516.
Ferguson, S. (2014, February 25). Michael Moran evaluates Lourdes miracle reports. BBC News. Retrieved online: ww.bbc.com/news/world-europe-26334964
Flavahan, W., Gaskell, E., Bernstein, B. (2017). Epigenetic plasticity and the hallmarks of cancer. *Science, 357*(6348), eaal2380.
Follett, S. (1999). *Ted Kaczynski Unabomber interview 1999.* YouTube. https://www.youtube.com/watch?v=o6mYuNd6uhY
Gadagkar, R., & Joshi, N. (1985). Colony fission in a social wasp. *Current Science, 54,* 57–62.
Gerson, C., & Bishop, B. (2010). *Defeating cancer and other chronic diseases* (new ed.). Carmel, CA: Gerson Health Media.
Gilmore, M. (1995). *Shot in the heart.* New York, NY: Anchor.
Gordon, D. M. (1999). *Ants at work.* New York, NY: Free Press.
Grant, P., & Grant, B. (1985). Responses of Darwin's finches to unusual rainfall. In G. Robinson & E. del Pino (Eds.), *El Niño* (pp. 417-47). Quito, Ecuador: Charles Darwin Foundation.
Haidt, J. (2012). *The righteous mind.* New York, NY: Pantheon.
Harari, Y. N. (2015). *Sapiens.* New York, NY: HarperCollins.
Henry, J. (1992). Biological basis of the stress response. *Integrative Physiological and Behavioral Science, 27,* 66–83.
Henry, J., & Stephens, P. (1977). *Stress, health, and the social environment: A sociobiologic approach to medicine.* New York, NY: Springer.
Hinkle, L. (1974). The effect of exposure to culture change, social change, and changes in interpersonal relationships on health. In B. S. Dohrenwend & B. P. Dohrenwend (Eds.), *Stressful life events: Their nature and effects* (pp9-45). New York, NY: Wiley.
Holt, R. (2011). Survival and the family of extinction. *Family Systems, 8,* 143–161.
Horney, K. (1942). *The collected works of Karen Horney* (vol. 2). New York, NY: Norton.
Howard, H. (2012). *Mr. and Mrs. Madison's War.* New York, NY: Bloomsbury.
Huang, Y., Zaas, A., Rao, A., Dobigeon, N., Woolf, P., Veldman, N., (. . .), Hero III, A. (2011). Temporal dynamics of host molecular responses differentiate symptomatic and asymptomatic influenza A infection. *PLOS Genetics, 7,* 1–25.
Huler, S. (2004). *Defining the wind.* New York, NY: Crown.
Jackson, J. H. (1932). *Selected writings of John Hughlings Jackson* (Vol. 2). J. Taylor (Ed.). London: Hodder and Stoughton.
Johnston, D. (1998, April 29). In Unabomber's own words, a chilling account of murder. *New York Times.*

Kandel, E. (1983). Metapsychology to molecular biology: Explorations into the nature of anxiety. *American Journal of Psychiatry, 140,* 1277–1293.
Kaplan, J. T., Gimbel, S. I., & Harris, S. (2016). Neural correlates of maintaining one's political beliefs in face of counterevidence. *Scientific Reports, 6,* 39589, http://doi.org/10.1038/srep 39589.
Karr, M. (1995). *The Liars' Club.* London, Penguin Books
Kerr, M. E. (1980) Emotional factors in physical illness, a multigenerational perspective. *The Family,* 7:59-66.
Kerr, M. E. (1988). Chronic anxiety and defining a self. *Atlantic Monthly, 262*(3), 35–58.
Kerr, M. E. (1992). Physical illness and the family emotional system: Psoriasis as a model. *Behavioral Medicine, 18,* 101–113.
Kerr, M. E. (2008). Why do siblings often turn out very differently? In A. Fogel, B. King, & S. Shanker (Eds.), *Human development in the 21st century: Visionary policy ideas from systems scientists* (pp. 206-15). Cambridge, UK: Cambridge University Press.
Kerr, M., & Bowen M. (1988). *Family evaluation: The role of the family as an emotional unit that governs individual behavior and development.* New York, NY: Norton.
Keynes, R. (2001). *Darwin, his daughter, and human evolution.* New York, NY: Riverhead.
Kipling, R. (1926). *We and They.* kipling society.co.uk.
Kors, A. (1998). *Birth of the modern mind: The intellectual history of the 17th and 18th centuries.* Chantilly, VA: Teaching Company.
Kovaleski, S. (1997, January 20). Kaczynski letters reveal tormented mind. *Washington Post.*
Kovaleski, S., & Adams, L. (1996, June 16). A stranger in the family picture. *Washington Post.*
LeDoux, J., & Pine, D. (2016). Using neuroscience to help understand fear and anxiety: A two-system framework. *American Journal of Psychiatry, 173,* 1083–1093.
Lee, Y. (2005). Pathogenesis of *Helicobacter pylori* infection. *Korean Journal of Gastroenterology, 46,* 159–165.
Libby, P. (2018). *Is inflammation the link between all disease.* Fourth International Vatican Conference. The Cora Foundation, Neww York, N.Y.
Livio, S. K. (2017, June 11). . Two years after parents' Nash deaths, son of "A Beautiful Mind" John Nash has one regret. Retrieved from NJ.com
Lysiak, M. (2013). *Newtown: An American tragedy.* New York, NY: Gallery Books.
MacLean, P. D. (1990). *The triune brain in evolution.* New York, NY: Plenum.
Mailer, N. (1979). *The executioner's song.* New York, NY: Grand Central.
Marshall, B., & Warren, J. (1984). Unidentified bacilli in the stomach of patients with gastritis and peptic ulceration. *Lancet, 323,* 1311–1315.
Mason, J. W. (1959). Psychological influences on the pituitary-adrenal cortical system. *Recent Progress in Hormone Research* 15:345-389.
McArthur, Tom, ed. (1992). *The Oxford companion to the English language.* Oxford, UK: Oxford University Press.
McEwen, B. (2002). *The end of stress as we know it.* New York, NY: Dana Press.
McGoldrick, M., Gerson, R., & Shellenberger, S. (1985). *Genogram: Assessment and intervention.* New York, NY: Norton.
Meares, R. (1999). The contribution of Hughlings Jackson to an understanding of dissociation. *American Journal of Psychiatry, 156,* 1850–1855.
Merton, R. K. (1948). The self-fulfilling prophecy. *Antioch Review, 8,* 193–210.
Moberg, K. U. (2011). *The oxytocin factor.* London: Pinter & Martin.

Mukherjee, S. (September 27, 2017). What we learn when two ruthless killers, heart disease and cancer, reveal a common route. *New York Times*.
Nasar, S. (1998). *A beautiful mind*. New York, NY: Simon & Schuster.
National Institute of Alcohol Abuse and Alcoholism (2018) *Genetics of Alcohol Use Disorder*
Osler, W. (1910). The factor that heals. *British Medical Journal, 18*, 1470–1472.
Panksepp, J. (1998). *Affective neuroscience*. New York, NY: Oxford University Press.
Panksepp, J. (2010). Affective neuroscience of the emotional brain mind: Evolutionary perspectives and and implications for understanding depression. *Dialogues in Clinical Neuroscience, 12*, 533–545.
Papez, J. W. (1937). A proposed mechanism of emotion. *Archives of Neurology and Psychiatry, 38*, 725–743.
PBS. (2002). A brilliant madness: A mathematical genius decent into madness *American Experience*, episode AMER 6409. Retrieved October 1, 2004, from PBS Home Video shop.pbs.org.
Pert, C. (1997). *Molecules of emotion*. New York, NY: Scribner.
Powell, N., Sloan, E., Bailey, M., Arevalo, J., Miller, G., Chen, E.. (. . .), Cole, S. (2013). Social stress up-regulates inflammatory gene expression in leukocyte transcriptome via β-adrenergic induction of myelopoiesis. *Proceedings of the National Academy of Sciences of the United States of America, 10*, 16574–16579.
Prehn, R. (2007). Does the immune reaction cause malignant transformation by disrupting cell-to-cell or cell-to-matrix communications? *Theoretical Biology and Medical Modelling, 4*, 16.
Rabstejnek, C. (Retrieved June 2014) An overview of expressed emotion. www.Houd.info.
Rainville, P. (1997). Pain affect encoded in human anterior cingulate but not somatosensory cortex. *Science, 277*, 968.
Ridker, P., Everett, B.M., Thuren, T., MacFadyen, B., Chang. W., Ballantyne, C., (. . .) and CANTOS Trial Group (2017a). Antiinflammatory therapy with cankinumab for atherosclerosis. *New England Journal of Medicine, 377*, 1119–1131.
Ridker, P., MacFadyen, J.G., Everett, B.M., Libby, P., Thoren, T., Glynn, R.J., and on behalf of the CANTOS trial group, (2017b). Effect of interleukin-1beta inhibition with canakinumab on incident lung cancer in patients with atherosclerosis: Exploratory results from a randomized, double-blind, placebo controlled trial. *Lancet, 390*, 1833–1842.
Selye, H. (1956). *The stress of life*. New York, NY: McGraw-Hill.
Shapiro, J. A. (1988). Bacteria as multicellular organisms. *Scientific American, 256*, 82–89.
Skinner, B. F. (1953). *Science and human behavior*. New York, NY: Simon & Schuster.
Sloman, S., & Fernbach, P. (2017). *The knowledge illusion*. New York, NY: Penguin Random House.
Smithers, D. (1962). An attack on cytologism. *Lancet, 274*, 493–499.
Solomon, A. (2014, March 17). The reckoning. *New Yorker*, retrieved online: https://www.newyorker.com/magazine/2014/03/17/the-reckoning
Stanovich, K. (1993). Dysrationalia. *Journal of Learning Disabilities, 26*(8), 501–515.
Stanovich, K. E. (2009). *What intelligence tests miss: The psychology of rational thought*. New Haven, CT: Yale University Press.
Stigum, B. P. (2003). *Econometrics and the philosophy of economics*. Princeton, NJ: Princeton University Press

Struhl, K. (2010). A transcriptional signature and common gene networks link cancer with lipid metabolism and diverse human diseases. *Cancer Cell, 17,* 348–361.
Thomas, E. (1996, April 22). Blood brothers. *Newsweek,* pp. 28–34.
Thomas, L. (1974). *Lives of a cell.* New York, NY: Macmillan.
Toman, W. (1961). *Family constellation.* New York, NY: Springer
Walker, D., Toufexis, D., & Davis, M. (2003). Role of the bed nucleus of the stria terminalis versus amygdala in fear, stress, and anxiety. *European Journal of Pharmacology, 28,* 199–216.
Warthin, A. (1913). Heredity with reference to carcinoma. *Archives of Internal Medicine, 12,* 546–555.
Weinberg, R. (2007). *The biology of cancer.* New York, NY: Garland
Wiener, N. (1948). *Cybernetics: Or control and communication in the animal and the machine.* Cambridge, MA: MIT Press.
Williams, G. (1966). *Adaptation and natural selection.* Princeton, NJ: Princeton University Press.
Wilson, E. O. (1975). *Sociobiology: The new synthesis.* Cambridge, MA: Belknap Press.
Wilson, E. O. (1998). *Consilience: the unity of knowledge.* New York, NY: Knopf.
Wilson, E. O. (2014). *The meaning of human existence.* New York, NY: Liveright.
Wohlleben, P. (2015). *The hidden life of trees.* Vancouver, BC: Greystone.
Zahalka, A. (2017). Adrenergic nerves activate an angio-metabolic switch in prostate cancer. *Science, 358,* 321–326.

Index

A *Beautiful Mind*, 223, 273.
   see also Nash, John
Abel Prize, 291
"A Brilliant Madness," 273
ACC activity. *see* anterior cingulate cortex (ACC) activity
Ackerman, D., 39, 99
action
   emotional/feeling system in motivating, 48
action–reaction process
   as part of emotional fusion, 213–14
active genes, 298
activity(ies)
   anxiety-binding, 114
acute anxiety
   chronic anxiety *vs.*, 171
   described, 109, 171
   fear and, 171
Adam, L., 233
adaptation
   capacity for, 109, 110
   defined, 109
adaptive behavior
   defined, 7
adaptive capacity
   chronic anxiety and, 110
adolescence
   degree of emotional separation in parent–offspring relationship during, 99

dominant-adaptive (deferential) interactions in, 34–35
emotional conflict in parent–child relationship during, 33–36
triangle interactions in, 34–35
of Unabomber, 232–33, 233f
adolescent(s)
   parental triangle in functioning of, 33–36
   peer group influences on, 35–36
adolescent rebellion, 34–36
   as reactive distancing, 34
adult dysfunctional child
   unresolved attachment between mother and, 39
Age of Enlightenment, 323, 324, 353
alcoholism
   causes of, 77–78
   epigenetics in, 77
alliance(s)
   cooperative, 16
allostasis, 314–15
   defined, 111
allostatic load, 314–15
American Family Therapy Association, 327
"ancestral tools for living," 283

anger
   of Unabomber, 231–32
Annual Family Symposium at Georgetown University Family Center, 328
anterior cingulate cortex (ACC) activity, 324–25
anticipation
   defined, 304
   phenomenon of, 304–5
anticipatory anxiety
   defined, 109
antisocial acts
   of psychopath, 240
anxiety
   acute *see* acute anxiety
   acute *vs.* chronic, 171
     see also acute anxiety; chronic anxiety
   anticipatory, 109
   binding of, 26, 26f
   changes in functional level of differentiation related to, 73
   chronic *see* chronic anxiety
   dealing with, 44
   defined, 109
   described, 108
   emotional reactivity and, 68–69
   functional shifts in individuality-togetherness balance related to, 73

anxiety (*continued*)
  impact on functioning, 170–71
  interlocking triangles and, 14
  internalized *vs.* externalized, 109
  outsider carrying, 16–17, 16*f*
  recognizing one's own, 90
  self and, 44
  social system–related, 51
  stress response system and, 108
  triangle in binding, 32
  triggers of, 90
anxiety-binding activities
  in stabilizing family system, 114
anxiety-driven distancing, 43
anxiety-driven emotionality
  poorly counterbalanced by reason, reflection, and principle, 50
anxiety-driven emotional process
  as silent killer, 23
  triangle as, 16
anxiety-driven emotional reactivity, 68–69, 120, 297
anxiety-driven interactions, xvii
anxiety-driven symptom process
  in society, 159
anxiety-driven togetherness, 98*f*, 99–101
  cutting off as part of, 146–47
  toning down, 100
anxiety reducer(s)
  capacity to maintain self in relationships as, 47–48
anxious overinvestment of mother in child, 40–41
anxious relationship system, 172
approval
  threats to, 112, 112*f*, 113

Arevalo, J., 299–300
argument(s)
  avoiding, 33
Aristotle, 141
Asperger's syndrome, 265
atavistic
  defined, 317
atherosclerosis
  biological processes in pathogenesis of, 297
  chronic inflammation in, 298
Atlantic Monthly, 234
attachment
  emotional *see* emotional attachment
  unresolved *see* unresolved attachment
attachment theory, xv
attention
  perception of adequate, 112, 112*f*, 113
  perception of inadequate, 112, 112*f*, 113
attitude(s)
  chronic anxiety triggered by, 110–11
  "love conquers all," 82
autonomy
  isolation for, 231
avolition
  defined, 332
awareness
  of multigenerational emotional process, 185
  triadic, 177
awareness of awareness
  self-awareness *vs.*, 49

Bacon, F. Sir, 323
bacteria
  social behavior of, 8
balance
  differentiation-togetherness, 73
  individuality-togetherness *see* individuality-togetherness balance
  relationship, 71

Barrett, Nichole, 242, 253–55, 257
Barzun, J., 150, 154–55, 157
basic level of differentiation, xxiii, 56
  of self, 331
Bateson, G., 327, 328
Beaufort wind force scale
  development of, 8
behavior(s)
  adaptive, 7
  of bacteria, 8
  childlike, 138
  in defining and maintaining self, xviii
  natural science of, 95–96
  oppositional, 51
  systems thinking applied to, xv
being
  conviction and courage in moving toward new way of, xx
  intellectual knowledge with emotional experience of, 185
belief(s)
  common, 67
  discrepant, 52
  emotion in resistance to changing one's, 182
  strongly held, 182
"belief papers," 50
Belsky, D., 315–17, 316*f*
Benditt, E., 307
Benson, H., 326, 329
Bernard, C., 305, 334
bias(es)
  confirmation, 31, 141
  binding of anxiety, 26, 26*f*
biological processes
  in all diseases, 297
biparental care
  among mammalian species, 38
blame
  Bowen theory and feelings of, 24
blended family, 123, 123*f*
Bleuler, E., 272
Bluebeard, 119–21

INDEX

body(ies)
  emotional operating systems in, 72
bodymind
  described, 72
Bonner, J.T., 211, 322
Book of Nature, 323
Bowen Center for the Study of the Family, 50, 138
Bowen family systems theory
  interlocking concepts of, xvi
Bowen–Kerr Interview Series, 328
Bowen, M., xiv–xvi, xxv, xxvi, 22–26, 39, 40, 44, 46, 50, 56, 60, 64, 69, 90–91, 93–96, 106, 111, 121, 127, 133, 135, 142–44, 147, 149, 150, 154, 157, 158, 165–67, 175, 180, 183, 186, 198, 199, 215, 217, 218, 221, 241, 320, 322–24, 326–29, 332, 333, 337, 348, 350
  as "uncoached coach," 167
Bowen theory
  applied to families in public eye, 223–94 see also specific families
  applied to societal emotional process, 158–59
  basis of, xiii
  concept of "self" of, xvi–xvii
  in conceptualizing relationship processes that regulate emotional functioning of individuals, 12
  core concepts in, 1–162 see also specific types
  critique of, 197
  defined, 166
  derivation of, 211
  described, xiv–xvii, 166, 211
  as description of what people do, 166

differentiation of self and, xiv
  emotional systems in, 7–12
  in facilitating process of differentiation, 211–21
  feeling that blame is placed on one in, 24
  operationalizing, 24
  patterns of interaction of, 22
  regulatory processes and, 12
  triangles in, 13, 27–28, 27t, 28f, 177
  unidisease in, 173
Bowen Theory Academy, 126
Bowen theory–based therapy
  conventional therapy vs., 35
  described, 213–14, 213f
Bowlby, J., xv, xvi
Boysen, S., xxi
brain
  emotional system of, 11, 11f
  functions of, 53, 55
  intellectual system as function of, 53
  mechanism of emotion in, 141
  solid self as function of, 55
brain functioning
  brain structure vs., 273
brain structure
  brain functioning vs., 273
brain system(s)
  in intellectual system, 53
Bricker, 274f, 275, 277–78, 280, 281, 285
bridging the cutoff, 143
Brigham and Women's Hospital, 298
Broadway gang, 249
Bushnell, B., 254
Bushnell, M., 324

Caccioppo, J., 299–300
calming effect
  on relationships, 212–13
  researching one's own family as, 183
calming oneself, 69
cancer
  chronic inflammation in, 298
Cannon, W., 305
"Can't live him, can't live without him," 12
CANTOS Trial Group, 298–99
Carnegie Institute of Technology, 276
Carnegie Mellon University, 300
Carolin, J., Father, 329
Carrier, B., 324
Carrier Clinic, 287, 289
cause-and-effect thinking, xv–xvi, 3f
  as default mode, 6
  described, 5
  in fostering guilt or denial, 24
  functional facts of relationship process and, 96
  letting go of, xvi
  as obstacle to seeing patterns of emotional functioning, 22
  systems thinking vs., 3, 54
causing
  playing part in vs., 24
CBS News, 237, 273
change(s)
  epigenetic, 306
child focus
  evolution in shaping, 38–39
childlike behavior
  sibling position–related, 138
children
  differentiation of self in relationship to, 147
chronic anxiety, 108–18
  absorber of, 110
  acute anxiety vs., 171

chronic anxiety (continued)
  adaptive capacity and, 110
  attitudes triggering, 110–11
  causes of, 110–11
  clinical symptoms resulting from, 118
  dealing with, 144–45
  defined, 109
  degree of disturbance in symptomatic individual's important relationship systems related to, 292, 292f
  described, 171
  family conflicts related to, 298
  family group therapy in reducing, 211–12
  in family systems, 114–18, 115f, 114f
  fluctuation of, 117
  internalization of, 297–321 see also unidisease; unidisease concept of John Nash, 273–74, 273f, 282
  level of, 110
  in marital relationship, 40
  market for, 173–74
  in multigenerational transmission process, 124
  pseudo-self as basis for reducing, 58
  recognition of, 173–74
  reducing, 174–75
  in relationships, 111–18, 112f, 114f, 115, 172
  as "silent killer," 172
  in symptom development, 118
  system-generated, 23, 110
chronic anxiety–driven functional dysfunction schizophrenia as, 292, 292f
chronic anxiety–driven unrealistic expectations, 185

chronic inflammation, 298
  social stress and, 172
chronic stress, 173
chronic stress response, 13
Churchill, W., 75, 292
clinical symptoms
  chronic anxiety and, 118
  link between patterns of emotional functioning and, 23
close-minded dogma
  conviction vs., 220
closeness
  emotional, 13
  threats to, 13
coach(es)
  Bowen as "uncoached," 167
  in differentiation of self, 220
  in Kerr family vignette, 186
  in process of differentiation, 201–10, 205f
  "uncoached," 167
coaching
  case example, 201–10, 205f
  in process of differentiation, 201–10, 205f
cognitive dissonance
  lack of, 52
cognitive functioning
  feelings in, 48
cognitive process(es)
  emotion's grip on, 50
  emotions vs., 53
Cognitive Revolution, 176
Cohen, S., 300–1
Cole, S., 299–300
Collins, M., 5
Columbia University, 299
comfortable courtship phase
  of relationship, 82, 82f
common beliefs, 67
communication(s)
  in defining and maintaining self, xviii
concept of "self"
  of Bowen theory, xvi–xvii

confirmation bias, 31, 141
conflict(s)
  chronic anxiety and, 298
  emotional, 26–27, 27t, 28f, 31–36, 32f see also emotional conflict
  family, 298
  pseudo-self at root of, 329–30
Congress
  regressed features of, 156
conjoint marital therapy, 212–13
Conley, D., 127
consciousness
  self as manifestation of highest level of, 54
  of thinking and emotions, 49
Consilience: The Unity of Knowledge, 166
content thinking
  process thinking vs., 25
context dependence
  pseudo-self and, 52
conventional therapy
  Bowen theory–based therapy vs., 35
conviction
  close-minded dogma vs., 220
  in moving toward new way of being, xx
cooperation
  described, 65
cooperative alliances
  triangles vs., 16
core concepts
  in Bowen theory, 1–162
  see also specific types
counterbalancing
  of life forces of individuality and togetherness in parent-offspring relationships, 97
  of stress response, 320
courage
  in moving toward new way of being, xx

criticism
  of each other, 35
culture
  becoming unstable, 156
  described, 70
  emotional system influences and influenced by, xviii
cutoff
  bridging of, 143
  emotional, 143–48 see also emotional cutoff
  as part of anxiety-driven togetherness process, 146–47
  between siblings, 146
cybernetics, xiv

Daily News, 259
Damasio, A., xix, 49, 112, 120
Darwin, C., 165–66
Davies, P., 317, 318
decadence
  pervasive societal changes reflecting, 150
DeCharms, R.C., 325
default mode
  cause-and-effect thinking as, 6
deferential interactions. see dominant-adaptive (deferential) interactions
de La Mettrie, J.O., 323
delinquency
  overly permissive family pattern and, 151–54, 152f–53f
denial
  cause-and-effect thinking in fostering, 24
developing "self"
  schizophrenia's impact on, 185
development
  parental triangle during, 95
de Waal, F., 79, 177
Diderot, D., 323, 353
differentiation

basic level of, xxiii, 56, 58–64, 60f, 331
basic vs. functional level of, 155–56, 155f
described, 70
emotional functioning at different basic levels of, 58–64, 60f
functional level of see functional level of differentiation
Kaczynski's level of, 236–37
poor, 50
process of, 163–221 see also specific components and process of differentiation
pseudo-self as basis for increasing person's functional level of, 58
reflected in stability of intimate relationships, 125
variable of, 125–26
differentiation of self, xvi, 45–64, 108
  as adult in one's family of origin, 166
  as attractive to family, 168
  benefits of, 165, 166
  Bowen theory and, xiv
  coach in, 220
  continuum of basic levels of, 131–32, 131f
  described, xviii, xxiv–xxv, 108, 127–28
  emotional maturity and, 127
  facilitating, 213
  in human relationship systems, 220
  importance of, 220
  lack of, 6
  Lanza and, 47
  levels of, 47
  as more than psychological process, 54
  moving toward goal as part of, 146–47

in relationship to spouse and children, 147
research on one's family in, 179–85
differentiation of self scale, 60
differentiation-togetherness balance
  in relationships, 73
discrepant beliefs
  pseudo-self and, 52
disease(s)
  biological processes in, 297
  gene networks in, 298
disequilibrium
  punctuated, 33
dissonance
  cognitive, 52
distance
  described, 143 see emotional distance; emotional distancing
distancing
  anxiety-driven, 43
  communication in subtle/not so subtle ways, 43–44
  reactive, 34
divorce(s)
  recording on family diagram, 122–23, 123f
doing
  saying vs., 23
dominance hierarchies
  in species living in social groups, 28–29
dominant-adaptive (deferential) interactions, 26–31, 27t, 28f, 29f
  in adolescence, 34–35
  described, 65
doublethink
  defined, 52
  pseudo-self and, 52
Duncan, G., 324–25
Durst, R., 5
Dvorak, H., 302
dynamic equilibrium of triangles
  variant of, 18

dysfunctional child
  unresolved attachment between mother and, 39
dysrationalia
  defined, 149
Eagleman, D., 49
Eggers, D., 223
ego fusion
  mechanisms to control intensity of, 24
El Niño, 159–60
emotion(s), 120
  brain and, 141
  cognitive processes vs., 53
  consciousness of, 49
  control of, 49
  decoupling from thinking, xxv
  grip on cognitive processes, 50
  impact on mental processes, 141–42
  impact on thinking, xxiii
  in resistance to changing one's beliefs, 182
  thinking with, 49
emotional attachment
  parent–offspring, 98f, 99–100
  sibling variations related to, 101–2
  unresolved, 198–99, 231
emotional closeness
  poorly differentiated people and, 14
  profound need for, 13
  undifferentiated people and, 14
  well-differentiated people and, 14
emotional conflict, 26–27, 27t, 28f, 31–36, 32f
  anchored in emotional system, 31
  in marriage, 31–32, 32f
  in parent–child relationships, 33–36
emotional cutoff, 143–48
  bridging of, 143
  described, 143
  emotional distance vs., 143
  emotional fusion vs., 146–47
    example of, 145
    gradations of, 145
    as part of anxiety-driven togetherness process, 146–47
    between siblings, 146
  emotional distance, 24, 27, 27t, 28f, 43–45
    described, 43
    emotional cutoff vs., 143
    in emotional functioning, 17
    open relationship vs., 44
    pattern of, 43
  emotional distancing
    example of, 26, 26f
  emotional dysfunction
    psychoses and, 240
  emotional experience of being
    intellectual knowledge with, 185
  emotional/feeling system, 47–48
    in motivating action, 48
  emotional flavor, 120
  emotional flow
    through generations, 126
  emotional forces
    networks of, 22
    through family system, 8
  emotional functioning
    assessment of, 49–50, 119
    balance between intellectual functioning and, 50
    Bowen theory in conceptualizing relationship processes that regulate, 12
    on continuum, xxiii–xxiv, 102
    criteria in assessing, 49–50
    described, 124–25
    emotional distance in, 17
    facilitating link between evolutionary biologists and Bowen theory's idea of, 26–27
    of family members, xvii
    of Gary Gilmore, 256–58, 256f
    individual variation in, 47
    interplay between intellectual and emotional systems in, 47
    longevity related to, 125
    lower-level, 50
    parallels between observation of similar patterns in other species and, 26
    patterns of, 22–45, 49–50
      see also patterns of emotional functioning
    in present and past generations, 119
    as product of evolution and embedded in emotional system, 26
    regression in, 47
  emotional fusion
    action–reaction process as part of, 213–14
    anchored in emotional system, 25
    emotional cutoff vs., 146–47
    emotional programming and, 100
    factors in determining, 55–57
    in marriages, 282
  emotional history
    of family memories of living members in enhancing, 181–82
  emotional immaturity
    described, 127–28
  emotional intensity, 198
    of family interactions, xxiv
  emotional interdependence between parents, 40
  emotionality
    anxiety-driven, 50
    rationality vs., xxiii

reasoning vs., 48
emotional logic, 91
"emotionally competent stimuli," 112
emotionally difficult situations
  engage in, 175–76
emotionally influenced intuitions, 141
emotional maturity
  described, 127
  differentiation of self and, 127
  genetic basis for, 127
  high level of intelligence vs., 127
emotional neutrality, 198
  in reducing chronic anxiety, 174–75
emotional objectivity, 89–94
  capacity for, 89
  case example, 89–93
  development of increased, 89–93
  functional facts in, 90
  functioning position in, 91–92
  in reducing chronic anxiety, 174–75
emotional operating systems
  in body, 72
emotional process(es)
  action–reaction process as part of, 213–14
  anxiety-driven, 16, 23
  described, 4
  family-of-origin, 18
  in financial crisis of 2007–2008, 160–61
  in Kaczynski family, 230
  in Lanza family, 259–60
  multigenerational, 121, 185
  in process of differentiation, 168–70, 169f
  societal, 149–62 see also societal emotional process; societal regression(s)

sources of, 149
transmission across generations, 130–31
triangle pattern of, 14
emotional programming, 37, 95–107, 339
  components of, 95
  in context of interplay between counterbalancing life forces of individuality and togetherness in parent-offspring relationships, 97
  described, 95
  emotional fusion and, 100
  gene expression and, 95
  in parental triangle during development, 95
emotional/psychic energy
  in relationships, 80–81, 80f
emotional reactivity, 33
  anxiety-driven, 68–69, 120, 297
emotional regression(s), 65–78, 150, 154–55
  biological roots in, 159–60
  causes of, 68
  defined, 65
  ending of, 156–58
  example of, 66–67
  family emerging from, 157
  in family system, 232–33, 233f
  fundamental process in, 156
  in ground finches of Galapagos Islands, 159–60
  individuality-togetherness balance and, 79–88
  in Kaczynski family, 231–32
  in U.S., 157
emotional reinforcement

from marital relationship, 40
emotional response
  to connecting with past, 183
emotional roots
  of triangles, 177
emotional separateness
  in marital relationship, 197–99
emotional separation
  described, 39
  in parent–offspring relationship during adolescence, 99
emotional shock wave, 116–17
emotional system(s), 48
  being in contact with, but outside of, 69
  in Bowen theory, 7–12
  of brain, 11, 11f
  characteristics of, xviii
  emotional conflict anchored in, 31
  in emotional functioning, 47
  emotional fusion anchored in, 25
  evolution and, 7–12
  influences and influenced by feeling states, psychological states, and culture, xviii
  logic of, 91
  molecule of, 13–21
  phylogenetic histories impact on, 7
emotional system disorders, 240
emotional system process
  example of, 8–9
emotional unit
  family functioning as, xvii, 46
energy
  emotional/psychic, 80–81, 80f
Engblom, C., 302–3
environmental factors
  in alcoholism, 77–78

Environmental Protection Agency (EPA), 149
envy
  womb, 281–82
EPA. *see* Environmental Protection Agency (EPA)
epigenetic changes, 306
epigenetics
  in alcoholism, 77
  described, 95
epinephrine
  stress and, 172
esophageal ulcers
  Helicobacter pylori and, 314
Everett, B.M., 298–99
evolution
  emotional system and, 7–12
  in shaping child focus, 38–39
expectation(s)
  about one's family, 184–85
  chronic anxiety–driven unrealistic, 185
externalized anxiety
  internalized anxiety *vs.*, 109

fact(s)
  functional *see* functional fact(s)
failure to lift off syndrome, 145
families in public eye, 223–94
  Bowen theory applied to, 223–94 *see also specific families*
family(ies). *see also specific families*
  of Adam Lanza, 259–71 *see also* Lanza, Adam (Sandy Hook shooter); Lanza family
  blended, 123, 123f
  defining self in, xxi
  differentiation of self as attractive to, 168

emerging from regression, 157
emotional functioning
  assessment of, 49–50
emotional functioning in present and past generations of, 119
emotional history of, 181–82
emotional intensity of interactions within, xxiv
as emotional unit, 46
expectations about one's, 184–85
Freudian theory
  extended to, xv
functioning as emotional unit, xvii
of Gary Gilmore, 239–58 *see also* Gilmore, Gary
group therapy in reducing chronic anxiety in, 211–12
Kaczynski, 230, 331–54 *see also* Kaczynski, Ted (Unabomber)
of origin *see* family of origin
reactivity to, 183–84
research on, 179–85
schizophrenia and, 272–94 *see also* Nash, John; schizophrenia
studying one's own, 331–54 *see also* studying one's own family
trees and, xiii
universality of difficulties related to, 184–85
Family Center, 218
family conflicts
  chronic anxiety and, 298
Family Constellation, 133, 140
family diagram(s), 119. *see also specific types and families*
  defined, 121, 122f
  described, 121, 122f, 334
  divorces recorded on, 122–23, 123f

of family of origin, 333–51, 333f, 342f, 345f, 346f *see also specific families*
function of, 121
of multigenerational family emotional process, 126–32, 126f, 128f, 130f, 131f
of Nash and Larde families, 274–75, 274f
purpose of, 334
remarriages recorded on, 122–23, 123f
three-generational, 122, 122f
family difficulties
  universality of, 184–85
family dynamics
  sibling position in, 139
Family Evaluation, 69, 221
family group therapy, 211–12
  in reducing chronic anxiety in family, 211–12
family history
  calming effect of, 183
  multiple versions of, 181
family interactions
  emotional intensity of, xxiv
family members
  emotional functioning of, xvii
  systems thinking related to, xvi
family movement, 46
family of origin
  differentiation of self as adult in, 166
  progress in, 179–85
  researching one's, 179–85
  unresolved attachment to, 145
  viewed in larger context, 184
family of origin diagram, 333–51, 333f, 342f, 345f, 346f. *see also specific families*

family-of-origin emotional process, 18
family of origin relationships
  as problematic, 183
"family organism," xv
family pattern(s)
  overly permissive, 151–54, 152f–53f
family process
  psychotic-level, 212
family projection process, 36, 105
family relationship system
  person's functioning position in, 23
Family Research Conference, 147, 166
family stress response, 318–19, 318f
Family Study Project, 102
  books on, xv
  of NIMH, xv, 211–21
family system(s)
  anxiety-binding activities in stabilizing, 114
  chronic anxiety in, 114–18, 115f, 114f
  emotional forces through, 8
  emotional regression in, 232–33, 233f
  example of, 114–17, 114f, 115f
  relationships in stabilizing, 114
  in symptom development, 23
family systems theory
  Bowen's, xiv
family therapists
  responsibilities of, 165
family therapy, 211–12
  multiple, 219
  with one person, 219–20
  as way of thinking, 220–21
Family Therapy in Clinical Practice, 165, 166
fear
  acute anxiety and, 171

Federal Reserve, 161
feeling(s)
  described, 48
  in normal cognitive functioning, 48
  from principle to, 156
  of rejection, 13
  thinking vs., 170–71
  thoughts vs., 49
feeling process
  intellectual process vs., 48–49
feeling state(s), 48
  counterbalancing of, 69
  emotional system influences and influenced by, xviii
feeling system
  intellectual system impact of, 75
  overriding objective judgments, 238
Fernbach, P., 329–30
financial crisis of 2007–2008
  emotional process related to, 160–61
Five Easy Pieces, 145
Flavahan, W., 306–7, 318
flip-flopping
  defined, 220
force(s)
  emotional, 8, 22
  functional facts about "unseen," 324
  togetherness, xviii
Framo, J., 147
free will, 45
Freudian theory, 46
  extended to family, xv
Freud, S., 6, 46, 165
Freud's theory, 165
From Dawn to Decadence, 150
functional dysfunction
  chronic anxiety–driven, 292, 292f
  schizophrenia as, 273
functional fact(s)
  about "unseen forces," 324
  described, 90

in emotional objectivity, 90
examples of, 90
of relationship process, 96
in systems thinking, 5–6
of triangles, 13
functional level of differentiation, 73
  anxiety-driven decrease in, 155–56, 155f
  anxiety-related changes in, 73
  from birth until death, 351–52, 352f
functional separateness
  loss of, 72
functioning
  anxiety's impact on, 170–71
  cognitive, 48
  emotional see emotional functioning
  intellectual system, 50, 54
  intellectual vs. emotional, 50
  interdependent, xvii
functioning position
  described, 91–92
  examples of, 23 see anxiety-driven emotional process
  in family relationship system, 23
  in reinforcing prevailing pattern, 23
fusion
  ego, 24
  emotional see emotional fusion
  in relationships, 55–56, 72
  transference vs., 176

Gadagkar, R., 66
Galapagos Islands
  emotional regression in ground finches of, 159–60
gastritis
  Helicobacter pylori and, 310–11

gene(s)
  active, 298
  schizophrenia related to, 293
gene amplification, 304–5
gene expression
  emotional programming and, 95
gene networks
  in diseases, 298
general adaptation syndrome, 299
general systems theory, xiv, xv
generation(s)
  emotional flow through, 126
  transmission of emotional process across, 130–31
generation gap, 143
genetics
  in emotional maturity, 127
  schizophrenia and, 293
genogram, 119
Georgetown University Department of Psychiatry, xv, 91
Georgetown University Family Center, 133
  Annual Family Symposium at, 328
Georgetown University Hospital, 347
Georgetown University School of Medicine, xiv, 332, 333
"Germs," 300
Gilmore–Brown families
  family diagram of, 240–42, 241f
  playing out of life forces and patterns of emotional functioning in, 256–58, 256f
Gilmore family story, 239–58, 248f, 256f. see also Gilmore, Gary
Gilmore, Gary, 223, 239–58
  arrests of, 249–52
  family of, 239–58
  father of, 240–41, 241f, 245–52, 248f, 256, 256f
  "good" side of, 255
  mother of, 241f, 242, 245–56, 248f, 256f
  Nichole Barrett and, 241f, 242, 253–55, 257
  nodal events in life of, 242–44
  at OSCI, 243, 251, 252
  parental triangle, 248–49, 248f, 256f
  playing out of life forces and patterns of emotional functioning, 256–58, 256f
  reform school for, 249–50
  siblings of, 239, 242, 250
Gilmore, Mikal, 239, 250, 251, 254
Glynn, R.J., 298–99
goal orientation
  in differentiation of self, 146–47
Gordon, D., 7
gossip
  linguistic skills and, 176–77
gossip system
  as essential element of all human groups, 21
  as manifestation of triangle, 176–77
Grant, P., 159
Grant, R., 159
ground finches of Galapagos Islands
  emotional regression in, 159–60
group(s). see specific types, e.g., we-they groups
  gossip system as essential element of all, 21
  social, 28–29
group therapy
  family, 211–12
guilt
  cause-and-effect thinking in fostering, 24
  as product of relationship interaction, 92

Haidt, J., xxiii, 31, 45, 64, 70, 141, 258
Haley, A., 183
Harari, Y.N., 1, 176, 177
hard core, 331–32
Harvard University
  Unabomber at, 233–34
Hawkley, L., 299–300
health histories
  data about, 125
Helicobacter pylori
  esophageal ulcers related to, 314
  peptic ulcers and gastritis related to, 310–11
helicopter parenting, 151–54, 152f–53f
helplessness
  sibling position in, 138
high level of intelligence
  emotional maturity vs., 127
Hinkle, L., 60
Holt, R., 241
homeostasis, 305–7, 314–15
Homo dysrationalis, 161, 162
  from *Homo sapiens* to, 149
Homo sapiens
  described, 141
  to *Homo dysrationalis*, 149
Horney, K., 281
Huang, Y., 300
Huler, S., 8
human behavior
  natural science of, 95–96
  systems thinking applied to, xv
human being's nature
  reconciling strikingly contradictory sides of, 223
humankind
  as rational animal, 141
hypertension
  as "silent killer," 23, 172

IAS. see Institute for Advanced Study (IAS)
immaturity, 232
  emotional, 127–28

INDEX 371

in marriage, 36–38
maturity vs., 102–5, 103t
immediate family(ies)
  reactivity to, 183–84
impaired functioning
  relationship system in creating and maintaining, 23
"Implications of Bowen Theory for Catholic Theology," 329
"inborn predisposition," 67
individualism
  defined, 70
  rugged, 70
individualistic societies
  described, 70
individuality, 68
  characteristics of, 158
  defined, xviii–xix
  in parent–offspring relationships, 97
  togetherness vs., xviii
individuality-togetherness balance, 79–88, 158–59
  anxiety-related functional shifts in, 73
  basic level of, 73
  differences in, 71
  emotional regression and, 79–88
  in relationships, 73
individual thinking
  letting go of, 8
  to relationship thinking, 22
infant(s)
  mother–offspring relationship in survival of, 39–40
inflammation
  chronic, 172, 298
  social stress and, 172
Inflammation and Atherosclerosis: A Translational Tale, 297
insane
  from psychopath to, 240
insider(s)
  outsiders vs., 15, 15f

tension arising between, 17, 17f
instability
  of culture, 156
  of intimate relationships, 13
  of two-person system, 13, 14
Institute for Advanced Study (IAS), 279, 286, 287
integration of self
  degree of, 108
  described, 108
intellectual functioning
  balance between emotional functioning and, 50
intellectual knowledge
  with emotional experience of being, 185
intellectual process
  feeling process vs., 48–49
intellectual system, xviii, 45
  brain systems in, 53
  in emotional functioning, 47
  feeling system's impact on, 75
  as function of brain, 53
  intelligence vs., 53
  overlapping with intelligence, 53
  solid self and, 52–53
  variation in development of, xix
intellectual system functioning
  prefrontal cortex in, 54
intelligence
  emotional maturity vs., 127
  high level of, 127
  intellectual system overlapping with, 53
  intellectual system vs., 53
  rational thinking vs., 53
intensity
  described, 25
  emotional, xxiv, 198
interdependence
  emotional, 40

interdependent functioning
  described, xvii
interlocking psychopathology thinking
  systems thinking vs., xvi
interlocking triangles, 6, 14, 177
  anxiety related to, 14
  in Kerr family vignette, 194–97
  observing, 194–97
intermediary sibling position
  profile of, 136–37
internalized anxiety
  externalized anxiety vs., 109
intimate relationships
  data in assessing how differentiation is reflected in stability of, 125
  instability of, 13
  self in maintaining, 77
  unresolved attachment in, 77
intuition(s)
  described, 141
  emotionally influenced, 141
I-position, 52
isolation
  autonomy for, 231
isolation call, 38

Jackson, J.H., 54
Jefferson, T., Pres., 74
Jensen, M., 254
Johns Hopkins Hospital, 326
Johnson, S., 234, 236
Johnston, D., 234
Jones, J.E., 75
Joshi, N., 66
judgment(s)
  objective, 238

Kaczynski–Dombek family
  at time of Unabomber's arrest, 226–27, 226f
Kaczynski family
  emotional process in, 230

Kaczynski, Ted
(Unabomber), 55, 144,
223, 225–38
adolescence of, 232–33,
233f
anger of, 231–32
assistant professor of
mathematics at University of California,
Berkeley, 234
bombing attempts by,
235, 236
cabin in Montana, 235
change in family emotional processes during
adolescence of, 232–
33, 233f
college and graduate education, 233–34
emotional regression in
family of, 231–32
employment with father,
235–36
family events impacting,
236
family interactions of,
225–38, 226f, 228t, 230
family members, 227
family's worry after arrest
of, 226
graduate studies, 234
important events, 228–
29, 228t
injuries by, 226
isolation of, 231
leaving high school at
age 16, 232
low basic level of differentiation of, 236–37
mother's early relationship with, 229–32, 233f
murders by, 226
parents' employment,
227–28
powerful emotional
fusion between mother
and, 229–32, 233f
schizophrenia in, 230
skipping grades, 232
Kaczynski, Theodore Richard, 227

Kaczynski, Wanda Dombek,
227
Kandel, E., 108, 109
"Kaynbred," 268
Kerr family
Bowen theory applied to,
331–54 see also Kerr,
M.E.
family of origin diagram,
333–51, 333f, 342f,
345f, 346f
schizophrenia impact on,
331–54
studying one's own family, 331–54
Kerr family vignette,
179–99, 331–43. see
also Kerr family; Kerr,
M.E.
aftermath of brother's
suicide, 187–91
gaining more emotional
separateness in marital
relationship, 197–99
interlocking triangle
involving Dad years
after his death, 194–95
interlocking triangles
involving Mother and
nuclear family, 194–97
of process of differentiation, 179–99
research on family,
179–85
seeing important triangle, 191–93, 192f
seeing my unresolved
attachment to mother
replicated in my marriage, 187
value of coach, 186
Kerr, Kathy, 179, 218, 326,
346–47
Kerr, M.E., 44, 69–71, 138–
39, 144, 167, 175, 218,
303–5
Bowen theory applied to
family of, 331–54
brother's vulnerability to
schizophrenia, 336
family of origin diagram,
333–51, 333f, 342f,
345f, 346f
father of, 333f, 335–44,
342f
grandparents of, 333f,
334–37
mother of, 333f, 335–51,
342f, 345f, 346f
multigenerational
research on family of,
179–99 see also Kerr
family vignette
schizophrenia's impact
on, 331–54
schizophrenic brother
of, 333f–51, 333f, 342f,
345f, 346f
King, R., 261
Kipling, R., 14
knee-jerk opposition to others' points of view
pseudo-self and, 51
knee-jerk reactivity, 48
knowledge
intellectual, 185
Kors, A., 323
Kovaleski, S.F., 233

Lancet, 306
Lanza, Adam (Sandy Hook
shooter), 47, 145, 223,
259–71
alias of, 268
Asperger's syndrome in,
265
college years, 268
deterioration of behavior, 269
early years, 263–64
father of, 259–61, 260f,
264–66, 266f, 268–71
high school years,
267–68
middle school years,
265–67
mother of, 259–71, 260f,
266f
siblings of, 261–63, 266
Lanza–Chapman families
family diagram of, 260,
260f

Lanza family, 259–71. *see also* Lanza, Adam (Sandy Hook shooter)
  emotional processes in, 259–60
  family diagram of, 260, 260f
Larde, Alicia, 274f, 278–94, 284f, 290f, 292f
Lederer, H., xiv, xxvi
LeDoux, J., 171–72
Lee, Y., 310, 311f
Libby, P., 297–99, 301, 312
life adjustments
  in multigenerational transmission process, 128–29, 128f
life forces
  individuality and togetherness, 68
Lineweaver, C., 317, 318
linguistic skills
  gossip and, 176–77
Livio, S.K., 291
logic
  emotional, 91
longevity
  emotional functioning and, 125
"love conquers all" attitude, 82
"low-level self-regulation," 113
Lysiak, M., 259, 261, 266

MacLean, P.D., 38, 100, 141, 255
Madison, D., 73–76, 156–57
Madison, J., Pres., 73–76, 156
Madison, P., 157
Mailer, N., 223, 239, 240, 242, 255
mammalian species
  biparental care among, 38
marital relationship(s)
  chronic anxiety in, 40
  conjoint therapy for, 212–13
  emotional conflict in, 31–32, 32f
  emotional fusion in, 282
  emotional reinforcement from, 40
  emotional separateness in, 197–99
  immaturity in, 36–38
  stressors in, 82–88, 83f–85f, 87f
  tension in, 82–88, 83f–85f, 87f
  undifferentiation in, 36–38
  unresolved attachment replicated in, 187
marriage. *see* marital relationship(s)
Marshall, B., 310
Marshall University, 289–90
Mason, J.W., 299
Massachusetts Institute of Technology (MIT), 277, 279–81, 285
mass shootings, 259–71
maternal deprivation thinking, xv–xvi
maturity
  emotional *see* emotional maturity
  immaturity *vs.*, 102–5, 103t
McEwen, B., 108, 110–11, 314, 317
McFayden, J.G., 298–99
McLean Hospital
  Belmont, Massachusetts, 281
MCV Conference. *see* Medical College of Virginia (MCV) Conference
mechanism(s)
  defined, 25
  as "patterns of emotional functioning in a family," 24, 25
Medical College of Virginia (MCV) Conference, 215–19, 216f
Meissner, W.W., 121
"melancholic shutdown," 233

Menninger Clinic, xv, 93
mental process(es)
  emotions impact on, 141–42
mental symptoms
  source of, 297–98
Merton, R., 105
milieu intérieur
  concept of, 305
mindware
  defined, 53
MIT. *see* Massachusetts Institute of Technology (MIT)
Moberg, K.U., 320
molecule(s)
  of emotional system, 13–21
mother(s)
  anxious overinvestment in child, 40–41
  unresolved attachment between adult dysfunctional child and, 39
mother–offspring relationship
  in infant's survival, 39–40
movement
  family, 46
Mukherjee, S., 299
multigenerational emotional process, 121
  awareness of, 185
multigenerational family(ies)
  study of, 119–32 *see also* multigenerational transmission process
multigenerational family emotional process
  family diagram of, 126–32, 126f, 128f, 130f, 131f
multigenerational family emotional system
  interconnections of members in, 129–30, 130f
multigenerational family organism, 119–32. *see also* multigenerational transmission process

multigenerational transmission process, 119–32
  chronic anxiety in, 124
  data about health histories in, 125
  data about occupational experiences in, 125
  described, 121
  emotional flow in, 126
  example of, 130–31
  family diagram for, 119–32 see also family diagram(s)
  life adjustments in, 128–29, 128f
  natural systems thinking in conceptualizing, 119
  as perspective-promoting concept in Bowen theory, 120
  specific data collected for, 124
multiple family therapy, 219
Mulvihill, J., 126

Nasar, S., 273, 277
Nash and Larde families
  family diagram of, 274–75, 274f
Nash equilibrium, 277
Nash, John, 223, 272–94, 351. see also schizophrenia
  Alicia Larde and, 274f, 278–94, 284f, 290f, 292f
  chronic anxiety of, 273–74, 273f, 282
  college years, 274f, 276
  downhill spiral, 285–89
  early years, 275–76
  European travel by, 285–86
  father of, 274–75, 274f
  graduate school, 276–77
  homosexual lifestyle of, 277, 280
  hospitalization of, 286
  at IAS, 279, 286, 287
  mother of, 274f, 275

Nobel Prize in Economics, 277
  professional work–related issues, 279–80
  psychosis of, 283–85, 284f
  relationships of, 274f, 275, 277–79, 278f
  residency changes by, 276–92
  social interactions of, 277
  son of, 289–92, 292f
  spouse's pregnancy effects on, 281–83
  troubling years at MIT, 280–281
  trying to solve Riemann hypothesis, 279–80
National Cancer Institute, 126
National Institute of Alcohol Abuse and Alcoholism, 77
National Institutes of Mental Health (NIMH), xv, 93
  Family Study Project of, xv, 211–21
  on functional facts of triangles, 13
naturally occurring systems
  described, 7–12
natural systems
  described, 7–12
natural systems thinking conceptualizing multigenerational process in, 119
nature
  human being's, 223
"networks of emotional forces," 22
neuropeptides, 327–28
neutrality, 120
  emotional, 174–75, 198
Newtown, 259
Newtown Middle School, 261
new way of being
  conviction and courage in moving toward, xx
New Yorker, 259

New York Times, 234, 299
  on Unabomber, 225
Nicholson, J., 145
NIMH. see National Institutes of Mental Health (NIMH)
NIMH Family Study Project, xv, xvii, xix, 39
Nineteen Eighty-Four, 52
Nobel Prize, 291
non-Bowen theory–based technique, 214
nonspecific stress response, 299
norepinephrine
  stress and, 172
Northwestern University
  bombing attempts at, 235, 236
nuclear family ego mass
  relationship system in, 24

objective judgments
  feeling system overriding, 238
objectivity
  emotional see emotional objectivity
  gaining, 332–33
  responses guided by, 48
occupational experiences
  data about, 125
Oedipus complex, 6
oldest brother of brother(s)
  profile of, 135
oldest brother of sister(s)
  profile of, 135
oldest sister of brother(s)
  profile of, 136
oldest sister of sister(s)
  profile of, 136
one-down relationship with parents, 35
oneself. see also self
  calming of, 69
only child
  profile of, 137
open relationship
  described, 44
  emotional distance vs., 44
  self in dealing with, 44

oppositional behavior
  pseudo-self and, 51
Oregon State Correctional
  Institution (OSCI),
  243, 251, 252
Orwell, G., 52
OSCI. *see* Oregon State
  Correctional Institution (OSCI)
Osler, W., Sir, 325–26
outsider(s)
  as carrying anxiety of
    triangle, 16–17, 16f
  insiders *vs.*, 15, 15f
overfunctioner(s)
  underfunctioners *vs.*,
    29–30, 29f
overfunctioning
  pattern of, xvii
overfunctioning-underfunctioning reciprocity,
    29–30, 29f
  in relationship, 57, 57f
overfunctioning-underfunctioning relationship
  views of, 51–52
overly permissive family
  pattern
  delinquency related to,
    151–54, 152f–53f

panic/grief system
  overactivity of, 283
panic system, 72
  overactivity of, 283
Panksepp, J., 48–49, 72, 283
Papez, J., 141
paranoid schizophrenia, 236
parent(s)
  emotional interdependence between, 40
  one-down relationship
    with, 35
  therapy sessions with,
    212
parental triangle
  during development, 95
  in functioning of adolescent, 33–36
  unresolved emotional
    attachment and, 231

parent–child relationships
  emotional conflict in,
    33–36
parenting
  helicopter, 151–54,
    152f–53f
  snowplow, 151–54,
    152f–53f
parent–offspring emotional
  attachment
  during course of child
    maturing biologically,
    98f, 99–100
parent–offspring
  relationships
  counterbalancing life
    forces of individuality and togetherness
    in, 97
  degree of emotional separation during adolescence, 99
partnering process, 80–81,
    80f
Pasteur, L., 334
pathology
  described, 298
patterns of emotional functioning, 22–45. *see also*
  emotional functioning; *specific types, e.g.,*
  emotional conflict
  activity level of, 108
  cause-and-effect thinking as obstacle to seeing, 22
  described, 25
  dominant-adaptive (deferential) interactions,
    26–31, 27t, 28f, 29f
  emotional conflict,
    26–27, 27t, 28f, 31–36,
    32f
  emotional distance,
    43–45
  in family, 24, 25
  link between clinical
    symptoms and, 23
  observing, 24
  sustaining of, 23
Payne, R., 50

peer group influences
  on adolescents, 35–36
people pretending to be
  something they are
  not, 51
peptic ulcers
  Helicobacter pylori and,
    310–11
personal vignettes
  on process of differentiation, 179–99, 331–43
Pert, C., 327–28
Pett, C., 302, 306
physical symptoms
  source of, 297–98
Pine, D., 171
placebo effect
  research on, 324–25
playing part in
  causing *vs.*, 24
polarizing conflicts
  pseudo-self at root of,
    329–30
political views
  sibling position's impact
    on, 138
poor differentiation
  difficulties resulting from,
    50
poorly differentiated people
  emotional closeness
    and, 14
poorly differentiated relationships, 112f, 113
position within family. *see*
  sibling position
Powell, N., 172, 300
predisposition(s)
  "inborn," 67
prefrontal cortex
  evolutionary development of, 54
  in intellectual system
    functioning, 54
Prehn, R., 302
preoccupation with status
  pseudo-self and, 51
Price, D., 324
Princeton University, 159,
  276–77, 291, 293
  IAS at, 279, 286, 287

principle(s)
  shift to feeling, 156
process of differentiation, 163–221. *see also specific components*
  Bowen theory in facilitating, 211–21
  case example, 200–10, 200f, 205f
  clinical example, 200–10, 200f, 205f
  coaching, 201–10, 205f
  described, 201
  discriminate between thinking and feeling in, 170–71
  engage in emotionally difficult situations in, 175–76
  initiation of, 201
  key ingredients in, 165–78
  maintain more of self with others in, 176–77
  method in, 211–21
  observe and think about emotional process in, 168–70, 169f
  personal vignettes of, 179–99 *see also* Kerr family vignette
  recognize impact of anxiety on functioning in, 171–75
  technique of, 211–21
  theoretical thinking and scientific inquiry in, 177–78
  theory of, 211–21
  value of coach in, 186
process thinking
  content thinking *vs.*, 25
programming
  emotional, 37, 95–107, 339 *see also* emotional programming
pseudo-self, 50, 124
  as basis for increasing person's functional level of differentiation and reducing chronic anxiety, 58
  borrowing and trading of, 81
  context dependence and, 52
  described, 50–51
  doublethink and, 52
  holding discrepant beliefs in, 52
  knee-jerk opposition to others' points of view and, 51
  as negotiable in relationship system, 51
  oppositional behavior and, 51
  people pretending to be something they are not, 51
  preoccupation with status and, 51
  at root of polarizing conflicts, 329–30
  solid self interplay with, 55–56, 56f
  solid self *vs.*, 50
psoriasis, 307–10, 308f, 310f
  manifestations of, 172–73
psychodynamic psychotherapy
  limitations of, xix–xx
psychological process(es)
  differentiation of self as more than, 54
psychological state(s)
  emotional system influences and influenced by, xviii
psychopath
  antisocial acts of, 240
  to insane, 240
psychosis(es). *see also* schizophrenia
  emotional dysfunction and, 240
  of John Nash, 283–85, 284f
"psychosomatic information network," 328
psychotherapy
  psychodynamic, xix–xx
psychotic-level family process
  therapy session with, 212
punctuated disequilibrium, 33

Queen Mary, 285
Queen Victoria, 54

Rainville, P., 324–25
Rand Corporation, 277
rational animal
  humankind as, 141
rationality
  emotionality *vs.*, xxiii
rational thinking
  as aspect of ability to function as self, 54
  intelligence *vs.*, 53
  problems associated with, 53
reactive distancing
  adolescent rebellion as, 34
reactivity
  emotional *see* emotional reactivity
  to families, 183–84
  knee-jerk, 48
readiness to help
  sibling position in, 137
reason
  processes shattering ability to, 272
reasoning
  emotionality *vs.*, 48
rebellion
  adolescent, 34–36
reciprocal relationship
  togetherness-driven fusion process, 72–73
reciprocity
  relationship, 96–97
recognition
  of anxiety, 90
reflection
  responses guided by, 48
regression(s)
  in Congress, 156
  emotional *see* emotional regression
  in emotional functioning, 47

ending of, 156–58
examples of, 65–67
family emerging from, 157
features of, 159
in human relationship system, 65–66
periods of, 67
in relationships, 84–85, 84f
societal, 149–62 see also societal emotional process; societal regression(s)
system, 65–67
regulatory processes
Bowen theory and, 12
reinforcement
emotional, 40
rejection
feelings of, 13
relationship(s)
calming effect on, 212–13
capacity to maintain self in, 47–48
chronic anxiety in, 111–18, 112f, 114f, 115f
comfortable courtship phase of, 82, 82f
defining self in, xxi
differentiation of self in, 147
differentiation-togetherness balance in, 73
emotional/psychic energy in, 80–81, 80f
emotional separateness in, 197–99
factors impacting, 172
fusion in, 55–56, 72
guilt as product of, 92
individuality-togetherness balance in, 73
intimate see intimate relationships; marital relationship(s)
loss of self in, xix
marital see marital relationship(s)
mother–offspring, 39–40
one-down, 35

open, 44
overfunctioning-underfunctioning, 51–52, 57, 57f
parent–offspring, 97
poorly differentiated, 112f, 113
as problematic, 183
regressed, 84–85, 84f
self in, xix
in stabilizing family system, 114
well-differentiated, 112f, 113
relationship balance
tilting of, 71
relationship oriented, 59
relationship pressure
solid self in resisting, 55
relationship process(es)
functional facts of, 96
in regulation of emotional functioning of individuals, 12
relationship reciprocity
case example, 96–97
relationship system(s), 10
anxious, 172
chronic anxiety's effects on, 172, 292, 292f
compromised position in, 172
in creating and maintaining impaired functioning, 23
defining self in, xxi
differentiation of self in, 220
in nuclear family ego mass, 24
pseudo-self as negotiable in, 51
regression in, 65–66
in shaping functioning of members, 23
relationship thinking
individual thinking to, 22
relative(s)
importance of talking to many close and distant, 182

remarriage(s)
recording on family diagram, 122–23, 123f
resolution
described, 292f, 293
response(s)
emotional, 183
objectivity in, 48
reflection in, 48
responsibility(ies)
of family therapists, 165
Rider College, 289
Ridker, P., 298–99
Riemann hypothesis
trying to solve, 279–80
Roman Catholic Church, 324
Roosevelt, F., Pres., 75
Roots, 183
roots experiences, 179–85
Rose, R., 299–300
rugged individualism, 70

Sanctuary of Our Lady of Lourdes, 324–26
Sandy Hook Elementary School
Newtown, Connecticut, 259–71
Sandy Hook shooter. see Lanza, Adam (Sandy Hook shooter)
San Quentin Prison, 246
Santayana, G., 119, 120
Sapiens: A Brief History of Humankind, 1, 176
saying
doing vs., 23
Scheflen, A., 327–28
schizophrenia
brother's vulnerability to, 336
as chronic anxiety–driven functional dysfunction, 292, 292f
clinical course of, 272–94
conceptualization of, 272
described, 331–54
differences in people with, 331–32

schizophrenia (*continued*)
  family and social contexts related to, 272–94 *see also* Nash, John
  as functional dysfunction, 273
  functional level of differentiation from birth until death, 351–52, 352f
  genetics and, 293
  hard core patients with, 331–32
  impact on developing "self," 185
  from individual and family vantage points, 272–94
  Kerr family impact of, 331–54
  in Kerr's brother, 331–54, 333f, 342f, 345f, 346f *see also* Kerr family; Kerr, M.E.
  negative symptoms of, 331
  paranoid, 236
  positive symptoms of, 331
  questions dominating existence of, 106
  recovery from, 223
  siblings vulnerable to, 102
  suicide related to, 187–91, 230, 332
  symptoms of, 331
  as thought disorder, 272–94
  triangles and, 338, 342f
  in Unabomber, 230
  unresolved attachment and, 39
schizophrenic(s)
  functional level of differentiation from birth until death, 351–52, 352f
  mothers of, 337
Scientific American, 229
scientific inquiry
  defined, 178

described, 178
in process of differentiation, 177–78
second-guessing, 35
seeking network
  diminished arousal of, 283
self
  ability to maintain, xvi–xvii
  anxiety and, 44
  basic level of, 45
  basic level of differentiation of, 331
  being more of, xx
  borrowing and lending of, 58
  calming of, 69
  capacity to maintain in relationships, 47–48
  communications and behaviors in defining and maintaining, xviii
  components of, 54
  concept of, xvi–xvii
  conceptualizing of, xvi
  in dealing with open relationship, 44
  defined, xvi
  defining in family or other relationship system, xxi
  degree of integration of, 108
  described, 332–33
  developing, 185
  differentiation of *see* differentiation of self
  difficulty in maintaining, 18–21, 19f, 20f
  evolving of, 54
  loss in relationships, xix
  in maintaining intimate relationships, 77
  maintenance with others, 176–77
  as manifestation of highest level of consciousness, 54
  in one's family of origin as adult, 166

pseudo-, 50
rational thinking as aspect of ability to function as, 54
in relationships, xix
self-regulation in maintaining, xviii–xix
solid *see* solid self
variation in, xix
self-awareness
  awareness of awareness vs., 49
self-fulfilling prophecy, 105
self-regulation
  "low-level," 113
  in self maintenance, xviii–xix
separateness
  emotional, 197–99
  functional, 72
separation
  emotional, 39, 99
Seyle, H., 299
shock wave
  emotional, 116–17
Shot in the Heart, 239, 250
"shutdown"
  melancholic, 233
sibling(s)
  of Adam Lanza, 261–63, 266
  cutoffs between, 146
  in different triangles, 102–5, 103t, 103f
  emotional attachment impact on, 101–2
  of Gary Gilmore, 239, 242, 250
  vulnerable to schizophrenia, 102
sibling position, 133–42
  in childlike behavior, 138
  family dynamics in, 139
  in helplessness, 138
  impact on political views, 138
  intermediary, 136–37
  oldest brother of brother(s), 135
  oldest brother of sister(s), 135

oldest sister of brother(s), 136
oldest sister of sister(s), 136
only child, 137
person's functioning
  related to, 134–42
  in readiness to help, 137
  therapists' knowledge about, 138
  twins, 137
  youngest brother of brother(s), 135
  youngest brother of sister(s), 135
  youngest sister of brother(s), 136
  youngest sister of sister(s), 136
"silent killer"
  anxiety-driven emotional process as, 23
  chronic anxiety as, 172
  hypertension as, 23, 172
similarity principle, 79
simulation processes, 53–54
60 Minutes, 237, 273
Skinner, B.F., 95–97
Sloman, S., 329–30
Smithers, D., Sir, 306, 307
snowplow parenting, 151–54, 152f–53f
social behavior
  of bacteria, 8
social context
  vulnerability to, 156
social groups
  dominance hierarchies in species living in, 28–29
social network
  of trees, xiii
social stress
  chronic inflammation related to, 172
social symptoms
  source of, 298
social system
  anxiety over one's status in, 51

social units of unrelated people
  triangling process in, 14
societal emotional process, 149–62. see also societal regression(s)
  Bowen theory applied to, 158–59
  described, 149
societal regression(s), 149–62. see also societal emotional process
  described, 149–50, 162
  ending of, 156–58
  features of, 159
society(ies)
  anxiety-driven symptom process in, 159
  individualistic, 70
  regressions in, 156–58
  sociocentric, 70
Sociobiology: The New Synthesis, 26
sociocentric societies
  described, 70
solid self, xxiii
  assessment of, 54–55
  components of, 52–53
  described, 52
  as function of brain, 55
  increasing, 179
  intellectual system and, 52–53
  measure of, 76–77
  principles anchored in, 51
  pseudo-self interplay with, 55–56, 56f
  pseudo-self vs., 50
  in resisting relationship pressure, 55
Solomon, A., 259–62, 270
spiritual
  defined, 323
  described, 323
spouse(s)
  differentiation of self in relationship to, 147
  in unresolved attachment, 77
Stanovich, K., 53–54, 149

status
  preoccupation with, 51
Stephens, P., 51
Stier, E., 274f, 275, 277–79, 278f
Stigum, B., 141
stress
  chronic, 173
  chronic inflammation related to, 172
  epinephrine and, 172
  norepinephrine and, 172
  social, 172
stressor(s)
  in marriage, 82–88, 83f–85f, 87f
  system-generated chronic anxiety and, 110
stress response
  activation of, 13, 315f
  chronic, 13
  counterbalancing of, 320
  family, 318–19, 318f
  nonspecific, 299
stress response system
  anxiety and, 108
strongly held beliefs
  challenges to, 182
Struhl, K., 298
"stuck-togetherness," xviii
studying one's own family, 331–54
  Bowen theory applied to, 331–54 see also Kerr family; Kerr, M.E.; schizophrenia
  family of origin diagram, 333–51, 333f, 342f, 345f, 346f
  purpose of, 332–33
subgroup(s)
  formation of, 14
"Subjectivity, Homo sapiens, and Science," 322
suicide
  aftermath of brother's, 187–91
  schizophrenia and, 230, 332
Sung, C., 299–300

supernatural phenomena
  towards systems concept
    of, 322–30
symbiosis
  defined, 39
symptom(s)
  chronic anxiety in development of, 118
  clinical, 118
symptomatic offspring
  therapy sessions with parents and, 212
symptom development
  family system in, 23
symptom process
  anxiety-driven, 159
system-generated chronic anxiety
  absorption of, 23
  stressors and, 110
system regression
  examples of, 65–67
systems concept of supernatural phenomena, 322–30
  toward, 322–30
systems thinking, xiv, 3–6, 3f
  in allowing one to be realistic about role in emotional process, 24
  application to human behavior, xv
  cause-and-effect thinking vs., 3, 54
  conceptualizing multigenerational process in, 119
  described, 5–6, 25
  functional facts in, 5–6
  group interactions through lens of, 25
  in helping to see world more as it really is, xxii
  as interaction of all variables, 24
  interactions between family members in describing, xvi
  interlocking psychopathology thinking vs., xvi

natural, 119
  in seeing larger picture, 24

talking
  calming effect on relationship, 212–13
tension
  between insiders, 17, 17f
  in marriage, 82–88, 83f–85f, 87f
The Atlantic Monthly, 221
The Executioner's Song, 223, 239, 240, 255
The Hidden Life of Trees, xiii, 165–66
theoretical thinking
  in process of differentiation, 177–78
The Origins of Family Psychotherapy: The NIMH Family Study Project, xv
theory(ies). see also specific types, e.g., attachment theory
  attachment, xv
  Bowen family systems, xvi
  determinants of validity of, 322
  Freud's, 165
  general systems, xiv, xv
  of process of differentiation, 211–21
The Oxytocin Factor, 320
"the past does not cause the problem in the present," 9
therapist(s)
  responsibilities of, 165
therapy sessions
  with parents and symptomatic offspring, 212
  with psychotic-level family process, 212
  videotapes of, 217–18
"The Reckoning," 259
The Righteous Mind, xxiii
The Scale of Nature, 322
"the systems miracle," 294

The Theoretical Structure of the Catholic Church, 329
"The Wilderness Years," 292
thinking
  cause-and-effect see cause-and-effect thinking
  consciousness of, 49
  with emotion, 49
  emotion decoupling from, xxv
  emotion's impact on, xxiii
  family therapy as way of, 220–21
  feeling vs., 170–71
  individual, 8
  individual to relationship, 22
  maternal deprivation, xv–xvi
  natural systems, 119
  process vs. content, 25
  rational, 53, 54
  systems see systems thinking
  systems vs. cause-and-effect thinking, 3
  systems vs. interlocking psychopathology, xvi
  theoretical, 177–78
Thomas, L., 300, 312
Thoren, T., 298–99
thought(s)
  feelings vs., 49
thought disorder
  schizophrenia as, 272–94
threat(s)
  types of, 112–13, 112f
three-generational family diagram, 122, 122f
Todd, J., 74
Todd, P., 74, 77–78
Todd, W.T., 74
togetherness, 68
  anxiety-driven, 98f, 99–101, 146–47
  characteristics of, 158
  essence of, 71

individuality vs., xviii
  in parent–offspring relationships, 97
  toning down, 100
togetherness force, xviii, 72
Toman, W., 133–35, 139–40
"tough love" approaches, 154
Towards a Systems Concept of Spiritual Phenomena, 328
Towards a Systems Concept of Supernatural Phenomena, 328
transference
  fusion vs., 176
transmission of emotional process across generations
  example of, 130–31
tree(s)
  families and, xiii
  social network of, xiii
Trenton State Hospital, 286
triadic awareness, 177
triangle(s), 6, 36–43. see also triangle pattern
  in adolescence, 34–35
  as anxiety-driven emotional process, 16
  in Bowen theory, 13, 27–28, 27t, 28f, 177
  cooperative alliances vs., 16
  as cornerstone of four patterns, 27, 28f
  described, 177
  dynamic equilibrium of, 15–18, 15f, 16f
  dynamic process of, 16–17, 16f, 17f
  emotional programming in parental, 95
  emotional roots of, 177
  of emotional system, 13–21
  in enabling people to bind anxiety, 32
  evolutionary roots of, 177
  in formation of we-they groups, 14

functional facts of, 13
of Gary Gilmore, 248–49, 248f, 256f
gossip system as manifestation of, 21, 176–77
impairment of children through, 41–43
interlocking see interlocking triangles
in Kerr family vignette, 191–93, 192f
learning how to track paths of, 18–21, 19f, 20f
less differentiated, 102–5, 103t, 103f
more differentiated, 102–5, 103t, 103f
outsider as carrying anxiety of, 16–17, 16f
parental, 33–36, 231
as patterns of interaction, 22
schizophrenia and, 338, 342f
siblings in different, 102–5, 103t, 103f
in social units of unrelated people, 14
as "solution" to instability of two-person system, 14
as ubiquitous, 21
triangle pattern, 36–43. see also triangle(s)
  described, 36
  of emotional process, 14
triangling process
  described, 15–18, 15f–17f
  in social units of unrelated people, 14
tribalism
  subcortical roots of, 67
trigger(s)
  of anxiety, 90
  of chronic anxiety, 110–11
twins
  profile of, 137
two-person system
  instability of, 13, 14

ulcer(s)
  Helicobacter pylori and, 310–11, 314
Unabomber. see Kaczynski, Ted (Unabomber)
Unabomber Manifesto, 225, 236
"uncoached coach"
  Bowen as, 167
underfunctioner(s)
  overfunctioners vs., 29–30, 29f
underfunctioning
  pattern of, xvii
underfunctioning-overfunctioning. see overfunctioning-underfunctioning
undifferentiated people
  emotional closeness and, 14
undifferentiation
  degree of, 6
  in marriage, 36–38
unidisease, 297–321. see also unidisease concept
  in Bowen theory, 173
  described, 173
  illnesses associated with potentially pathogenic microorganisms, 310–14, 311f–13f
  for psoriasis, 307–10, 308f, 310f
unidisease concept, 297–321. see also unidisease
  chronic inflammation in cancer and atherosclerosis, 298
  development of, 303–21, 308f, 310f–13f, 315f, 316f, 318f
  research consistent with, 298–303
United States (U.S.)
  emotional regression in, 157
universality
  of family difficulties, 184–85

University of California,
    Berkeley, 234
University of Michigan, 234
University of Texas, 259
University of Washington,
    336
unrealistic expectations
    chronic anxiety–driven,
        185
unrelated people
    triangling process in
        social units of, 14
unresolved attachment
    described, 144
    emotional, 198–99
    examples of, 144–45
    to family of origin, 145
    in intimate relationships,
        77
    between mother and
        adult dysfunctional
        child, 39
    replicated in marriage,
        187
    schizophrenia and, 39
unresolved emotional
    attachment
    described, 198–99
    parental triangle and, 231

"unseen forces"
    functional facts about,
        324
unsolved attachment
    spouse and, 77
Utah Magazine, 245, 246
Utah State Hospital, 239

videotape(s)
    of therapy sessions, 217–18
von Bertalanffy, L., xiv
Vonnegut, K., 119–21
voodoo, 326–27
vulnerability
    to social context, 156

Wallace, M., 237, 273
Warren, J., 310
Warthin, A.S., 304
Washington Post, 233, 235
    on Unabomber, 225
Washington State, 336
"We and They," 14
Weinberg, R., 318
Weiner, N., 306
well-differentiated people
    balance between intel-
        lectual and emotional
        functioning in, 50

emotional closeness
    and, 14
well-differentiated relation-
    ships, 112f, 113
Western Connecticut State
    University, 268
we-they groups
    triangles in formation
        of, 14
"whisper of nature," 80
Whitman, C., 259–71
Wiener, N., xiv
Williams, G.C., 178
Wilson, E.O., 26, 67, 166
Wohlleben, P., xiii, 165–66
womb envy, 281–82
Woods, J.C., 239, 240

youngest brother of
    brother(s)
    profile of, 135
youngest brother of sister(s)
    profile of, 135
youngest sister of brother(s)
    profile of, 136
youngest sister of sister(s)
    profile of, 136

Zahalka, A., 301